PHOTOGRAPHIC ATLAS OF
THE HUMAN BODY

PHOTOGRAPHIC
ATLAS
OF THE HUMAN BODY

Branislav Vidić, S.D.

Professor of Anatomy,
Georgetown University Schools
of
Medicine and Dentistry,
Washington, D.C.

Faustino R. Suarez, M.D.

(1929-1983)

Associate Professor of Anatomy,
Georgetown University Schools
of
Medicine and Dentistry,
Washington, D.C.

with 413 illustrations

The C. V. Mosby Company

St. Louis   Toronto   1984

MOSBY

A TRADITION OF PUBLISHING EXCELLENCE

Editor: Samuel E. Harshberger
Assistant editor: Anne Gunter
Manuscript editor: Marjorie L. Sanson
Book design: Kay M. Kramer
Cover design: Diane M. Beasley
Production: Gail Morey Hudson, Mary Stueck, Margaret B. Bridenbaugh

Printed in the United States of America

The C.V. Mosby Company
11830 Westline Industrial Drive, St. Louis, Missouri 63146

Library of Congress Cataloging in Publication Data

Vidić, Branislav.
Photographic atlas of the human body.

    Bibliography: p.
    Includes index.
    1. Anatomy, Human—Atlases. I. Suarez,
Faustino R., 1929-   II. Title.
QM25.V5 1984   611'.0022'2   83-13251
ISBN 0-8016-5244-8

C/VH/VH 9 8 7 6 5 4 3 2 1   01/A/094

Preface

The recognition of human structure was no doubt the origin of the eternal medical dilemma, the normal versus the abnormal. However, despite monumental scientific effort over the centuries to depict the minute variations in human anatomy, concepts of a normal form are divided even at the present time because of a great deal of uncertainty.

Anatomy is essentially a visual subject that concerns a number of functional systems. Each system is further subdivided into integral parts, each part being made of tissues, tissues of cells, cells of subcellular organelles, organelles of molecular subunits, and so on. An anatomical entity, however, is pedagogically regarded as a composite of regions that most frequently represent conventional topographical, rather than functional, units (e.g., parotid region, posterior triangle of neck, anterior compartment of arm, posterior abdominal wall, sole of foot). It must be recognized from the beginning of a study that an anatomical structure (organ, blood vessel, nerve, muscle, bone, or other) is not always confined to only one anatomical region. Therefore it may be necessary to explore several regions to appreciate morphologically a structure as a whole, this being particularly true of the tubular systems (e.g., intestines, airways, urinary tract) and the cranial or spinal nerves (e.g., vagus, radial, sciatic). Only after an anatomical unit has been fully physically perceived as a whole and as it relates to other structures should the conceptual evaluation of this structural function be commenced. Functions of the relevant anatomical units should subsequently be integrated with one another gradually until the morphology and function of an entire system, and then of the whole body, are completely established. Hence an anatomical study encompasses two pedagogical steps in succession: first the analytical and then the synthetic.

The anatomical analysis results in a gradually expanding appreciation of the human structure by a sequential dissection of regions. This process is fundamental in providing the morphological data for the subsequent conceptual elaboration, the synthesis of material into a functionally meaningful entity. Although dissection is generally accepted as the most ancient method implemented in the analytical study of an anatomical subject, it has survived the scrutiny of doubt and the test of time throughout the history of medicine. The dissection by anatomy students is recognized as an essential pedagogical experience even in contemporary curricula for the understanding of fundamental body composition and function, for the differential assessment between the normal and the abnormal form, and furthermore for an optimum physical treatment of disease conditions.

The methodology of dissection, as currently implemented, is based on some inherent limitations. It is a lengthy procedure that cannot be condensed indiscriminately and still provide a sufficient quantity of structural demonstration. The progress of dissection requires that numerous important elements be removed or partially damaged and consequently that the essential anatomical relationships be distorted. This is particularly disadvantageous for the future review of a dissected region, since many superficial elements are deliberately taken away for exploration of the deeper regional layers or skeletal structures. In the head region, for example, and somewhat less so in the thorax, abdomen, pelvis, and perineum, a regional dissection requires an almost entire sequential destruction and removal of local anatomical structures, resulting in the loss of referential material for the subsequent review. This specific aspect of the practical work in anatomy imposes a considerable demand on the student to absorb the entire anatomical wealth of an area just during the course of that regional dissection. Furthermore, a dissector must be well informed beforehand about the technical procedures of every specific dissection to satisfactorily demonstrate the required anatomical structures of that particular region. This is especially important in the current educational systems because of an unfavorably high number of students per instructor and an unfavorably low number of hours per course. For dissection to remain the most effective pedagogical tool of the anatomical study, the following two sets of conditions should be satisfied.

Preview

Before a dissection is begun, the students must be instructed about the following: how the dissection is to be technically done; what structures are to be observed in a region; in which dissecting sequence the structures are to be demonstrated; which structures are to be preserved intact as the referential points for the subsequent dissection; which structures are to be cut, reflected, or removed to gain access to deeper layers.

Review

The method of dissection should maximally preserve the anatomical elements of a dissected area. Irrespective of the technical approaches that may be selected to satisfy this requirement, however, every dissecting procedure causes considerable damage to or distortion of relationships among the regional structures. This inherent limitation of the methodology may be compensated for by using, in addition to the still preserved cadaveric structures, various visual aids or memory to review an anatomical region either immediately following the dissection or at a later time.

With these two sets of requirements in mind—the

need for preview and review of dissected structures as an effective learning methodology in the anatomical sciences—the concept of this atlas was born more than a decade ago. Since then the original idea has been subjected to innumerable exposures to anatomical and medical instructors all over the world, to clinical educators in practically all fields of medicine, and most important to many generations of students. Needless to say, each encounter has shed light on new pedagogical implications and consequently modified somewhat the mosaic of the evolving idea. The process of changing has never ended, nor will it end in the future as the new challenges are met.

The atlas has been prepared for all those in need of visual anatomical information, whether it be the surface anatomical structures, dissectable soft tissue structures, bony elements, joints, or the relationships of structures in any particular topographical layer. The anatomical structures are consistently identified in accordance with the International Nomenclature, *Nomina Anatomica*, ed. 4, 1977, or its English translation. For ease of usage and consistency of presentation all bilaterally symmetrical regions are demonstrated only from the right side of the body. The description of each major subdivision of the body (i.e., head and neck, upper limb, thorax, abdomen, pelvis, perineum, lower limb) is preceded by a presentation of the skeletal elements of that specific region. This system was adopted because skeletal anatomy can be studied independently of the cadaveric material, and this knowledge could subsequently be used as the topographical reference, from the beginning until the end of a regional dissection.

Each major body subdivision is further differentiated in a number of regions, which are arranged throughout according to the logical sequence of dissection. Anatomical elements of a region are successively presented from the surface inward. First, the surface anatomical details are ascertained on a living subject, and then the superficial (subcutaneous) and deep (deep to the regional fascia) regional structures are exhibited in the cadaveric material. The same cadaver was used for an entire regional dissection to maintain the same points of reference throughout and to establish the identical framework and magnification for all consecutive views. This technical aspect of the atlas is highly important in providing an easy and careful method of previewing and reviewing a body part. Photographs of all dissected layers within a region were taken from the same angle and distance and under the same lighting condition to obtain the identical visual perspective and color representation of the same structures in all consecutive views. The bony components and the internal structures of joints, together with the associated membranes, ligaments, bursae, deep muscles, nerves, and blood vessels, are grouped

at the conclusion of each respective major body compartment.

Some dissection views are accompanied by corresponding drawings, the proportion between the two being 1 to 1; these more clearly identify the important structures and relationships. In these cases it was possible to avoid obscuring the photographs with labels, an important consideration in the sequential, color-photographic presentation of human anatomy. In instances of less complex structural anatomy or relationships (e.g., surface anatomical views, bones, joints, and isolated organs) the photographs themselves were labeled and thus have no accompanying drawings.

The sequence of presentation is strictly enforced in both the regional views and the body segment regions. This system provides a logical continuity during the course of learning and subsequent reviewing of the topographical anatomy. The textual material, which was kept at a minimum, is included as a supplement to the graphic material, to establish an easy and logical flow from one dissecting view to the subsequent one and to point out some important features of the regional anatomy and clinical implications. For these reasons the text of each particular dissection is subdivided into Title, Specific remarks, General remarks, and References. *Title* provides the anatomical name of a structure or a region and the proper orientation as to the side from which such a structure or region is observed. *Specific remarks* are included wherever necessary to give a comprehensive survey of dissecting manipulations involved in obtaining a view from the previous one or in developing that view into the following one. *General remarks* emphasize only those structures or topographical relationships that are obviously important for the anatomical study and that may be clearly implicated in a variety of clinical circumstances. A list of *References* is provided at the end of each part as a source of more detailed literature on some anatomical structures, relationships, variations, functions, and diseases. The number preceding the references indicates the figure to which they refer. It is expected that the presentation and description of human anatomy in the sequence and style of this atlas will be an essential pedagogical tool for the preview of what is to be immediately dissected, or for the review of what was just dissected, or what has been dissected a long time ago.

Thomas C. Lee, M.D., Associate Professor of Surgery at Georgetown University School of Medicine, provided the essential advisorship for the technical composition of the atlas. The drawings were prepared by Peter Y. Stone, Medical Illustrator in the Department of Educational Media at Georgetown University Schools of Medicine and Dentistry. The photographs were taken by Dr. Faustino R.

Suarez. Technical advisorship by Bernard F. Salb, Manager, Photography Division of the Department of Educational Media at Georgetown University Schools of Medicine and Dentistry, was essential for the course of photographic work. Dissections of the intrapulmonary bronchial distribution (Figs. 166 and 167) and of the male pelvis (Figs. 212 and 213) were prepared by Saeed Marefat, junior student at Georgetown University School of Medicine. The anatomical terminology was reviewed and updated by Roy R. Peterson, Ph.D., Professor of Anatomy at Washington University School of Medicine in St. Louis. Members of The C.V. Mosby Company were, from the very beginning of the project, fully supportive of the basic idea on which the atlas was subsequently created. Their essential contributions toward the development and the completion of the project were constructive, stimulating, and inspiring without exception.

In Washington, D.C.
on November 16, 1983
Branislav Vidić

Contents

Part Six

PERINEUM

Part Seven

LOWER LIMB

Part One
HEAD AND NECK

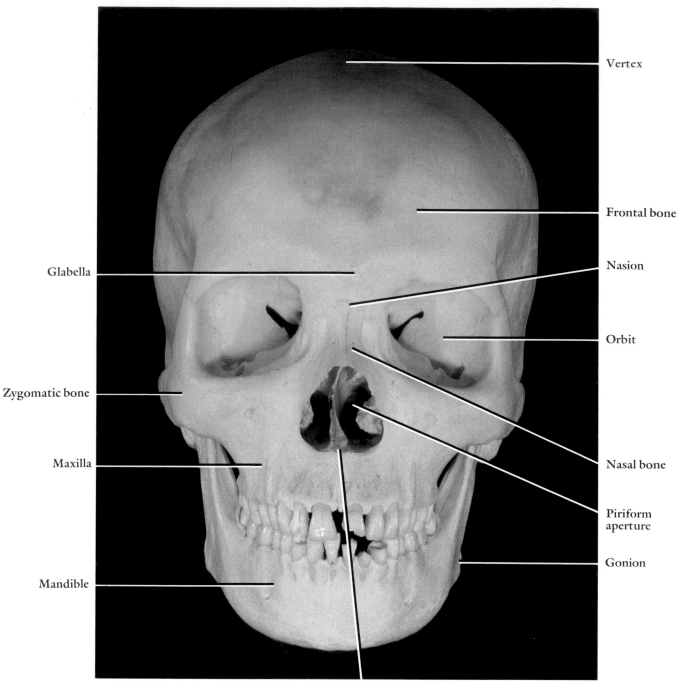

Vertex

Frontal bone

Nasion

Glabella

Orbit

Zygomatic bone

Nasal bone

Maxilla

Piriform aperture

Gonion

Mandible

Anterior nasal spine

Specific remarks: In this view several important communications between the inside of the skull and the facial region are shown: *supraorbital notch* within the *frontal bone,* *zygomaticofacial foramen* within the *zygomatic bone, infraor-* *bital foramen* within the *maxilla,* and *mental foramen* within the *mandible. Superior and inferior orbital fissures* communicate between the *middle cranial* and the *pterygopalatine fossae* and the *infratemporal fossa* and the *orbit,* respectively.

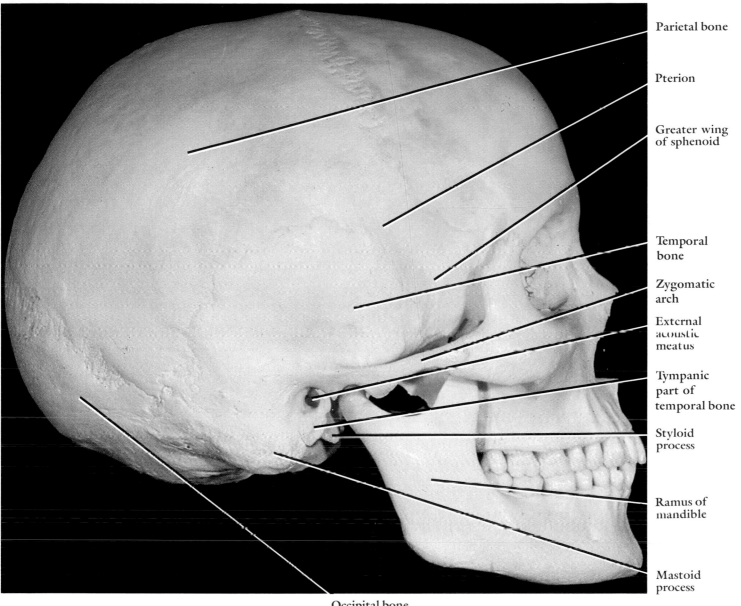

Parietal bone

Pterion

Greater wing of sphenoid

Temporal bone

Zygomatic arch

External acoustic meatus

Tympanic part of temporal bone

Styloid process

Ramus of mandible

Mastoid process

Occipital bone

Specific remarks: The *ramus of the mandible* supports two processes, the *coronoid* anteriorly and the *condylar* posteriorly. The *mandibular notch,* situated between these processes, communicates interiorly with the *infratemporal fossa.* The *condylar process* articulates with the *mandibular fossa of the temporal bone.*

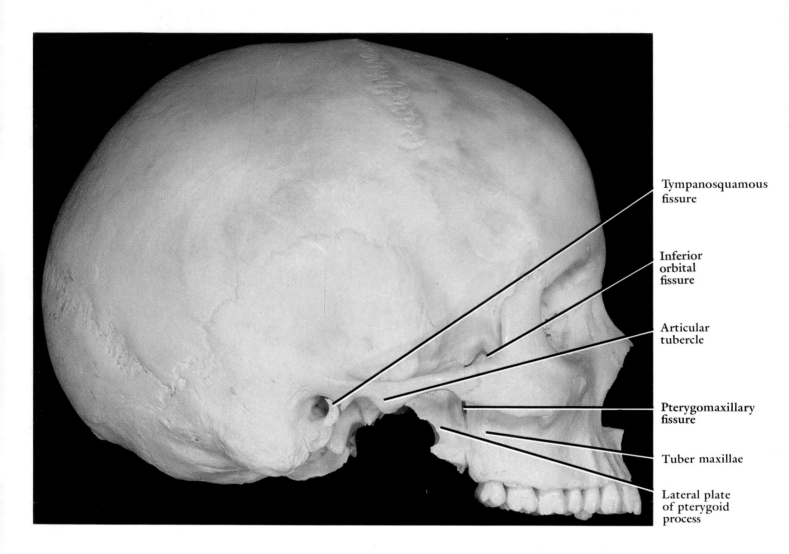

Tympanosquamous fissure

Inferior orbital fissure

Articular tubercle

Pterygomaxillary fissure

Tuber maxillae

Lateral plate of pterygoid process

Specific remarks: Three bony walls of the *infratemporal fossa* demonstrated in this view are the *tuber maxillae* anteriorly, the *lateral pterygoid plate* medially, and the *infratemporal surface of the greater wing* superiorly. The *pterygomax-illary fissure* opens interiorly into the *pterygopalantine fossa,* which still further interiorly communicates with the *nasal cavity* and *orbit* by way of the *sphenopalatine foramen* and *inferior orbital fissure,* respectively.

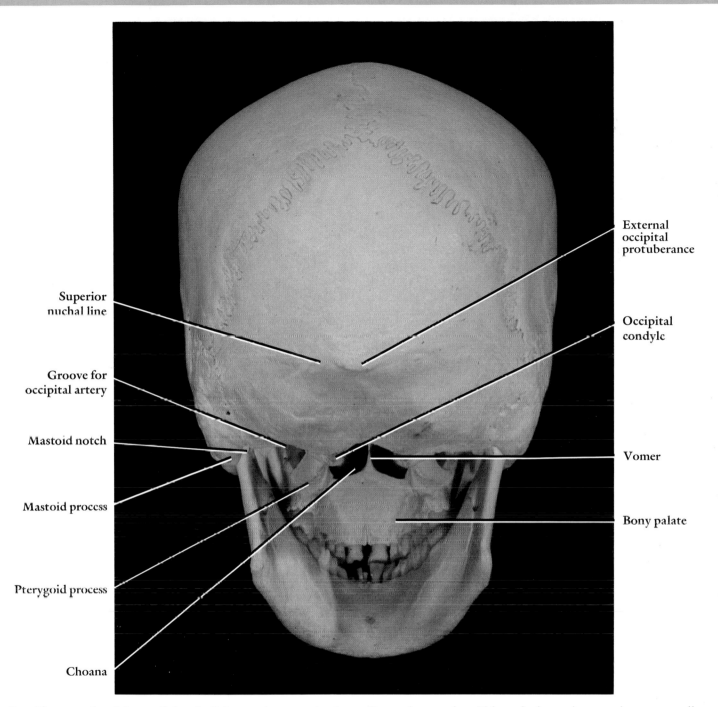

Superior nuchal line

Groove for occipital artery

Mastoid notch

Mastoid process

Pterygoid process

Choana

External occipital protuberance

Occipital condyle

Vomer

Bony palate

Specific remarks: Many of the skull bones (e.g., *parietal, occipital, temporal*) may be passed through by the *emissary veins*, which connect the *dural venous sinuses* with the superficial, extracranial venous system.

General remarks: Although the emissary veins are usually small, when there is a gradual obstruction of the *jugular foramen* they enlarge to shunt the blood from the sinuses to the outside of the skull.

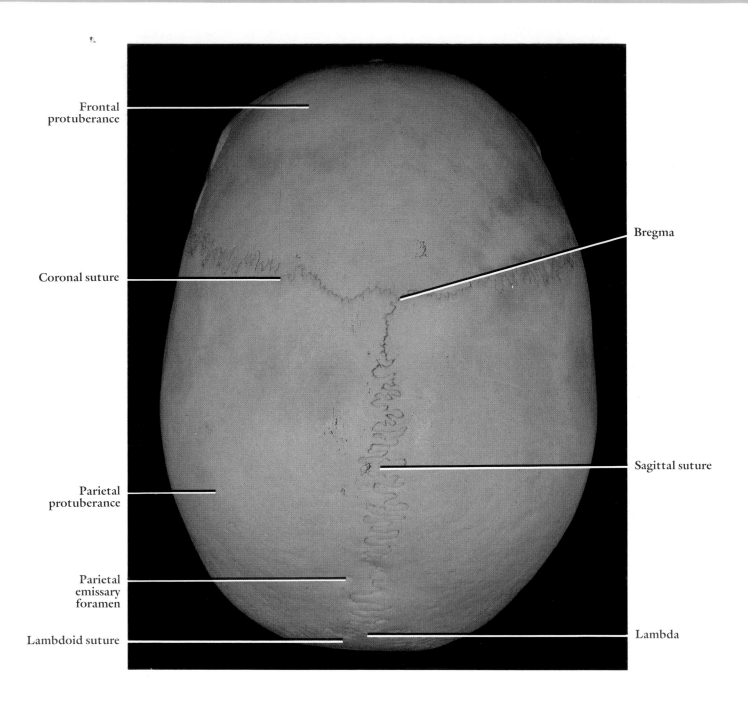

Frontal
protuberance

Bregma

Coronal suture

Parietal
protuberance

Sagittal suture

Parietal
emissary
foramen

Lambdoid suture

Lambda

General remarks: In a newborn the segments of the skull adjacent to the *bregma* and *lambda* are still membranous *(fontanelles)*. These segments provide a ready access to the *dural venous sinuses*, specifically to the *superior sagittal sinus* for taking a blood sample or for other intravenous procedures.

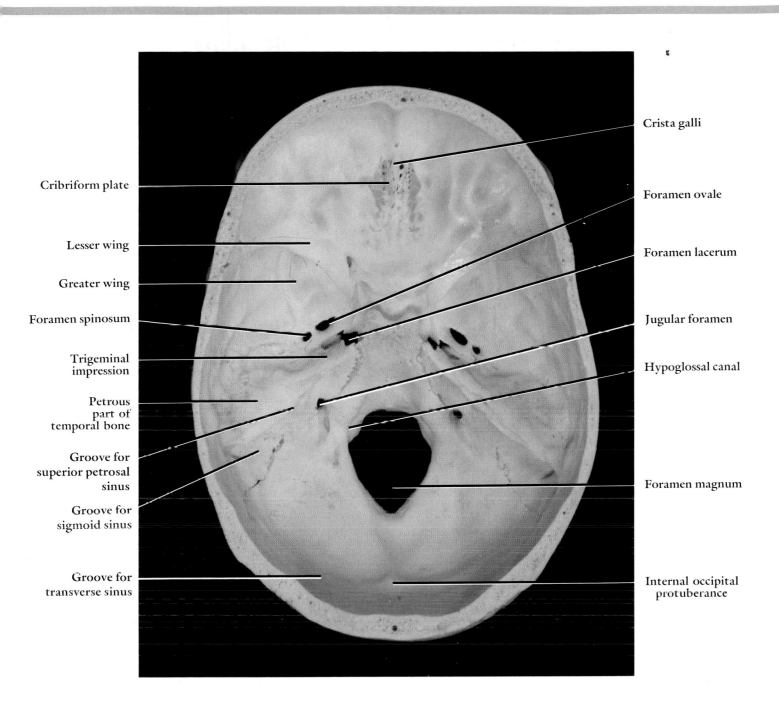

Crista galli

Cribriform plate

Foramen ovale

Lesser wing

Foramen lacerum

Greater wing

Foramen spinosum

Jugular foramen

Trigeminal
impression

Hypoglossal canal

Petrous
part of
temporal bone

Groove for
superior petrosal
sinus

Foramen magnum

Groove for
sigmoid sinus

Groove for
transverse sinus

Internal occipital
protuberance

Specific remarks: The skullcap (consisting of the *frontal, parietal,* and *occipital* bones) was separated from the skull and subsequently removed to obtain this view of the base of skull.

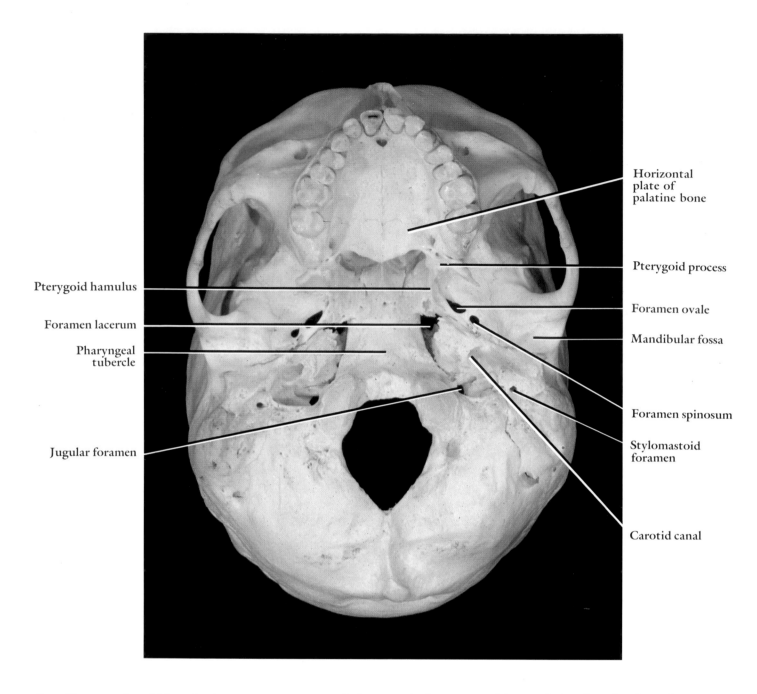

Pterygoid hamulus

Foramen lacerum

Pharyngeal
tubercle

Jugular foramen

Horizontal
plate of
palatine bone

Pterygoid process

Foramen ovale

Mandibular fossa

Foramen spinosum

Stylomastoid
foramen

Carotid canal

Specific remarks: Although the greater segment of the base of skull is accessible to inspection, the bony roof of the *nasal cavities* is obstructed in this view by the *hard palate*. This bony plate is pierced anteriorly by the unpaired *incisive fossa* from the nasal cavities and posteriorly by the

paired *greater and lesser palatine foramina* from the *pterygopalatine fossae*. Anteriorly and laterally the *palate* is surrounded by the *maxillary teeth* (two *incisors*, one *canine*, two *premolars*, and three *molars*). The free, posterior border of the bony palate shows at the midline the *posterior nasal spine*.

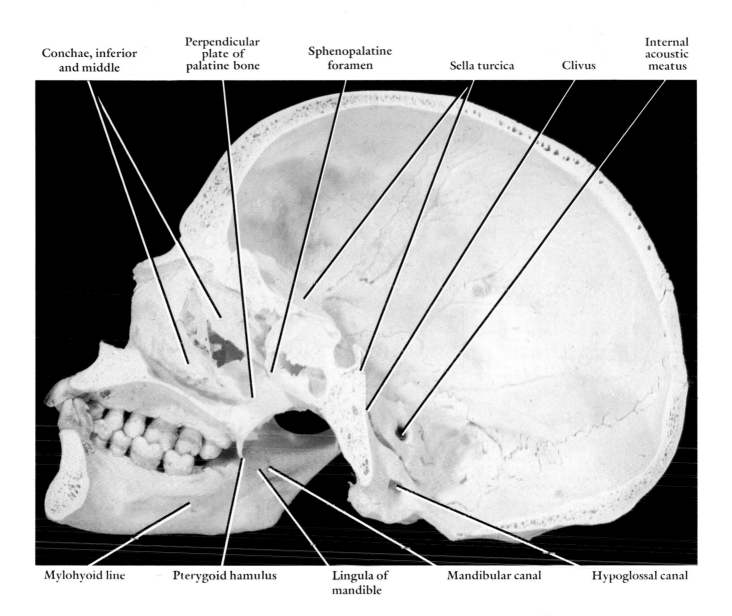

Conchae, inferior and middle

Perpendicular plate of palatine bone

Sphenopalatine foramen

Sella turcica

Clivus

Internal acoustic meatus

Mylohyoid line

Pterygoid hamulus

Lingula of mandible

Mandibular canal

Hypoglossal canal

Specific remarks: In this view the bony *nasal septum,* consisting of the *perpendicular plate of ethmoid bone* and the *vomer,* was removed for observation of the lateral bony wall of the *nasal cavity.*

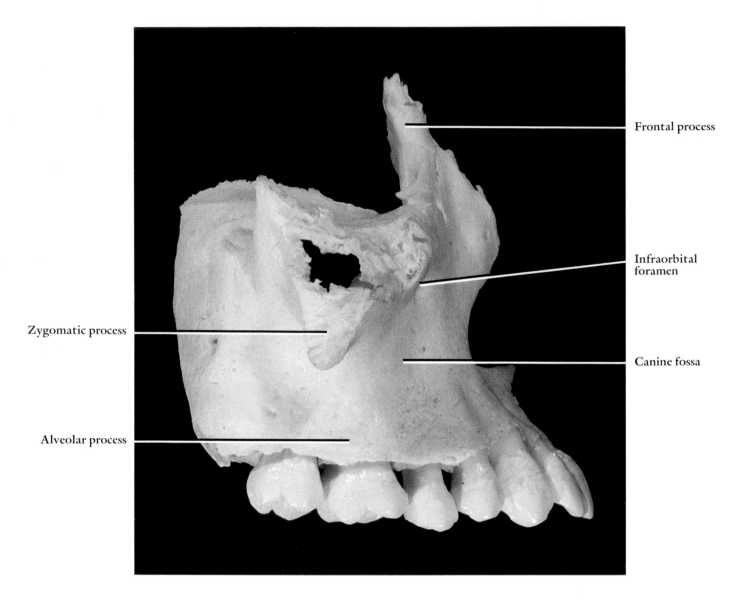

Frontal process

Infraorbital foramen

Zygomatic process

Canine fossa

Alveolar process

Frontal process

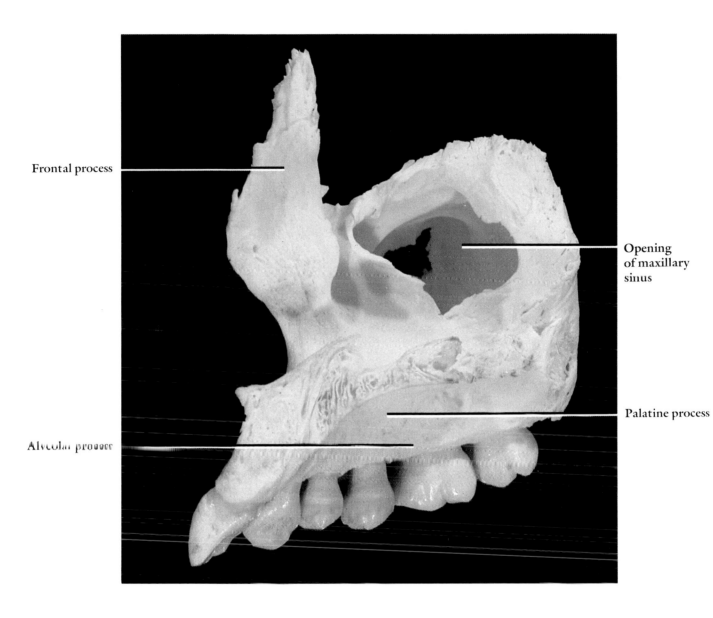

Opening
of maxillary
sinus

Palatine process

Alveolar process

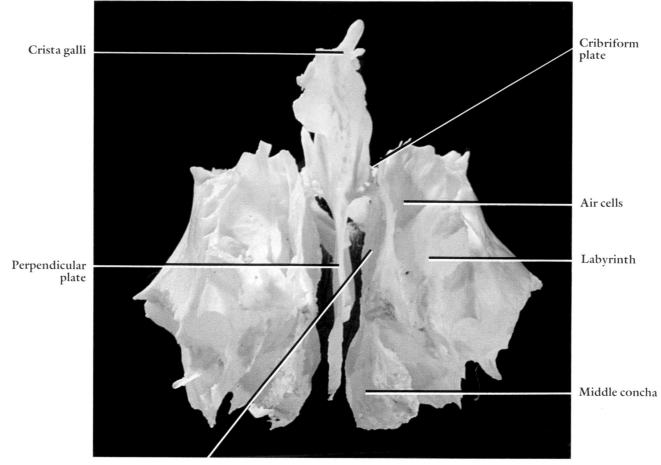

Crista galli

Cribriform plate

Air cells

Labyrinth

Perpendicular plate

Middle concha

Superior concha

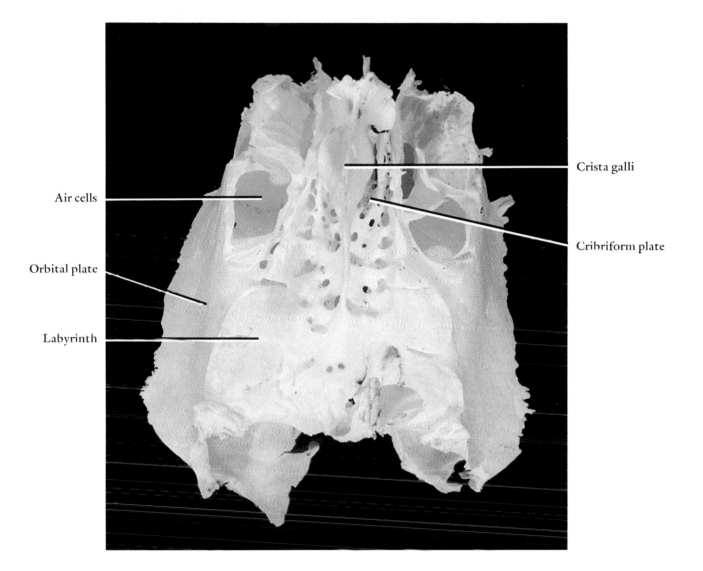

Air cells

Orbital plate

Labyrinth

Crista galli

Cribriform plate

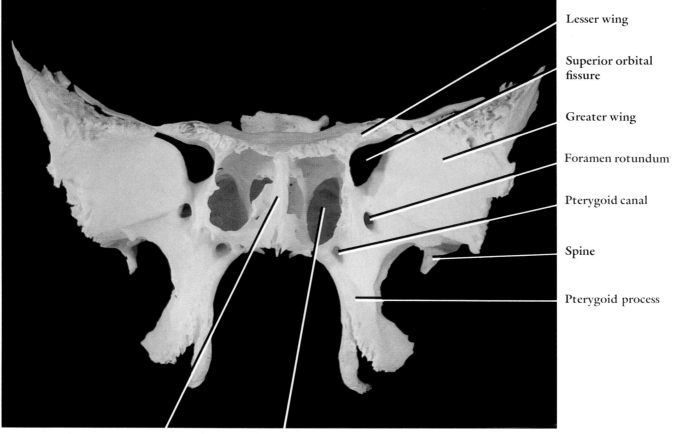

Lesser wing

Superior orbital
fissure

Greater wing

Foramen rotundum

Pterygoid canal

Spine

Pterygoid process

Sphenoid crest
and rostrum

Sphenoid sinus

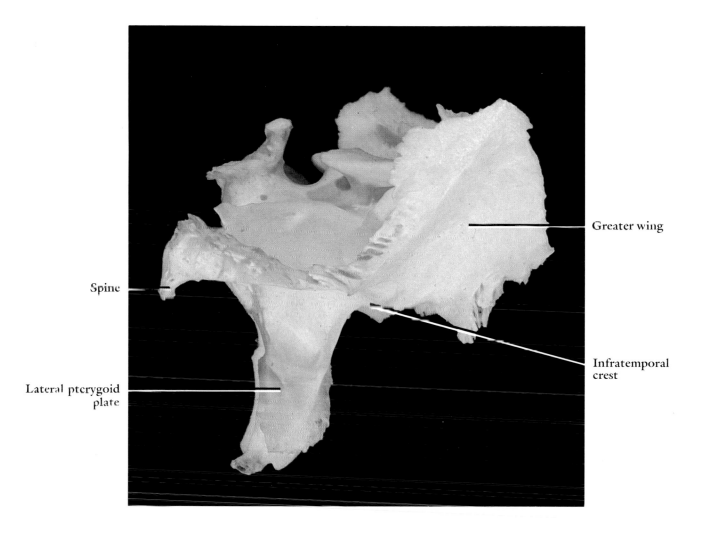

Greater wing

Spine

Infratemporal crest

Lateral pterygoid plate

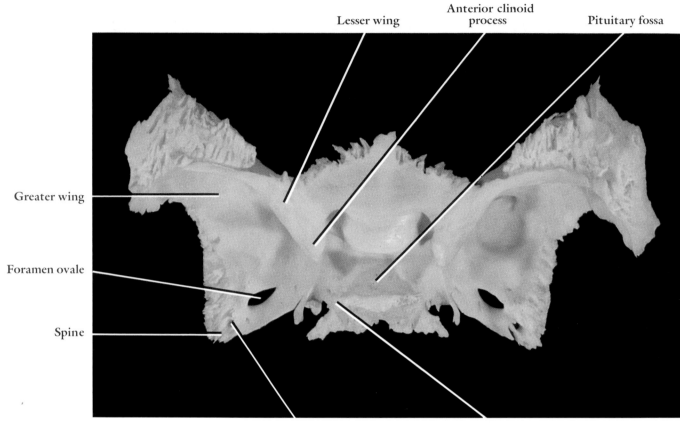

Lesser wing

Anterior clinoid
process

Pituitary fossa

Greater wing

Foramen ovale

Spine

Foramen spinosum

Posterior clinoid
process

Tympanosquamous
fissure

Postglenoid tubercle

Mandibular fossa

Squamous
part

Zygomatic process

External
acoustic
meatus

Articular tubercle

Mastoid
process

Tympanic part

Styloid process

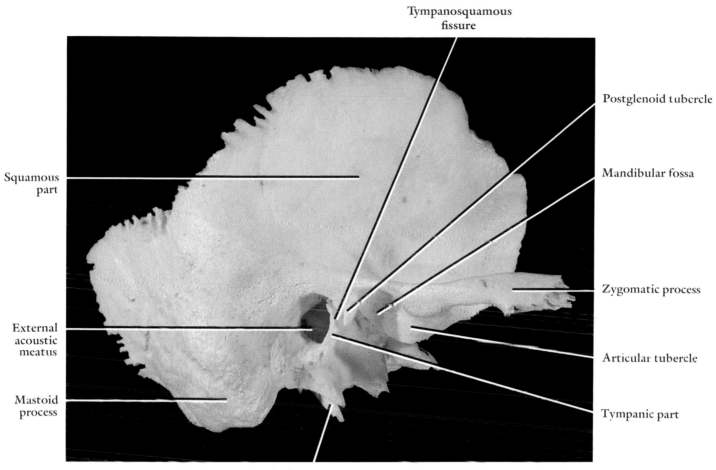

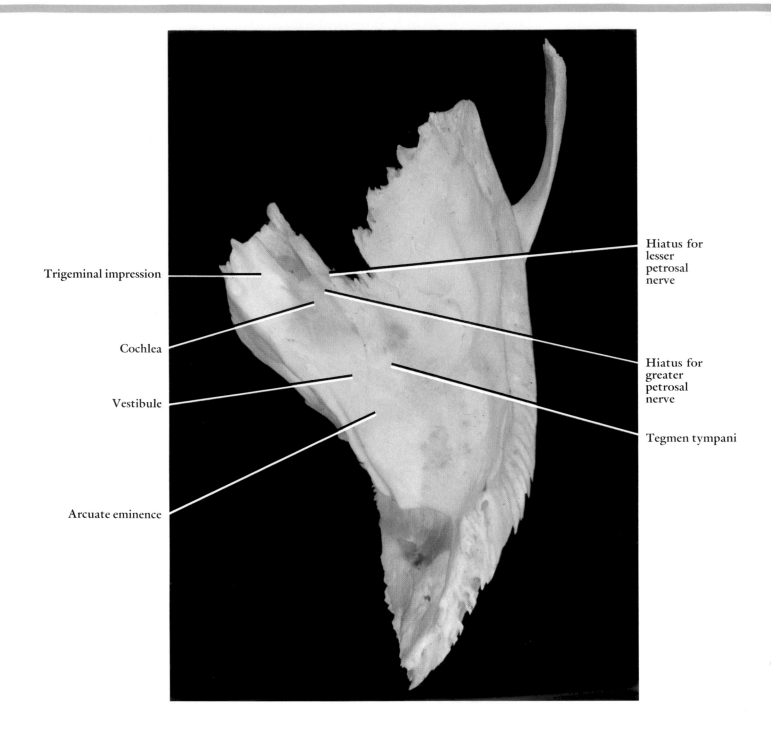

Trigeminal impression

Cochlea

Vestibule

Arcuate eminence

Hiatus for
lesser
petrosal
nerve

Hiatus for
greater
petrosal
nerve

Tegmen tympani

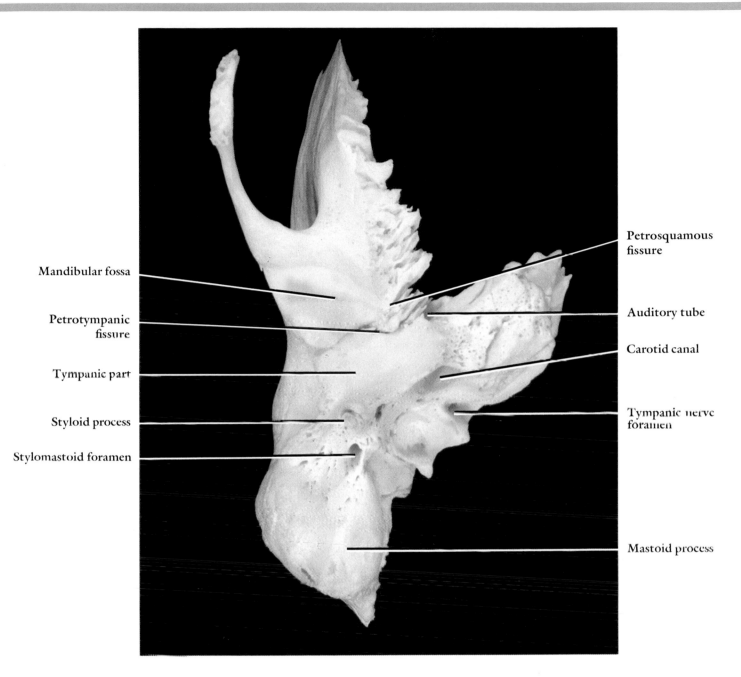

Mandibular fossa

Petrotympanic fissure

Tympanic part

Styloid process

Stylomastoid foramen

Petrosquamous fissure

Auditory tube

Carotid canal

Tympanic nerve foramen

Mastoid process

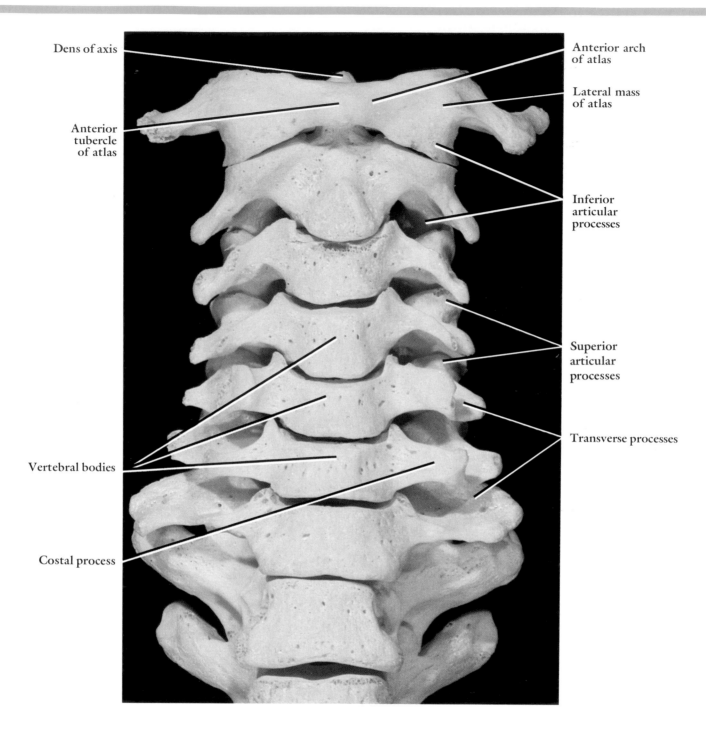

Dens of axis

Anterior arch of atlas

Anterior tubercle of atlas

Lateral mass of atlas

Inferior articular processes

Superior articular processes

Transverse processes

Vertebral bodies

Costal process

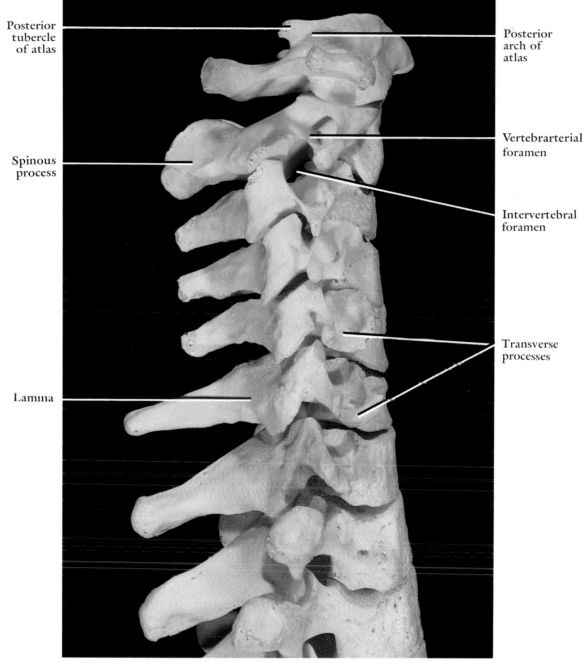

Posterior tubercle of atlas

Spinous process

Lamina

Posterior arch of atlas

Vertebrarterial foramen

Intervertebral foramen

Transverse processes

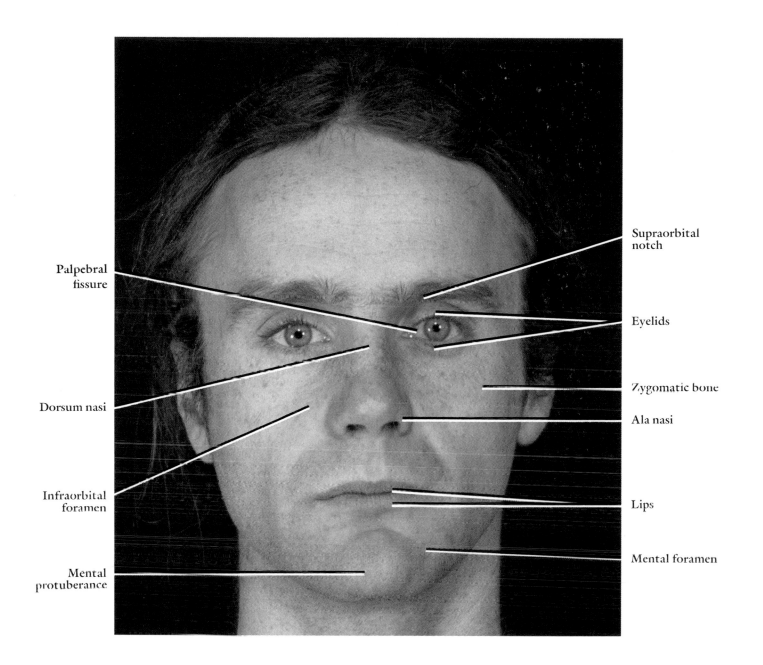

Palpebral fissure

Dorsum nasi

Infraorbital foramen

Mental protuberance

Supraorbital notch

Eyelids

Zygomatic bone

Ala nasi

Lips

Mental foramen

Specific remarks: The relief of the head reflects mostly the bony configuration (prominences, depressions, foramina, ridges, grooves) of the *skull* and the *mandible*. In the external nose, however, the cartilage supplements the bony framework to determine its superficial morphology. Two openings, the *oral* and *nasal*, represent the communications of the *digestive* and *respiratory tracts*, respectively, with the outside environment. The *palpebral opening* or *fissure* leads into the *conjunctival space* and hence provides an easy access for inspection of the transparent segment of the eyeball, the *cornea*.

General remarks: Most skeletal elements of the head, because of a relatively superficial position, are visible and/or digitally palpable. These also include the important communications *(supraorbital notch, infraorbital foramen, mental foramen)* that transmit the essential sensory nerve impulses from the facial skin to the central nervous system.

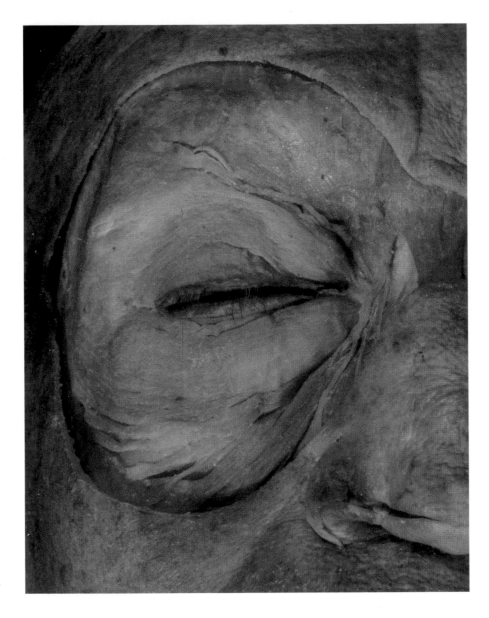

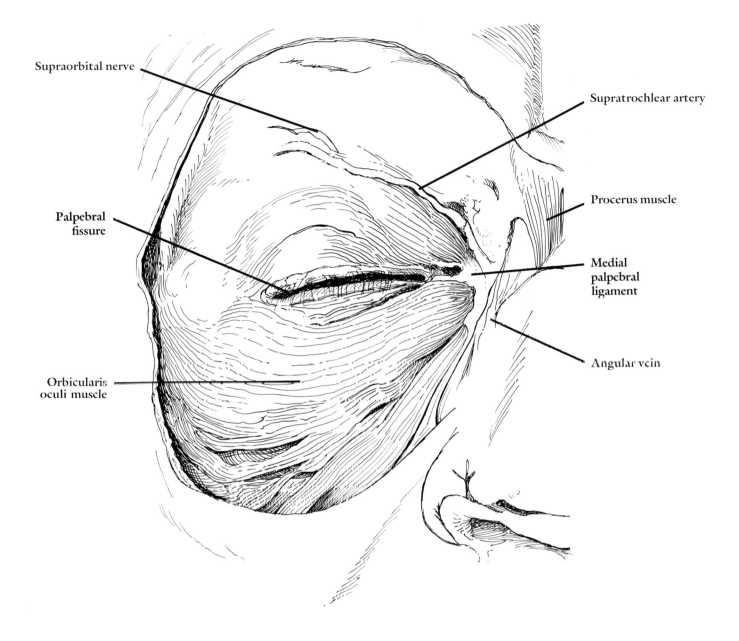

Supraorbital nerve

Supratrochlear artery

Palpebral fissure

Procerus muscle

Medial palpebral ligament

Orbicularis oculi muscle

Angular vein

Specific remarks: This muscle of facial expression has been brought into view first by incision of and subsequently by removal of all the skin around the *orbital margin*. One part of the muscle is contained within the *eyelids;* the other, peripheral, part overlaps the skeletal boundaries of the *orbit*. Attachments of the muscular fibers to the *palpebral ligaments,* especially to the medial palpebral ligament, are evident.

General remarks: This muscle, like most other muscles of facial expression, is characterized by subcutaneous position, absence of a distinct fascial covering, skin attachment, variability in size and extent, and innervation by the *facial nerve.*

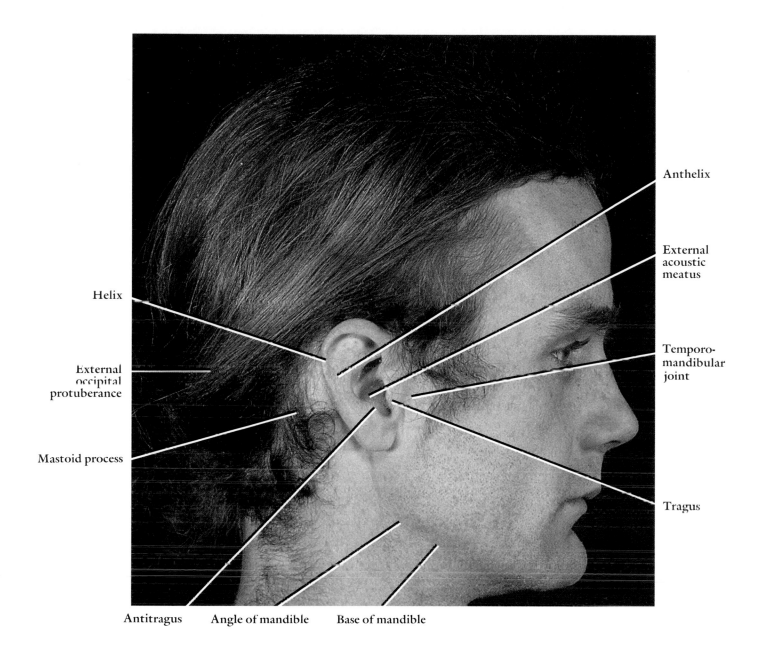

Anthelix

External
acoustic
meatus

Temporo-
mandibular
joint

Helix

External
occipital
protuberance

Mastoid process

Tragus

Antitragus   Angle of mandible   Base of mandible

Specific remarks: Some of the important skeletal landmarks here include the *angle of the mandible*, the *base of the mandible*, the *mastoid process*, the *external occipital protuberance*, the *superior nuchal line*, and the *temporomandibular joint* and its components. The external ear, with its cartilaginous support *(tragus, antitragus, helix, anthelix)* and the *lobule*, leads interiorly into first the *cartilaginous* and then the *osseous external acoustic meatus*. The *meatus* ends at the *tympanic membrane*.

General remarks: Because of a close relationship to the external acoustic meatus, the movements of the *mandibular head* in the *temporomandibular joint* are best appreciated by digital inspection via the meatus. Between the *temporomandibular joint* anteriorly and the tragus posteriorly, and immediately deep to the skin, the *superficial temporal artery* exits from the *parotid region* to become distributed primarily to the lateral aspect of the scalp.

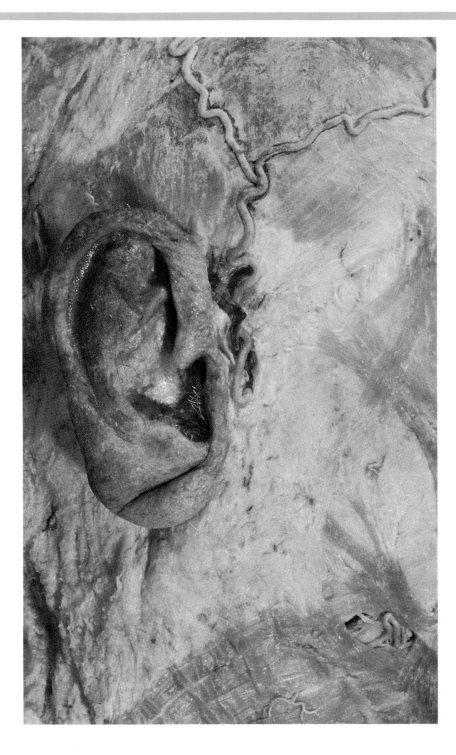

Specific remarks: Several muscles of facial expression *(anterior auricular, superior auricular, risorius, platysma, zygomaticus, orbicularis oculi)* are demonstrated to a greater advantage in the lateral view, after the skin has been carefully removed. The *parotideomasseteric fascia* is easily identifiable, in particular over the posterior segment of the parotid gland. Anteriorly, however, although the fascia continues to cover the *masseter muscle*, it gradually disorganizes as it approaches the *buccal panniculus adiposus*. The attachments of the platysma, risorius, zygomaticus, and orbicularis oculi muscles to the parotideomasseteric fascia are evident in this view.

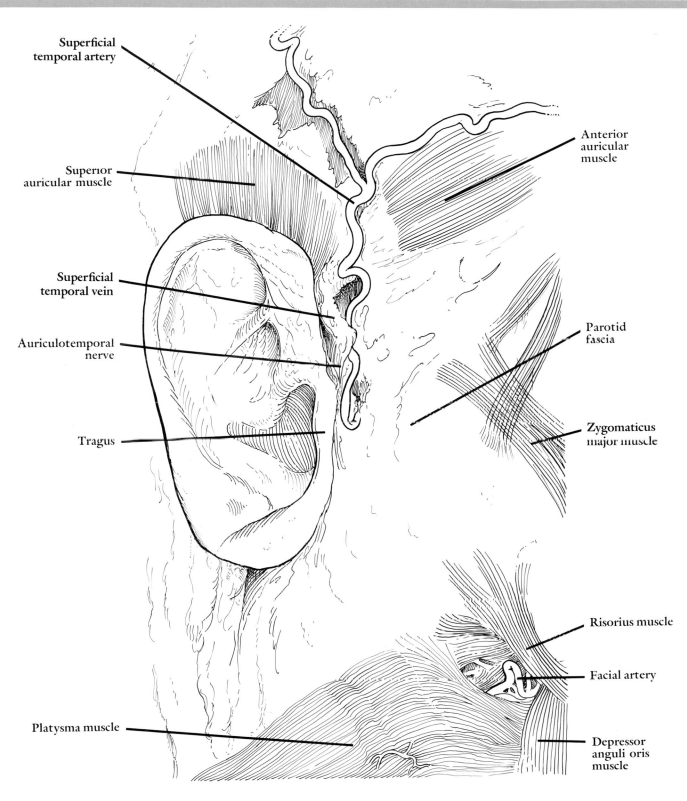

Superficial temporal artery

Superior auricular muscle

Superficial temporal vein

Auriculotemporal nerve

Tragus

Platysma muscle

Anterior auricular muscle

Parotid fascia

Zygomaticus major muscle

Risorius muscle

Facial artery

Depressor anguli oris muscle

General remarks: Two major arteries, the *facial* and *superficial temporal*, because of a relatively superficial position and a close relation to the underlying skeleton, are sometimes considered for (1) taking the pulse and (2) digital compression for peripheral hemorrhage. The *notch of the facial artery* at the base of the *mandible* and the root of the *zygomatic process of the temporal bone,* immediately anterior to the *tragus,* are specific levels for the respective arteries.

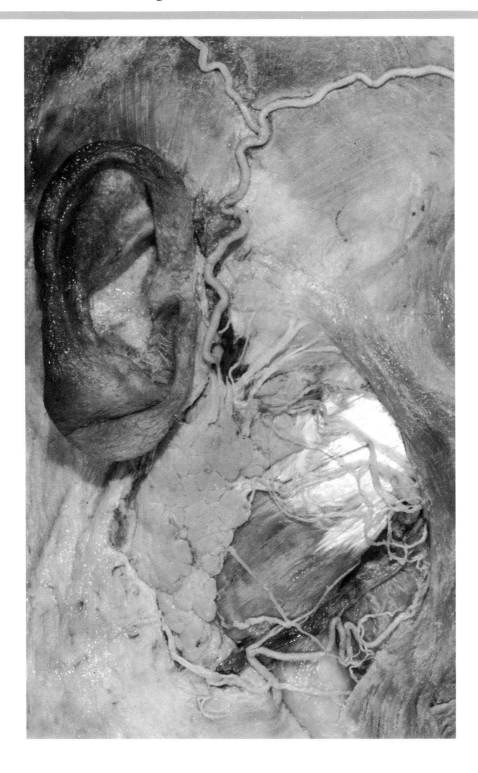

Specific remarks: The removal of the *parotideomasseteric fascia* proceeds best when the branches of the *facial nerve* are separated simultaneously because the latter branches pass through the *fascia* on their way from the *parotid region* into the face. At the same time the point of exit from and entry into the *parotid region* of the *superficial temporal vessels* and the *auriculotemporal nerve*, as well as the initial part of the *parotid duct*, may be demonstrated. Although the terminal distribution of branches of the facial nerve is quite specific, the course of and the interconnections among the same branches vary to a great extent from one individual to another.

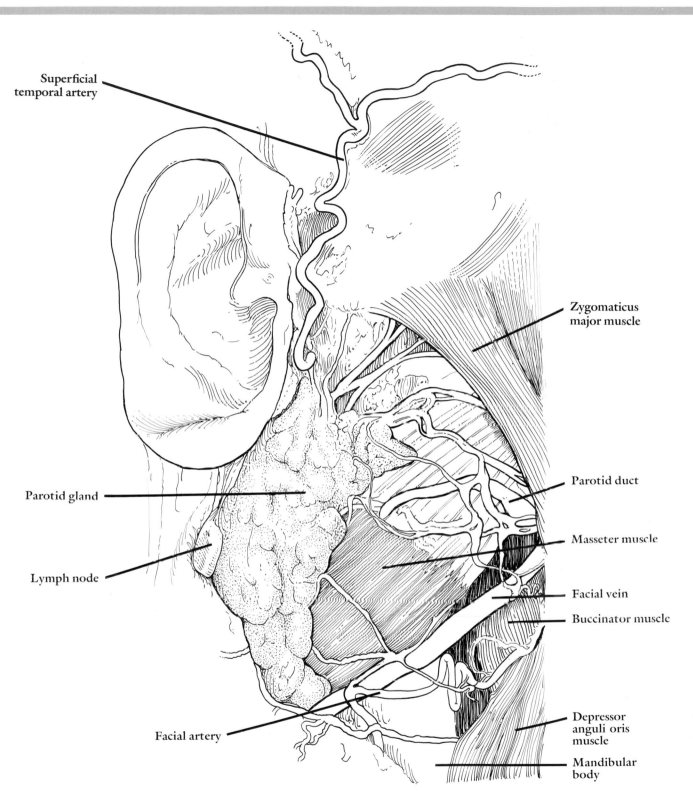

Superficial temporal artery

Zygomaticus major muscle

Parotid gland

Parotid duct

Masseter muscle

Lymph node

Facial vein

Buccinator muscle

Facial artery

Depressor anguli oris muscle

Mandibular body

General remarks: The *parotid duct* is usually projected on the surface along the middle third of a line drawn from the lower pole of the *auricular lobule* to the *external nares*. The duct is accompanied by several *branches of the facial nerve,* and it is paralleled by the *transverse facial vessels,* which are superior to it. The distribution of facial branches and the course of the parotid duct are important to consider while diagnosing or repairing traumatic damage, particularly of a vertical kind, to the face. The *parotid lymph nodes* drain the glandular lymph, as well as that from the skin, *eyelids, auricle,* and the *middle ear,* into either the *submandibular* or the *deep cervical lymph nodes.*

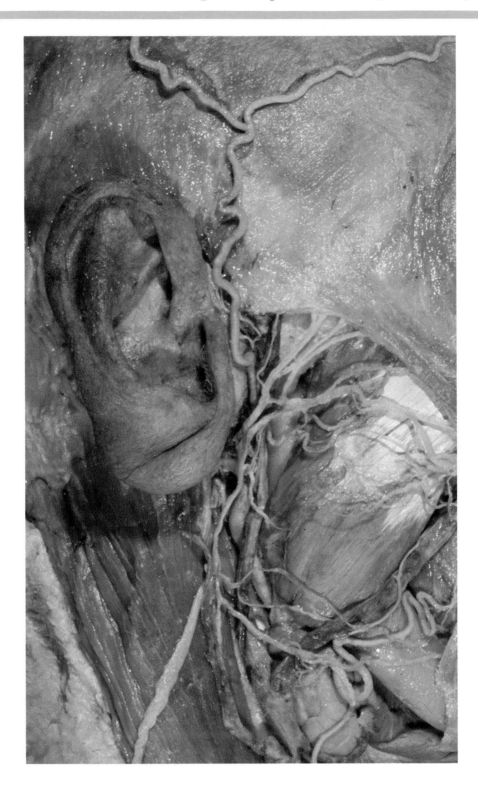

Specific remarks: The *parotid region* contains, in addition to the gland, several important nerves, nerve ramifications, and blood vessels that can be identified only after the glandular tissue has been systematically removed. Then the osteomuscular walls of the *parotid region* can also be appreciated.

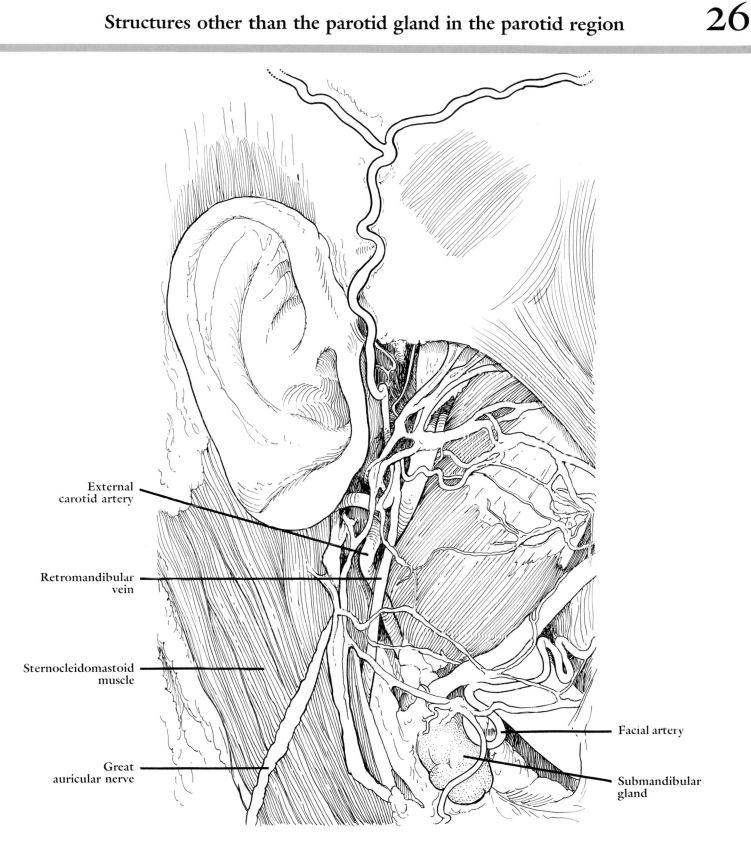

External carotid artery

Retromandibular vein

Sternocleidomastoid muscle

Great auricular nerve

Facial artery

Submandibular gland

General remarks: It was developmentally ascertained that the *facial nerve* makes several connections with other *cranial* and *cervical nerves (vagus, glossopharyngeal, trigeminal, auriculotemporal, great auricular, lesser occipital, transverse cervical)*. Although it is suspected that these nerves contribute to the proprioceptive innervation of muscles otherwise supplied by the *facial nerve*, the functional aspect of the connections is not completely clear. The *parotid gland* has a close relationship with the *transverse process of the atlas*. This topographic proximity, in an extremely developed process, might simulate a tumor mass of the gland and be diagnosed and treated accordingly.

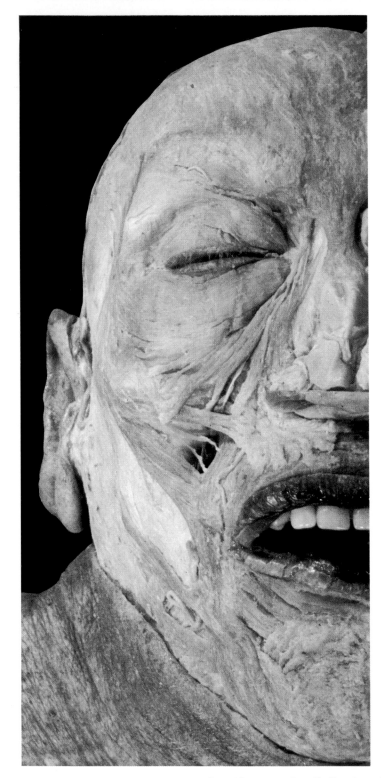

Specific remarks: Following the removal of skin and subcutaneous tissue, several characteristics of the muscles of facial expression can be observed: (1) attachment to the skin, especially well demonstrated for *levator labii superioris* and *depressor labii inferioris muscles;* (2) variations in size, shape, and position of these muscles, when several specimens are compared; and (3) absence of an organized fascia to separate these muscles from subcutaneous tissue.

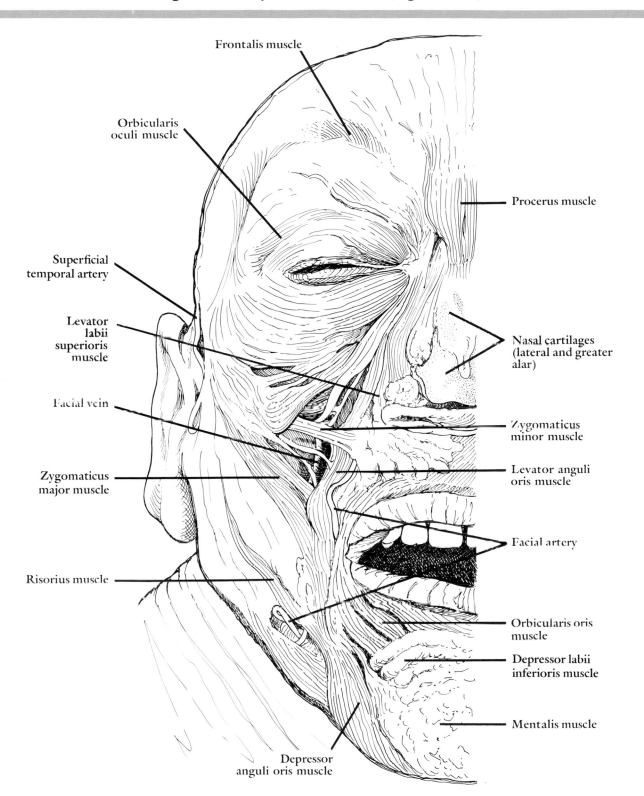

Frontalis muscle

Orbicularis
oculi muscle

Procerus muscle

Superficial
temporal artery

Levator
labii
superioris
muscle

Nasal cartilages
(lateral and greater
alar)

Facial vein

Zygomaticus
minor muscle

Zygomaticus
major muscle

Levator anguli
oris muscle

Facial artery

Risorius muscle

Orbicularis oris
muscle

Depressor labii
inferioris muscle

Mentalis muscle

Depressor
anguli oris muscle

General remarks: The relationship of *facial vessels* with the muscles is greatly variable. The *facial vein*, however, usually begins as the *angular vein* from the area adjacent to the *medial palpebral ligament*. The latter vein is connected to the *ophthalmic venous system* and thus to the *cavernous sinus* by way of the *supraorbital vein*. Because of the absence of valves in the *facial vein*, this pathway might play a role in transmitting an infectious agent from the facial region into the *dural venous sinuses*. The relationship of the *orbicularis oculi muscle* with the *medial palpebral ligament* is also important as an initial landmark during the exploration of the *lacrimal apparatus*.

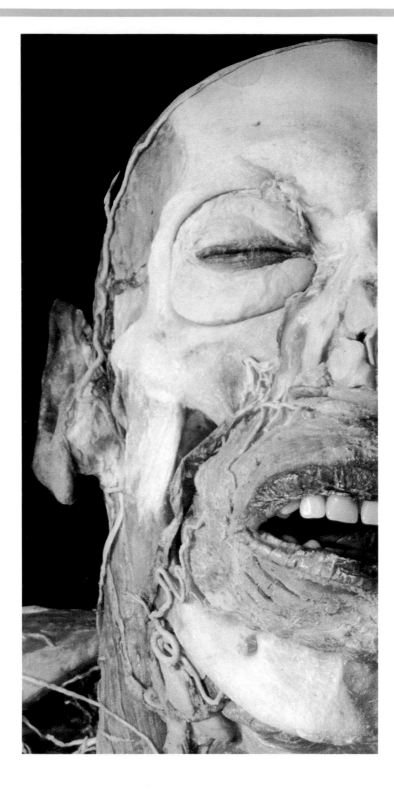

Specific remarks: Once all the facial muscles except the *orbicularis oris, levator anguli oris,* and *buccinator* are removed, the origin of the *levator anguli oris muscle* from the *maxilla,* immediately inferior to the *infraorbital foramen,* may be observed. The arteries, veins, and nerves that pass through the *supraorbital notch,* infraorbital foramen, and the *mental foramen* then can be demonstrated.

General remarks: In this view the middle segment of the *facial vein* is shown in close apposition to the *infratemporal space,* deep to the *masseter muscle* and the *ramus of the mandible.* Usually at this level the vein is connected to the *pterygoid venous plexus* by the *deep facial vein.* The *facial arteries* from both sides are connected across the midline by anas-

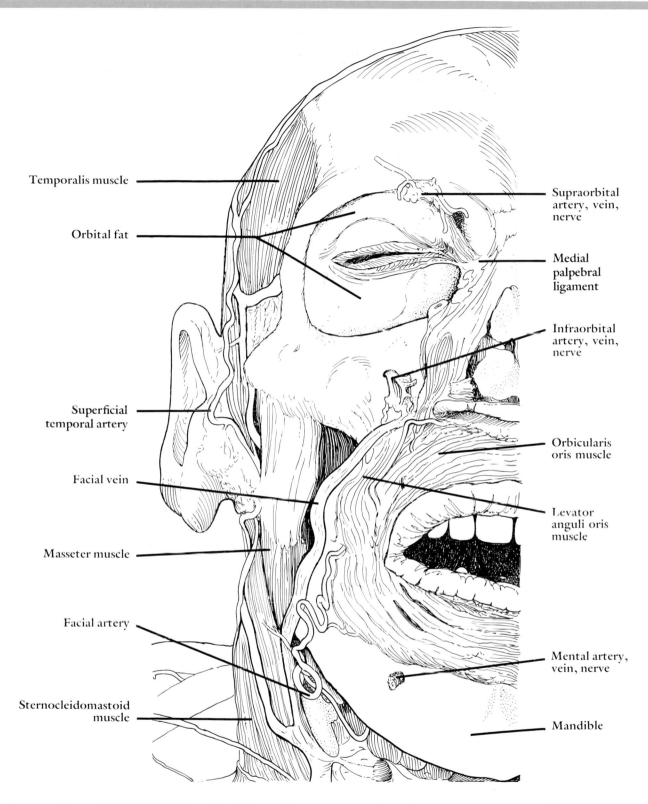

Temporalis muscle

Orbital fat

Superficial temporal artery

Facial vein

Masseter muscle

Facial artery

Sternocleidomastoid muscle

Supraorbital artery, vein, nerve

Medial palpebral ligament

Infraorbital artery, vein, nerve

Orbicularis oris muscle

Levator anguli oris muscle

Mental artery, vein, nerve

Mandible

tomosing *superior* and *inferior labial arteries*. These collateral pathways should be considered during therapeutic intervention within the labial areas. The exiting points of three main sensory nerves to the face from the skull—the *supraorbital, infraorbital,* and *mental*—are important anesthesiological landmarks. It is of interest to note that they occur along the same vertical plane of the skull. The three nerves, in addition to general sensory components to the facial skin, are thought to carry some afferent messages from the *muscles of facial expression,* in this instance from specializations other than the *muscle spindle.*

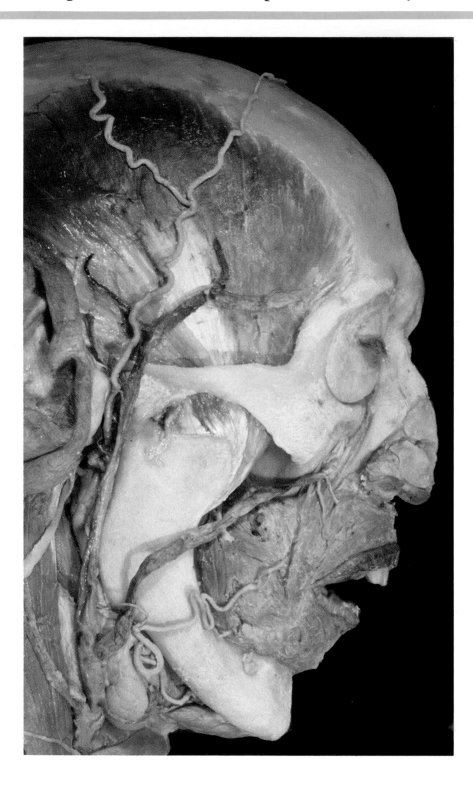

Specific remarks: To demonstrate the *temporomandibular joint* and the *temporalis muscle,* in particular the mandibular attachment of the muscle, the *masseter muscle* must be separated from the *zygomatic arch* and then reflected inferiorly. During this procedure the *masseteric blood vessels* and *nerve*

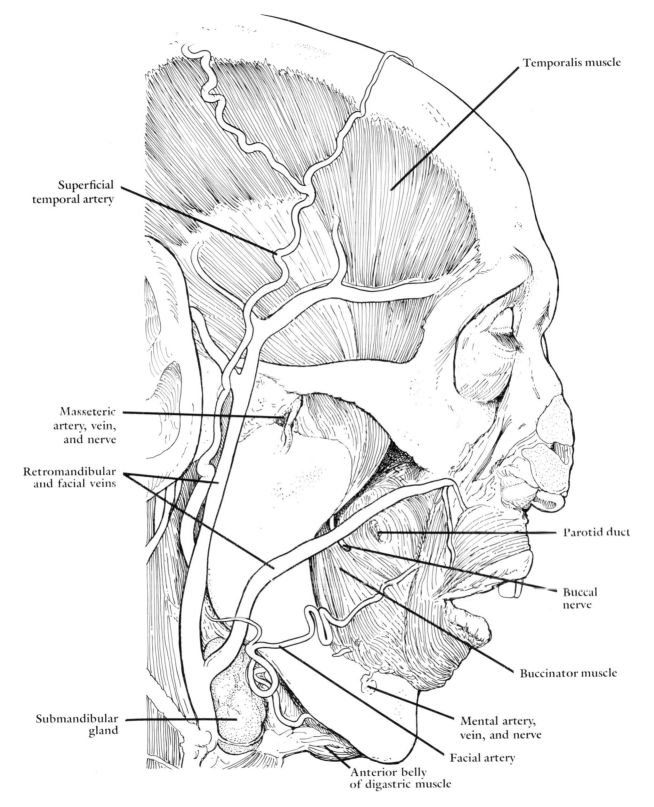

Temporalis muscle

Superficial
temporal artery

Masseteric
artery, vein,
and nerve

Retromandibular
and facial veins

Parotid duct

Buccal
nerve

Buccinator muscle

Mental artery,
vein, and nerve

Submandibular
gland

Facial artery

Anterior belly
of digastric muscle

are accessible as they emerge from the *infratemporal fossa* by way of the *mandibular notch* to penetrate into the deep aspect of the muscle. The *buccal nerve*, a *branch of the mandibular nerve*, also emerging from the infratemporal fossa, courses immediately deep and anterior to the tendon of the temporalis muscle and then branches off over the *buccinator muscle*. All the latter branches pass through the thickness of buccinator muscle before they become distributed entirely to the *mucosa of the oral vestibule*.

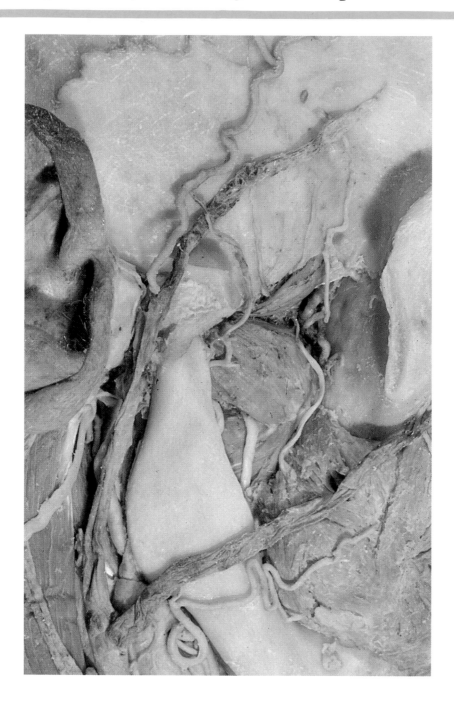

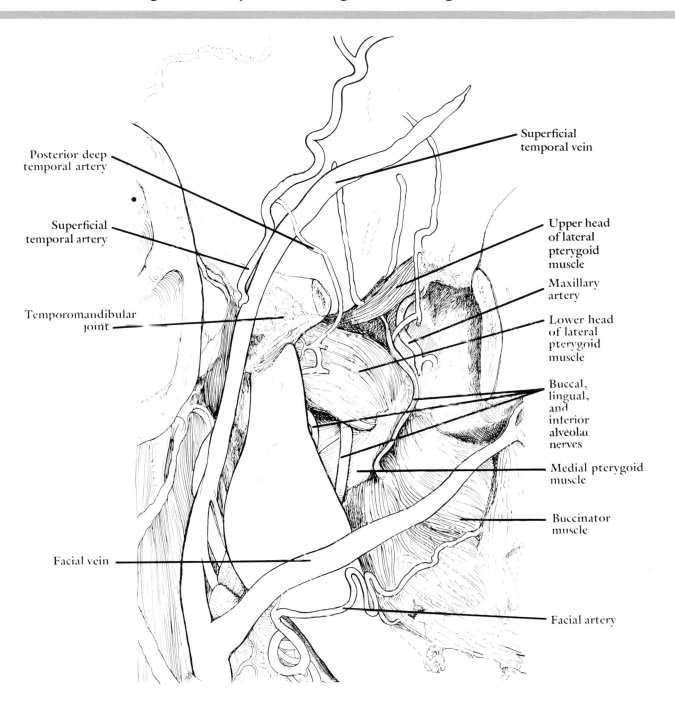

Posterior deep temporal artery

Superficial temporal artery

Temporomandibular joint

Facial vein

Superficial temporal vein

Upper head of lateral pterygoid muscle

Maxillary artery

Lower head of lateral pterygoid muscle

Buccal, lingual, and interior alveolar nerves

Medial pterygoid muscle

Buccinator muscle

Facial artery

Specific remarks: The content of the fossa is shown here after the *zygomatic arch, coronoid process* with *temporalis muscle,* and a part of the *mandibular ramus* have been removed. The *infratemporal fossa* contains two muscles of mastication, the *lateral* and the *medial pterygoid, maxillary artery* and branches, *maxillary vein* and tributaries (frequently the *pterygoid venous plexus* is present instead of veins), and the *mandibular nerve* and its branches. The *maxillary artery* courses superficial, or at times deep, to the *lateral pterygoid muscle,* approaches the *tuber maxillae,* and then enters the *pterygopalatine fossa* through the *pterygomaxillary fissure.*

General remarks: Because an aneurysm of the maxillary artery might occur where it is closely apposed to the tuber maxillae, the surgical exploration of such a condition is frequently made by way of the *maxillary sinus* (transmaxillary approach).

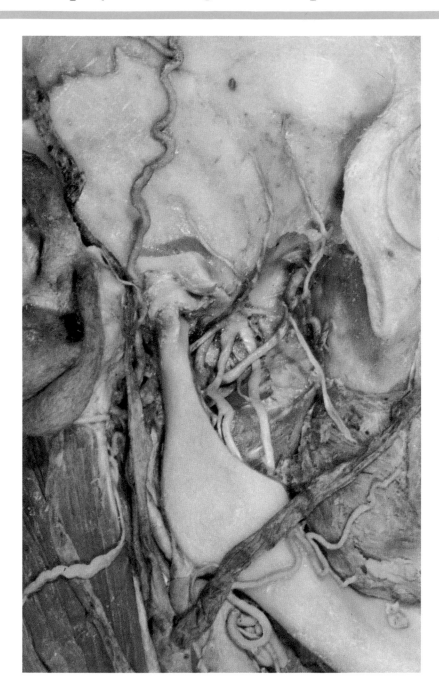

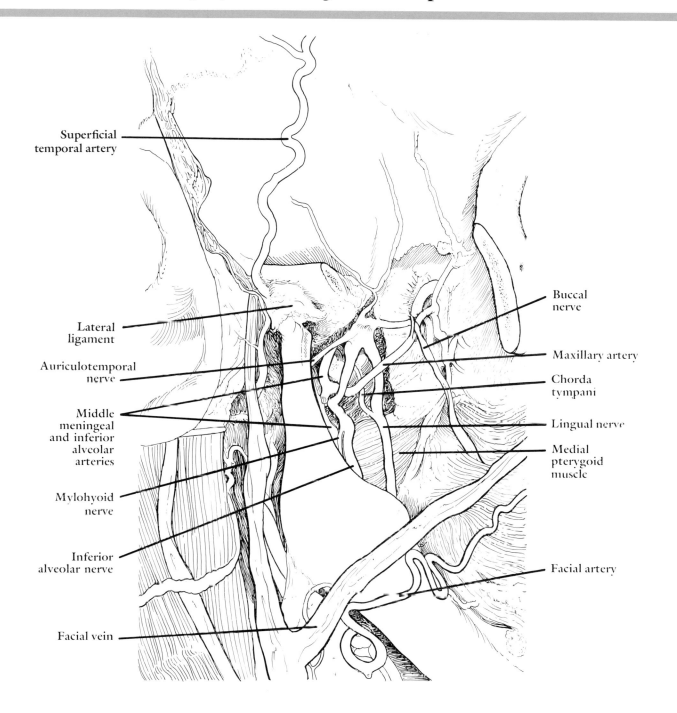

Superficial temporal artery

Lateral ligament

Auriculotemporal nerve

Middle meningeal and inferior alveolar arteries

Mylohyoid nerve

Inferior alveolar nerve

Facial vein

Buccal nerve

Maxillary artery

Chorda tympani

Lingual nerve

Medial pterygoid muscle

Facial artery

Specific remarks: Distribution of the *mandibular nerve* is demonstrated deep to the *lateral pterygoid muscle*, with the muscle being removed.

General remarks: The mandibular nerve, including all of the branches, might be blocked within the *infratemporal fossa*. For mandibular dental block anesthesia the *lingual, buccal,* and *inferior alveolar nerves* are reached just above the level of the *lingula*. The lingual nerve already contains at this level the *chorda tympani* as well as the *communicating branch of the otic ganglion* to the latter nerve. Functional significance of the communicating branch, however, is not sufficiently understood.

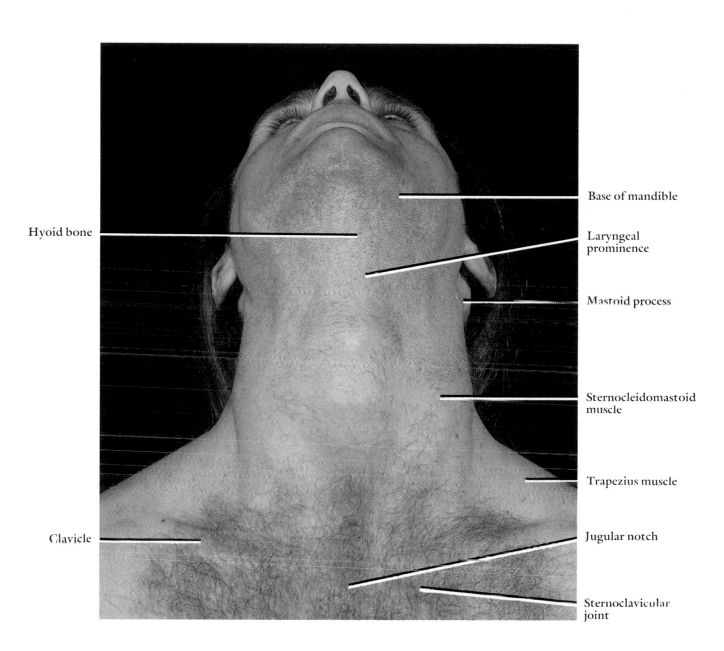

Hyoid bone

Clavicle

Base of mandible

Laryngeal prominence

Mastoid process

Sternocleidomastoid muscle

Trapezius muscle

Jugular notch

Sternoclavicular joint

Specific remarks: Topographic boundaries of the neck include the *base of the mandible* and the *mastoid process* superiorly; and the *manubrium sterni, sternoclavicular joint, clavicle,* and *acromioclavicular joint* inferiorly. Apart from the *cervical vertebral column* the skeletal elements, the *hyoid bone,* and the *laryngeal cartilages* are very mobile.

General remarks: The following structures are accessible to either visual or digital inspection: *facial artery, external* and *anterior jugular veins, sternocleidomastoid muscle, trapezius muscle, hyoid bone, thyroid cartilage, cricoid cartilage, trachea, common carotid artery, thyroid gland,* and *transverse process of C6 vertebra.*

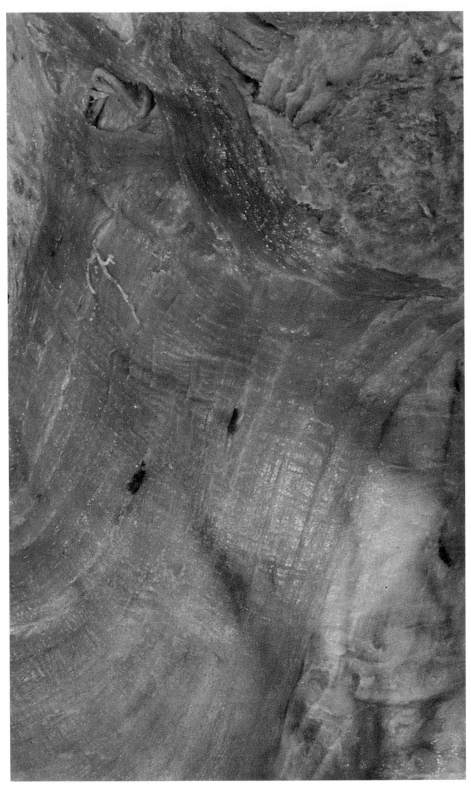

Specific remarks: This subcutaneous layer, unlike that of most other regions of the body, contains, in addition to a more or less developed connective tissue, a superficial muscle of facial expression, the *platysma,* and a number of subcutaneous veins and nerves. The veins, the most important of which are the *external* and *anterior jugular veins,* are

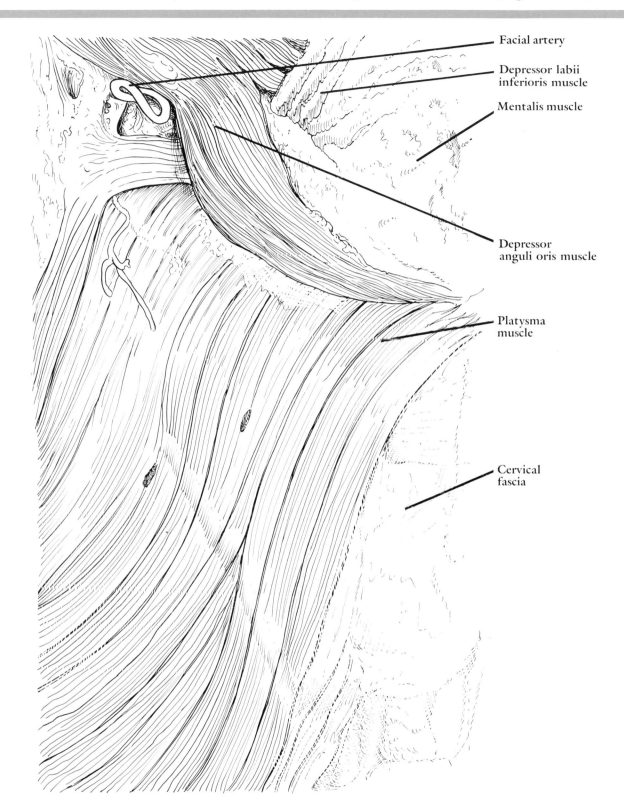

Facial artery

Depressor labii
inferioris muscle

Mentalis muscle

Depressor
anguli oris muscle

Platysma
muscle

Cervical
fascia

greatly variable in their sizes, relationships, and distributions. The cutaneous nerves of the region (*great auricular, lesser occipital, transverse cervical, supraclavicular*) all are derived from the *cervical plexus*. The nerve of the platysma, the *cervical branch of the facial nerve*, becomes subcutaneous at a point immediately below and deep to the *angle of the mandible*.

General remarks: Because of numerous connections between the subcutaneous and deep veins, the blood could be shunted preferentially from either system to the opposite one.

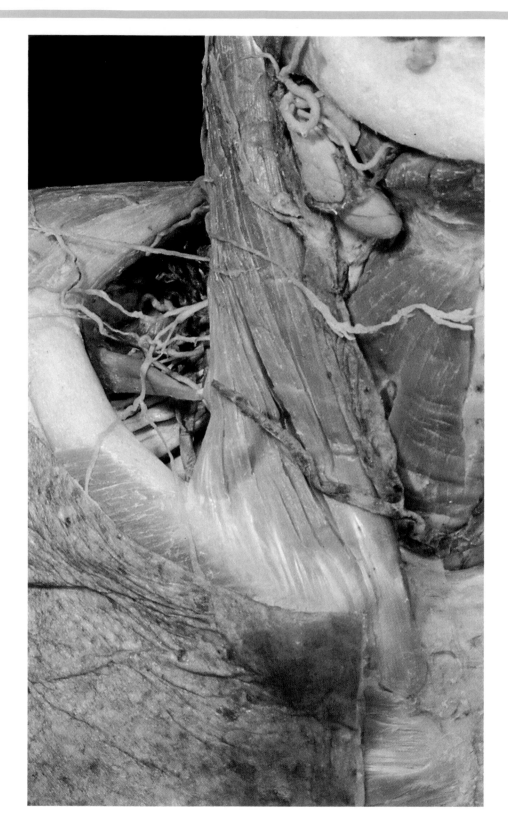

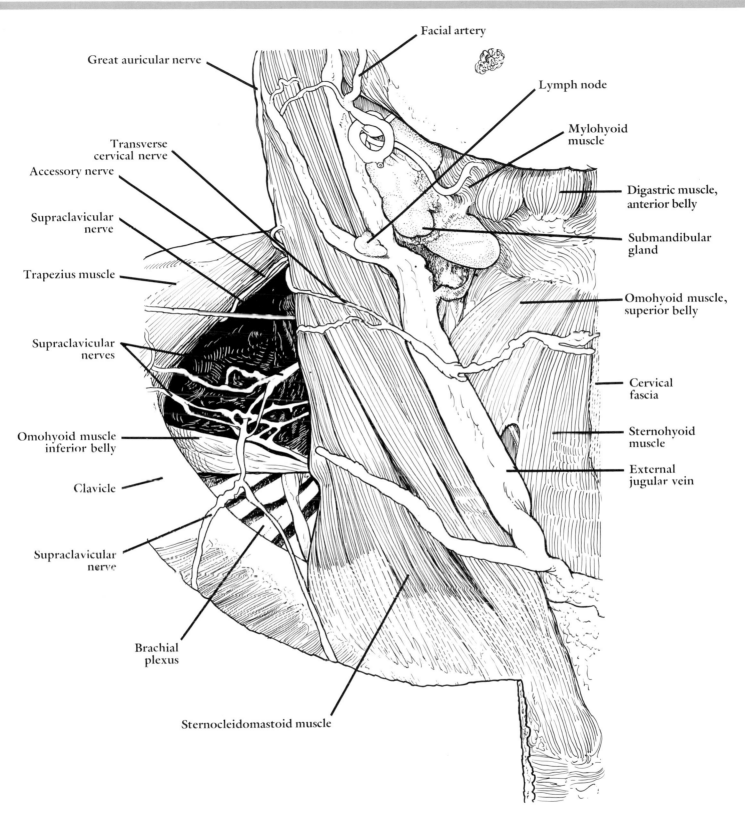

Specific remarks: Once the subcutaneous elements and the *superficial layer of the cervical fascia* are removed, a number of important topographical landmarks of the neck can be shown. The *sternocleidomastoid muscle* delimits the *anterior* and the *posterior triangles of the neck*. The anterior triangle is further subdivided by the *hyoid bone* into the *su-*

prahyoid and *infrahyoid regions*. In addition to muscles, blood vessels, and nerves the suprahyoid region contains the *submandibular salivary gland* and the associated lymph nodes. Major structures of the infrahyoid region are the *laryngeal skeleton* and the *thyroid gland*.

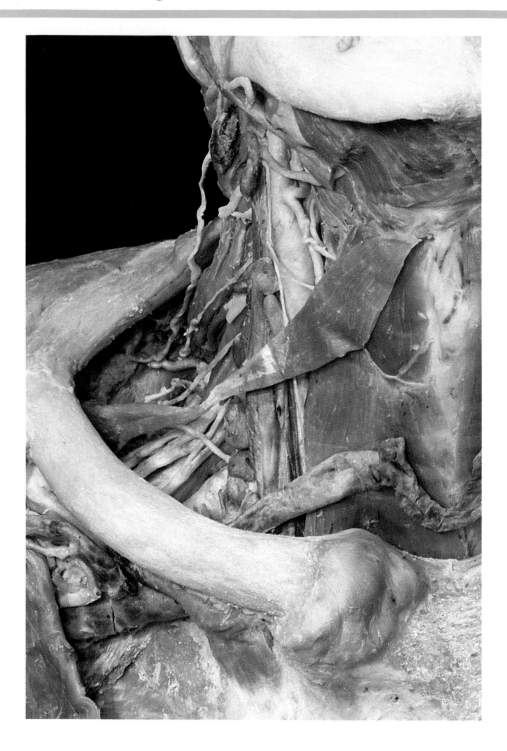

Specific remarks: The contents of the *carotid sheath*—the *common carotid artery* and *internal jugular vein* together with their respective branches and tributaries—are exposed deep to the *sternocleidomastoid muscle*. Deeper muscular layers in the *suprahyoid* and *infrahyoid regions* are also brought into this view, following the removal of the *digastric muscle*

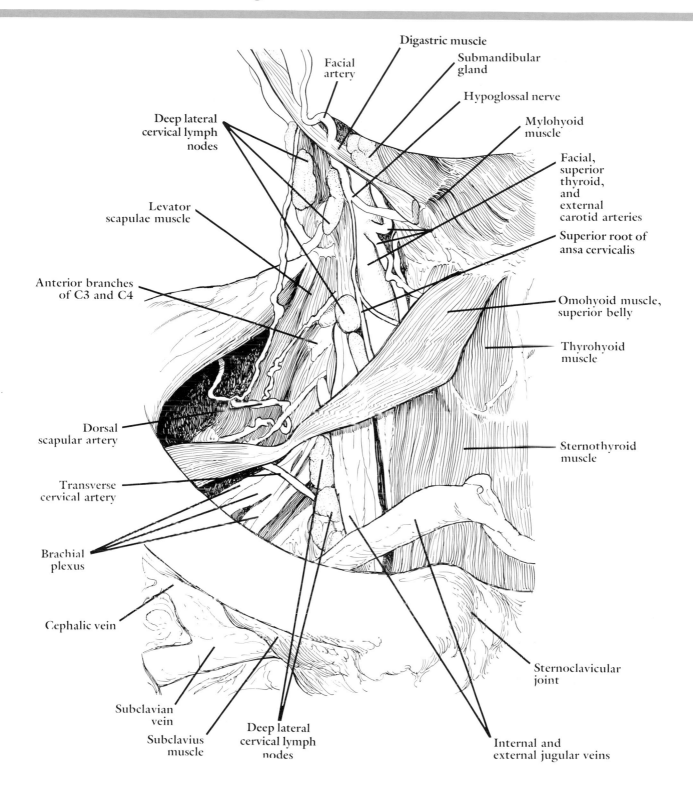

Digastric muscle

Facial artery

Submandibular gland

Hypoglossal nerve

Mylohyoid muscle

Deep lateral cervical lymph nodes

Facial, superior thyroid, and external carotid arteries

Superior root of ansa cervicalis

Levator scapulae muscle

Anterior branches of C3 and C4

Omohyoid muscle, superior belly

Thyrohyoid muscle

Dorsal scapular artery

Sternothyroid muscle

Transverse cervical artery

Brachial plexus

Cephalic vein

Sternoclavicular joint

Subclavian vein

Subclavius muscle

Deep lateral cervical lymph nodes

Internal and external jugular veins

and the *omohyoid* and *sternohyoid muscles,* respectively. Within the *posterior cervical triangle* several branches of the *subclavian artery, external branch of the accessory nerve,* and the components of the *cervical* and *brachial plexuses* are demonstrated.

General remarks: The main lymphatic flow from the head and neck proceeds along the *deep lateral cervical lymphatic chain* organized around the *internal jugular vein.* Two lymph nodes of this chain, the *jugulodigastric* and *juguloomohyoid,* are of particular topographic importance. They are related to the vein where it is crossed by the digastric and omohyoid muscles, respectively.

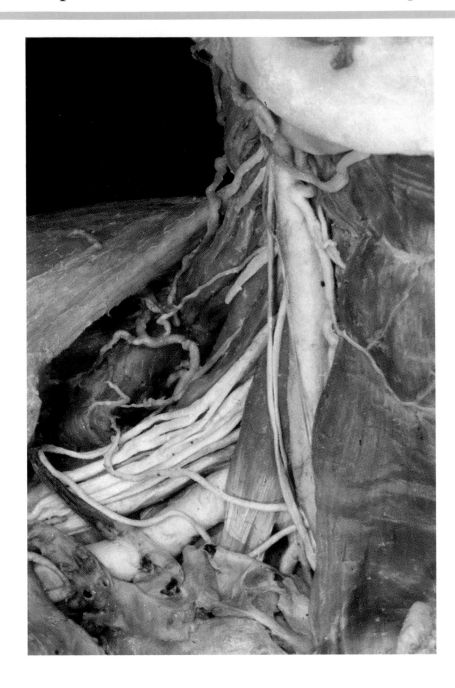

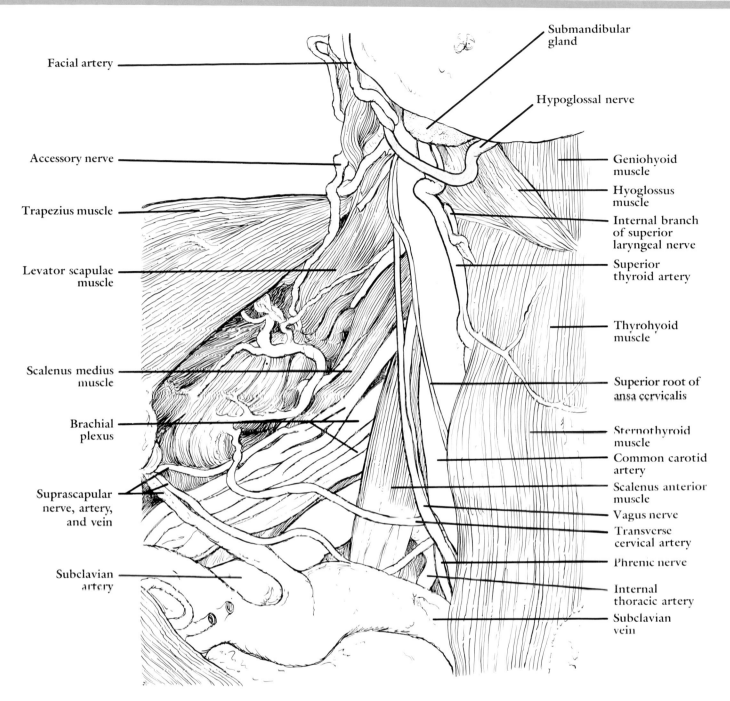

Facial artery

Accessory nerve

Trapezius muscle

Levator scapulae muscle

Scalenus medius muscle

Brachial plexus

Suprascapular nerve, artery, and vein

Subclavian artery

Submandibular gland

Hypoglossal nerve

Geniohyoid muscle

Hyoglossus muscle

Internal branch of superior laryngeal nerve

Superior thyroid artery

Thyrohyoid muscle

Superior root of ansa cervicalis

Sternothyroid muscle

Common carotid artery

Scalenus anterior muscle

Vagus nerve

Transverse cervical artery

Phrenic nerve

Internal thoracic artery

Subclavian vein

Specific remarks: The *hyoid bone, thyrohyoid membrane, larynx, thyroid gland,* and *trachea* are demonstrated deep to the *infrahyoid muscles;* the *lingual* and *hypoglossal nerves* and the *submandibular duct* are located deep to the *mylohyoid muscle.* The relationships of the structures at the root of the neck can best be demonstrated if the *clavicle* is first disarticulated at the *sternoclavicular joint* and then taken away.

General remarks: For the superficial exploration of the *posterior cervical triangle,* the *omohyoid muscle* and the *external branch of the accessory nerve* are important points of reference. At a deeper plane, however, the muscles of the floor of this triangle are equally useful for orientation in approaching the blood vessels and nerves of the region (e.g., *scalenus anterior muscle* for the *phrenic nerve,* and the *scalenus anterior* and *medius muscles* for the *brachial plexus* and *subclavian artery*).

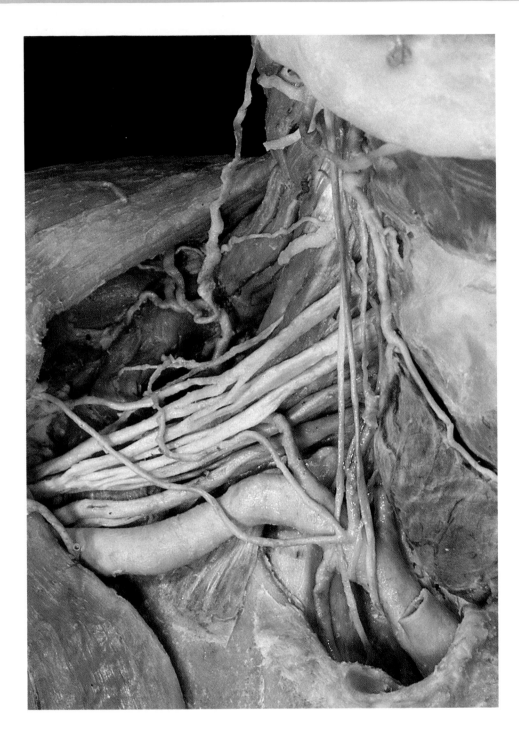

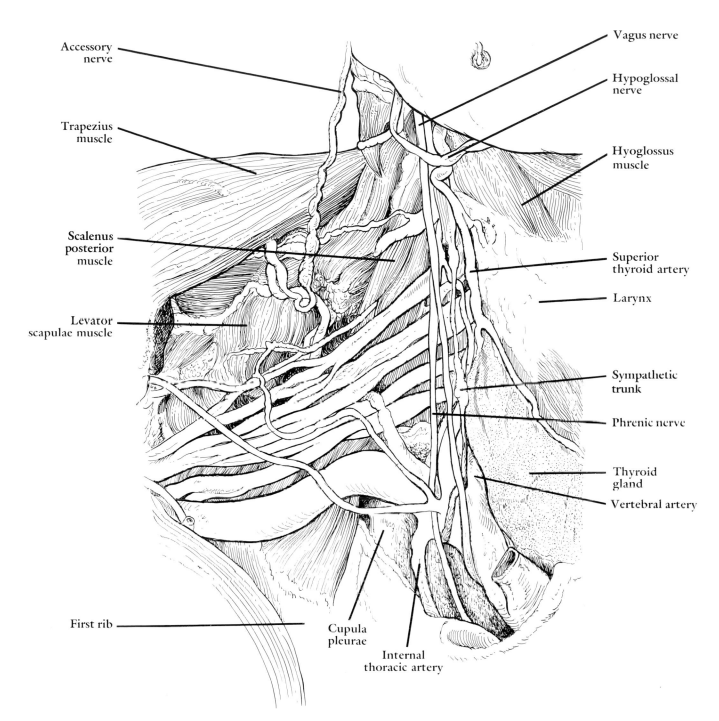

Accessory nerve

Trapezius muscle

Scalenus posterior muscle

Levator scapulae muscle

First rib

Cupula pleurae

Internal thoracic artery

Vagus nerve

Hypoglossal nerve

Hyoglossus muscle

Superior thyroid artery

Larynx

Sympathetic trunk

Phrenic nerve

Thyroid gland

Vertebral artery

Specific remarks: To best demonstrate the initial segment of the *subclavian artery* and its branches and roots of the *brachial plexus*, the *scalenus anterior muscle* must be displaced or removed. The anterior aspect of the artery is crossed by the *vagus* and *phrenic nerves* and by the anterior arm of the *ansa subclavia*. The right *vagus nerve* at this level gives off the *recurrent laryngeal nerve*, which turns first inferior and then posterior to the artery before it ascends toward the *larynx*. The *cervical sympathetic trunk* consists of a variable number of ganglia. The lowest of these, before

the *stellate ganglion*, gives off two branches that embrace the *subclavian artery* anteriorly and posteriorly *(ansa subclavia)* to end in the stellate ganglion. The *dome of the pleura* is topographically also included among the structures of the cervical root.

General remarks: On the side of the neck opposite to the one demonstrated herein the *thoracic duct* is closely related to the *vertebral blood vessels, thyrocervical trunk,* sympathetic trunk, phrenic nerve, and the right scalenus anterior muscle.

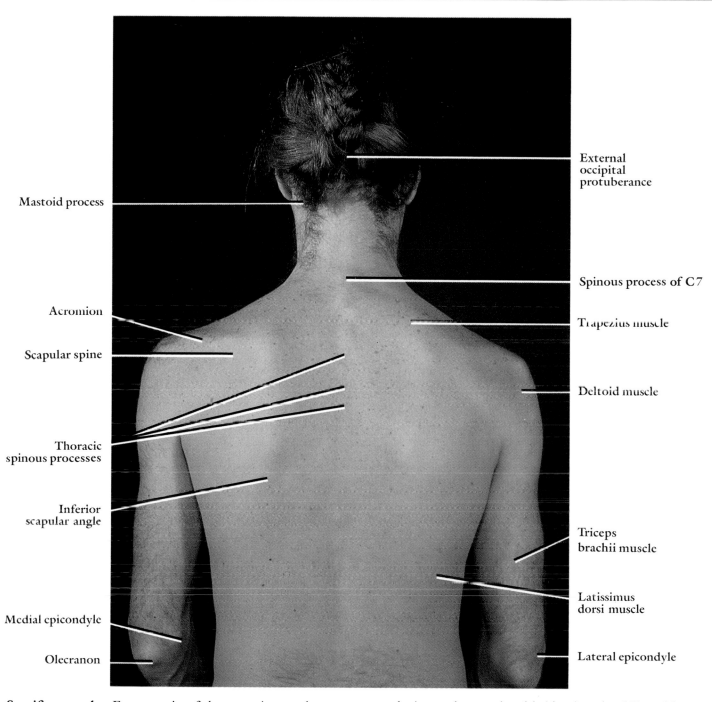

Mastoid process

Acromion

Scapular spine

Thoracic
spinous processes

Inferior
scapular angle

Medial epicondyle

Olecranon

External
occipital
protuberance

Spinous process of C7

Trapezius muscle

Deltoid muscle

Triceps
brachii muscle

Latissimus
dorsi muscle

Lateral epicondyle

Specific remarks: Free margin of the *trapezius muscle* represents the topographical borderline between the anterior and posterior compartments of the neck. Some of the bony landmarks in the posterior compartment include the *external occipital protuberance*, the *mastoid process*, and the *spine of the C7 vertebra*. On the posterior surface of the *thorax* and *arm* several muscles or muscular groups (*trapezius, latissimus dorsi, scapular muscles, deltoid, triceps brachii*) and bony landmarks (*acromion and scapular spine, inferior angle of the scapula, spines of thoracic vertebrae, ribs, glenohumeral joint, greater tubercle of the humerus, humeral shaft, epicondyles, elbow joint*) are identifiable by inspection and palpation. The thoracic landmarks are particularly important for percussion and auscultation of internal organs.

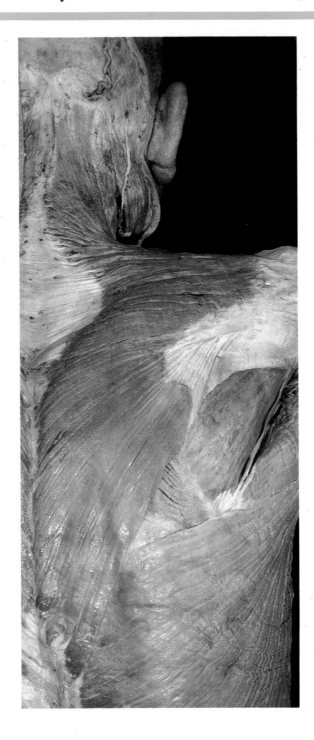

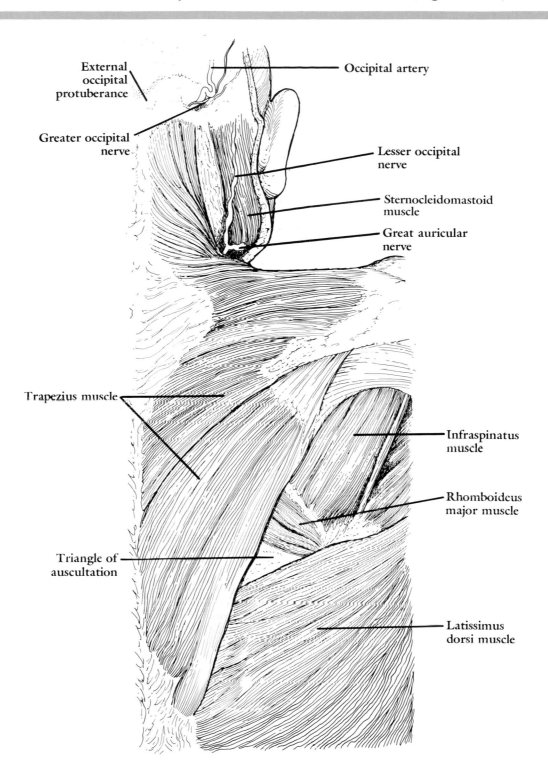

External occipital protuberance

Occipital artery

Greater occipital nerve

Lesser occipital nerve

Sternocleidomastoid muscle

Great auricular nerve

Trapezius muscle

Infraspinatus muscle

Rhomboideus major muscle

Triangle of auscultation

Latissimus dorsi muscle

Specific remarks: The *trapezius muscle* covers most of this region. The cephalic attachment of this muscle is characterized by the passage of the *greater occipital nerve (dorsal ramus of C2)* through its aponeurosis. It is from here that the nerve, together with the *occipital blood vessels,* becomes distributed throughout the subcutaneous layer and the skin of the *occipital region.* Between the *external occipital protuberance* and the *spine* of either the *C7* or *T1 vertebra* the *aponeurosis of the trapezius* is fused along the midline with the counterpart from the opposite side, thus contributing to the *ligamentum nuchae.* The muscle is perforated at various levels by the *dorsal rami of the spinal nerves,* which eventually terminate in the adjacent skin.

General remarks: Because of a relatively superficial position of the *greater occipital nerve,* prior to the division into the terminal branches, it is convenient to anesthetize the nerve at a point 1.5 cm lateral and inferior to the *external occipital protuberance.*

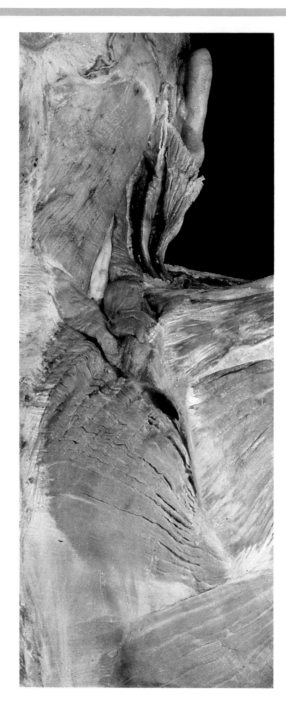

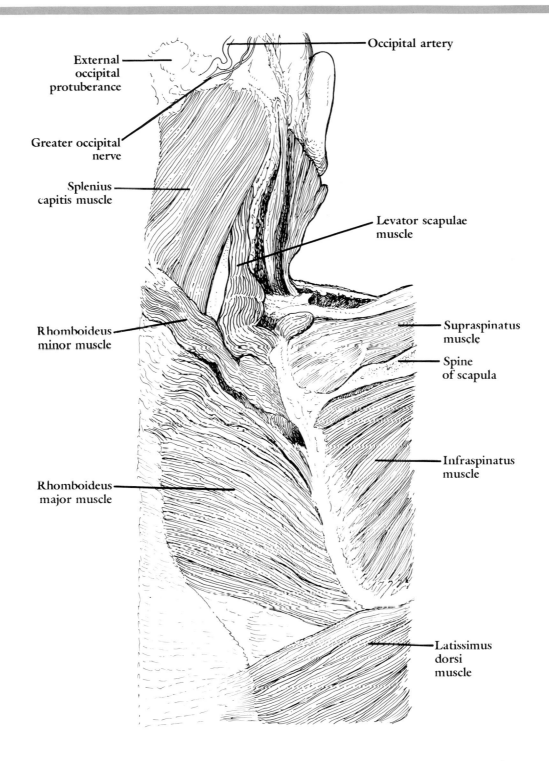

External occipital protuberance

Greater occipital nerve

Splenius capitis muscle

Rhomboideus minor muscle

Rhomboideus major muscle

Occipital artery

Levator scapulae muscle

Supraspinatus muscle

Spine of scapula

Infraspinatus muscle

Latissimus dorsi muscle

Specific remarks: Following the removal of the *trapezius muscle*, the fascia of this muscle, and the *deep layer of the cervical fascia*, several muscles in the region of the back of neck are demonstrated: *splenius capitis, splenius cervicis, rhomboids,* and *levator scapulae*. The upper part of the *aponeurosis of the splenius capitis muscle* fuses along the midline with the counterpart from the opposite side to contribute to the *ligamentum nuchae*. The *dorsal rami of the spinal*

nerves are also apparent here along the paramedian plane, as they course through this musculature on the way to the more superficial structures.

General remarks: Together with the *trapezius muscle*, the *rhomboids* and the *levator scapulae muscles* are important stabilizers of the shoulder joint. They all give support to the muscles that act directly on the *glenohumeral joint.*

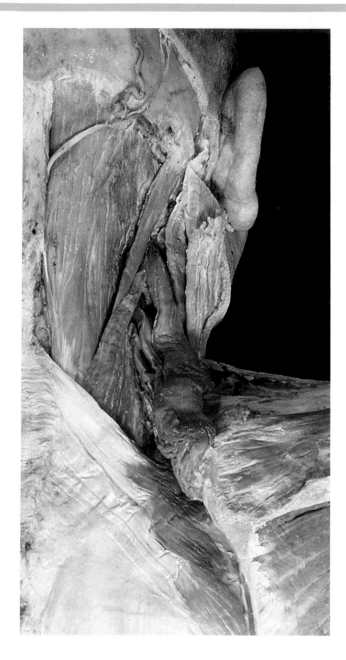

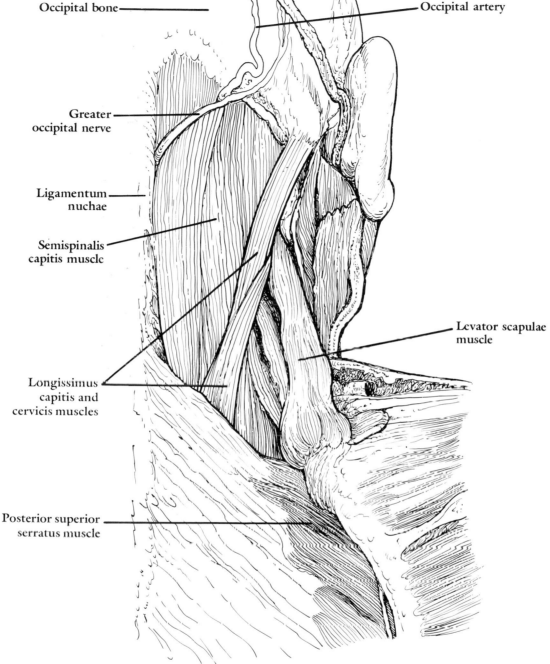

Occipital bone

Occipital artery

Greater occipital nerve

Ligamentum nuchae

Semispinalis capitis muscle

Levator scapulae muscle

Longissimus capitis and cervicis muscles

Posterior superior serratus muscle

Specific remarks: The *semispinalis capitis muscle* is the main component of this layer. Its origin from the *transverse processes of thoracic vertebrae* is obscured in this view by the *posterior superior serratus muscle*. While this origin is complex, consisting of several bundles or tendons, the muscle attaches as a whole to the *occipital bone*. The upper muscular part is perforated by the *dorsal ramus of the C2 nerve (the greater occipital nerve)*, and it is also closely related to the *occipital blood vessels*. The uppermost extension of the longissimus musculature, *longissimus capitis* and *longissimus cervicis*, is identified immediately lateral and deep to the *semispinalis capitis muscle*.

General remarks: The *semispinalis capitis muscles* usually act independently from one another. In some instances, however, their actions are to some extent combined by the way of accessory attachments of these muscles to the *ligamentum nuchae*.

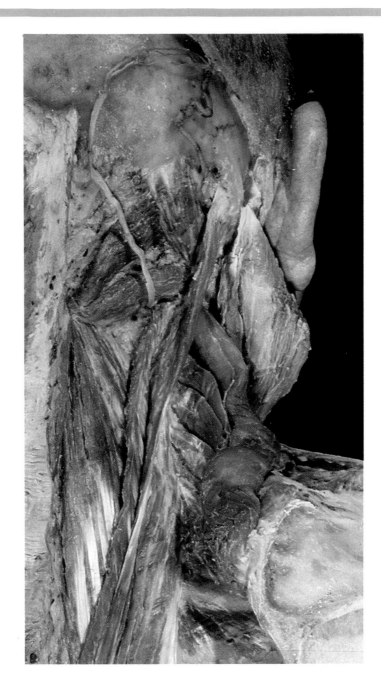

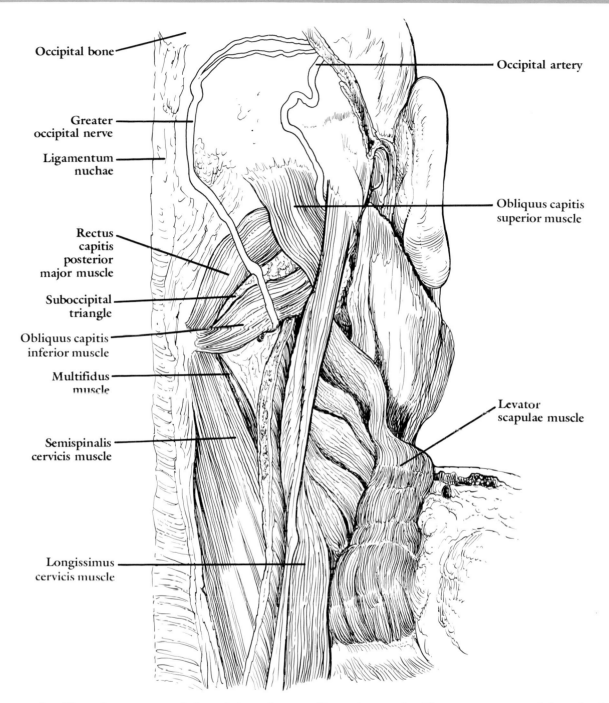

Occipital bone

Greater
occipital nerve

Ligamentum
nuchae

Rectus
capitis
posterior
major muscle

Suboccipital
triangle

Obliquus capitis
inferior muscle

Multifidus
muscle

Semispinalis
cervicis muscle

Longissimus
cervicis muscle

Occipital artery

Obliquus capitis
superior muscle

Levator
scapulae muscle

Specific remarks: The *spinons process of the axis* is an important topographical point because two deep muscles of this region (*semispinalis cervicis* and *multifidus*) and two muscles of the *suboccipital triangle* (*rectus capitis posterior major* and *obliquus capitis inferior*) originate from it. The third muscle of the triangle, the *obliquus capitis superior*, extends from the *transverse process of the atlas* to the *occipital bone*. The *greater occipital nerve* turns at this level typically inferior to the *obliquus capitis inferior muscle* before it becomes continuous with the corresponding ganglion.

General remarks: The narrow space of the *suboccipital triangle*, which leads to the *vertebral artery*, is occupied by connective tissue. The floor of the triangle is formed by the *posterior arch of the atlas* and the *posterior atlantooccipital membrane*. The *vertebral artery* courses superior to the *posterior arch*, and the *dorsal ramus of the C1 nerve*, which innervates all of the suboccipital muscles, emerges between the artery and the arch.

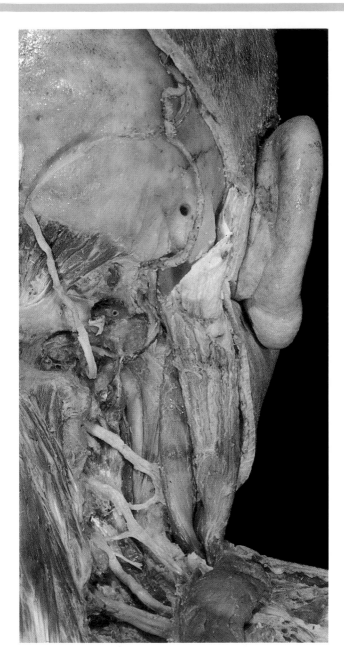

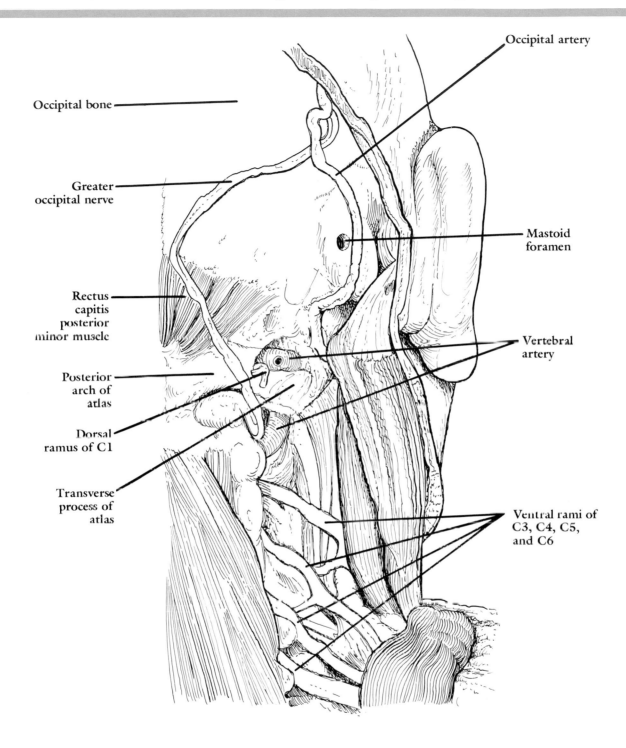

Occipital artery

Occipital bone

Greater
occipital nerve

Rectus
capitis
posterior
minor muscle

Posterior
arch of
atlas

Dorsal
ramus of C1

Transverse
process of
atlas

Mastoid
foramen

Vertebral
artery

Ventral rami of
C3, C4, C5,
and C6

Specific remarks: When three muscles of the *suboccipital triangle* (*rectus capitis posterior major* and *superior* and *inferior obliques*) are removed, the deep muscle of the region, the *rectus capitis posterior minor*, and the structures of the floor of the triangle can be seen. Along the floor the *posterior arch of the atlas*, the *posterior atlantooccipital membrane* superiorly, and the *ligamentum flavum* inferiorly are dis- sected out. The former membrane gives passage to the *vertebral artery* and the *dorsal ramus of the C1 nerve;* the latter membrane is perforated by the *ganglion* of the *C2 spinal nerve.* The course of the *vertebral artery* through the *vertebrarterial foramina* and the grouping of *ventral rami* of the *cervical spinal nerves* into the *cervical plexus* are partially demonstrated in this view.

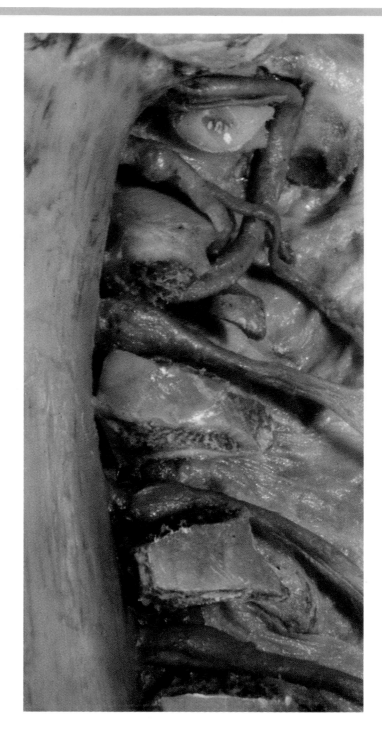

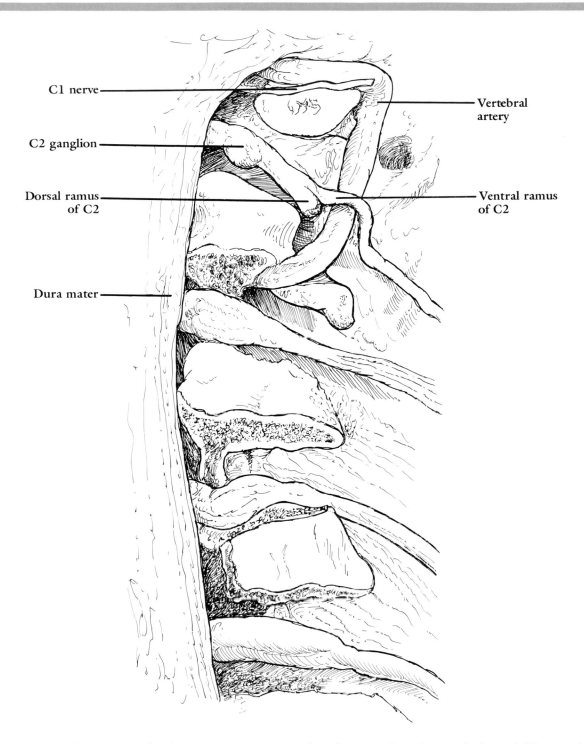

C1 nerve

C2 ganglion

Dorsal ramus
of C2

Dura mater

Vertebral
artery

Ventral ramus
of C2

Specific remarks: To demonstrate the deep structures contained within the *vertebral column,* the following steps are carried out: (1) all muscles from the back of neck are removed; (2) the *vertebral laminae,* together with the *spinous processes,* are removed; (3) the content of the *epidural space* (connective tissue and venous plexus) is removed from the posterior aspect of the *dura mater;* (4) the *intervertebral foramina* are enlarged posteriorly; and (5) several *vertebrarterial foramina* are opened posteriorly. Following such a dissection the extensions of the *dura mater* to the *spinal ganglia,* distribution of *spinal nerves* into the *rami,* grouping of the *ventral rami,* and the relationship of the *vertebral artery* to the *transverse processes* and the *spinal nerves* become apparent.

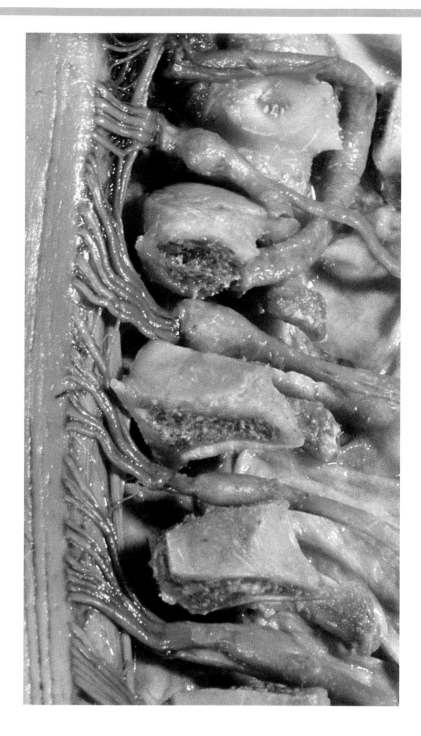

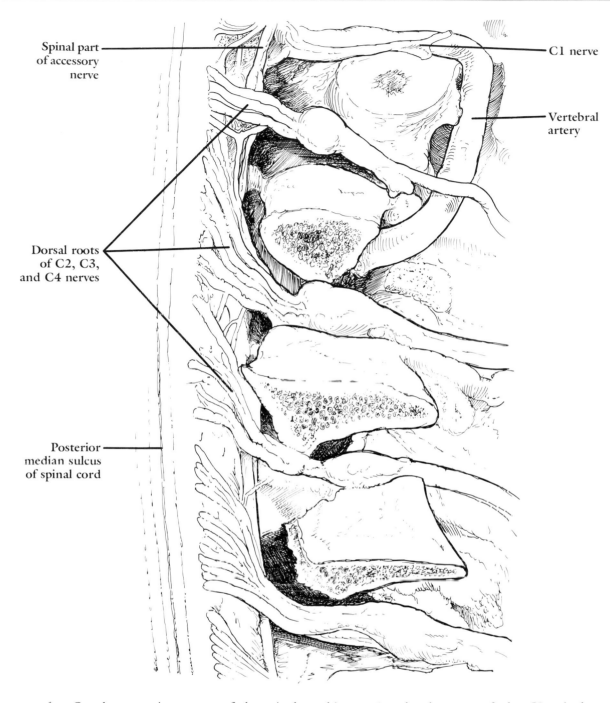

Spinal part of accessory nerve

C1 nerve

Vertebral artery

Dorsal roots of C2, C3, and C4 nerves

Posterior median sulcus of spinal cord

Specific remarks: On the posterior aspect of the *spinal cord*, which is shown here after the *dura mater* and *arachnoid* have been dissected away, the following structures can be identified: *posterior sulcus, spinal part of the accessory nerve, dorsal roots, ventral roots* and *dorsal root ganglia*. The horizontal segment of the *vertebral artery*, one that courses superior to the *posterior arch of the atlas*, has a close relation-ship to the *dorsal ramus of the C1 spinal nerve*. The relationship of the vertical segment of the same artery with the *ventral rami of cervical spinal nerves* is shown to a greater advantage, as are the ventral rami, which form the *cervical plexus* further laterally. Like the *ventral roots*, each group of *dorsal roots*, converging to a specific ganglion, emerges from a distinct segment of the *spinal cord*.

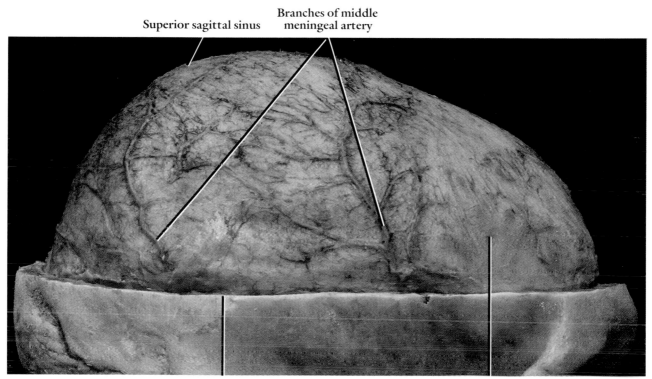

Superior sagittal sinus

Branches of middle meningeal artery

Cut surface of skull

Dura mater

Specific remarks: To obtain this view of the *dura mater,* the soft tissues and the bones of the skull have been cut horizontally just above the *superciliary arch* anteriorly, the *auricle* laterally, and the *external occipital protuberance* posteriorly. The bony layer was subsequently separated from the underlying *dura mater* and removed together with the scalp.

General remarks: The *middle meningeal artery* and its branches are distributed through a narrow layer enclosed between the *dura mater* and the inner table of the skull bones. Hemorrhage from this artery, or from a branch of it, leads to a compression of the cerebral surface and subsequently to various neurological disorders. In addition to the main artery, *accessory meningeal arteries* may sometimes develop.

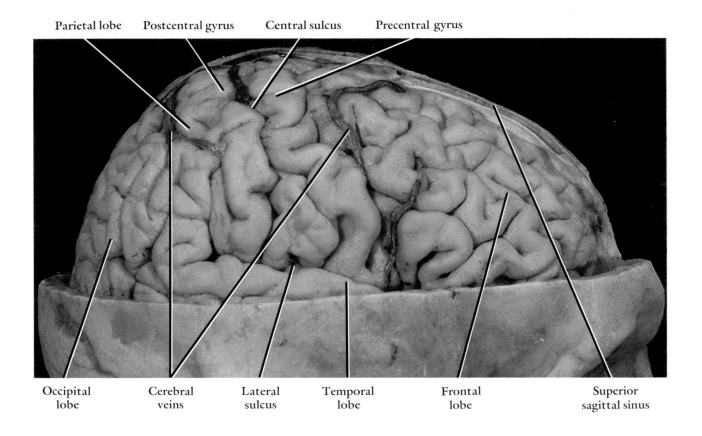

Parietal lobe   Postcentral gyrus   Central sulcus   Precentral gyrus

Occipital lobe   Cerebral veins   Lateral sulcus   Temporal lobe   Frontal lobe   Superior sagittal sinus

Specific remarks: To demonstrate the right *cerebral hemisphere* in situ, the appropriate segments of the *dura mater* and *arachnoid* have been removed. Branches of the cerebral venous system predominately join one another to finally empty into the *great cerebral vein*. Some branches, however, open individually into the neighboring *dural venous sinuses*. Because of this tributary contribution, the diameter of the *dural venous sinuses* increases steadily in the direction of the blood flow. In the case of the *superior sagittal sinus* that is anteroposteriorly.

General remarks: Some of the skull bones, which cover directly the *superior sagittal sinus*, are still membranous at birth (i.e., *frontal, parietal, occipital*). Because of this developmental characteristic, the *superior sagittal sinus* in newborns can be used for collecting blood samples for diagnostic purposes and administering drugs intravenously.

Inferior sagittal sinus   Falx cerebri   Superior sagittal sinus   Corpus callosum

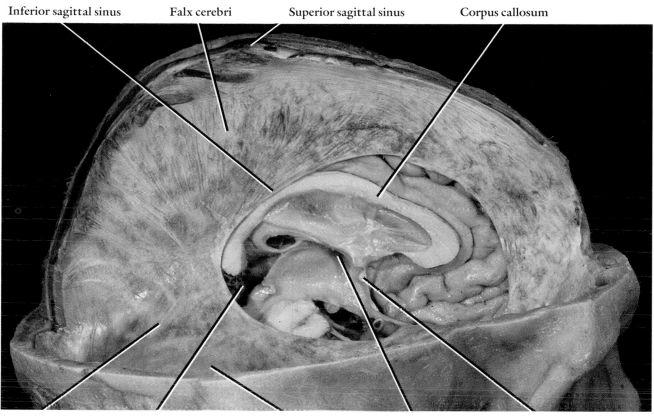

Straight sinus   Great cerebral vein   Tentorium cerebelli   Interventricular foramen   Anterior commissure

Specific remarks: In this specimen both the *anterior* and the *posterior cerebral commissures, optic chiasma, lamina terminalis, interthalamic adhesion,* and the *corpus callosum* have been cut sagittally to separate the two *cerebral hemispheres.* Subsequently the right *cerebral hemisphere* was separated from the midbrain and then removed. (In the course of this dissection the *falx cerebri* was preserved in situ.) The anterior end of the *falx cerebri* is attached to the *crista galli;* the posterior extension fuses with the *tentorium cerebelli,* whereby the *straight sinus* is formed. The superior and inferior margins of the *falx cerebri* contain the corresponding *sagittal sinuses.* The *superior sagittal sinus* empties directly into the *confluence of sinuses.* The *inferior sagittal sinus* receives the *great cerebral vein* to become the *straight sinus.* The latter sinus also empties into the *confluence of sinuses.*

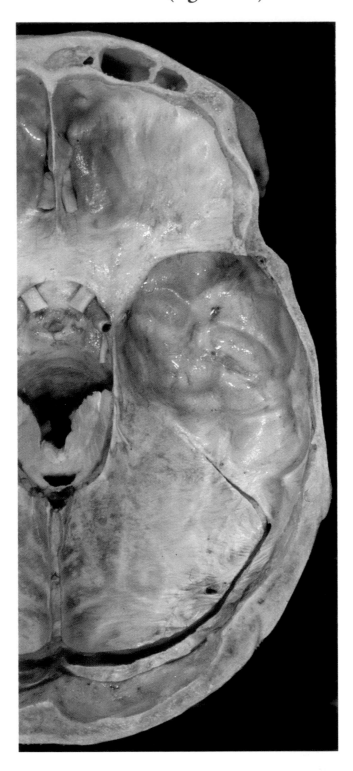

Specific remarks: To better demonstrate some of the formations by the *dura mater* (i.e., *cavernous sinus, straight sinus, tentorium cerebelli*), the previous specimen (Fig. 48) is viewed here from above, after the *falx cerebri* has been separated and removed from the *tentorium cerebelli* and the *crista galli*. Along the line of fusion between the *falx cerebri*

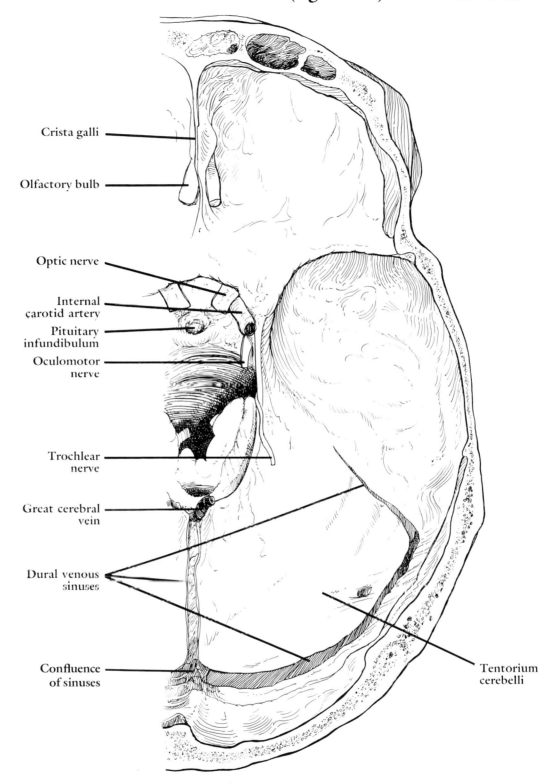

Crista galli

Olfactory bulb

Optic nerve

Internal carotid artery

Pituitary infundibulum

Oculomotor nerve

Trochlear nerve

Great cerebral vein

Dural venous sinuses

Confluence of sinuses

Tentorium cerebelli

and *tentorium cerebelli*, the *straight sinus* is now open. The circumference of the *tentorium cerebelli* attaches posteriorly to the *occipital bone* to enclose the *transverse sinus* and laterally to the superior margin of the *petrous part of the temporal bone* to enclose the *superior petrosal sinus*. The latter sinus communicates between the *transverse sinus* and the *cavernous sinus*, which is located on the lateral side of the *sella turcica*. Anteriorly, however, the *tentorium cerebelli*, together with the *dorsum sellae* and the *clivus*, gives passage between the supratentorial and infratentorial compartments of the *cranial cavity* to the brainstem.

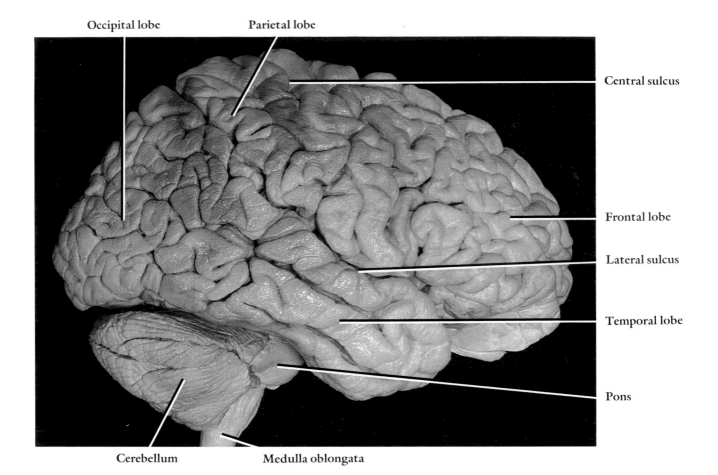

Occipital lobe   Parietal lobe

Central sulcus

Frontal lobe

Lateral sulcus

Temporal lobe

Pons

Cerebellum   Medulla oblongata

Specific remarks: To demonstrate the surface morphology of the brain, brainstem, and the *cerebellum,* the three meningeal layers and the superficial blood vessels have been removed. The *cerebral hemisphere* is divided into several lobes (*frontal, parietal, temporal, occipital*) by way of two major sulci, the *central* and the *lateral.* Each lobe is further subdivided into a number of *gyri* by way of the secondary order *sulci.*

General remarks: From a functional point of view the *cerebral cortex* contains numerous areas (e.g., *sensorimotor, visual, acoustic,* and *ectosylvian*) that are confined within the morphological subunits, the gyri.

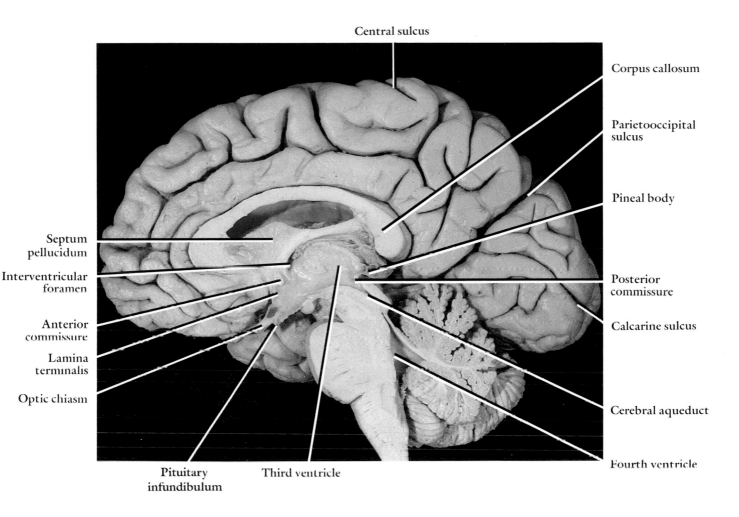

Central sulcus

Corpus callosum

Parietooccipital sulcus

Pineal body

Septum pellucidum

Interventricular foramen

Anterior commissure

Lamina terminalis

Optic chiasm

Posterior commissure

Calcarine sulcus

Cerebral aqueduct

Fourth ventricle

Pituitary infundibulum

Third ventricle

Specific remarks: This view, which has been obtained by separation of the two halves of the central nervous system organs along the midsagittal plane, demonstrates the major connections between the two *cerebral* and the two *cerebellar* hemispheres. In addition to the structures on the medial cerebral surface, the internal structures of the brainstem, the walls of the *third* and *fourth ventricles,* and the *cerebral aqueduct* are shown.

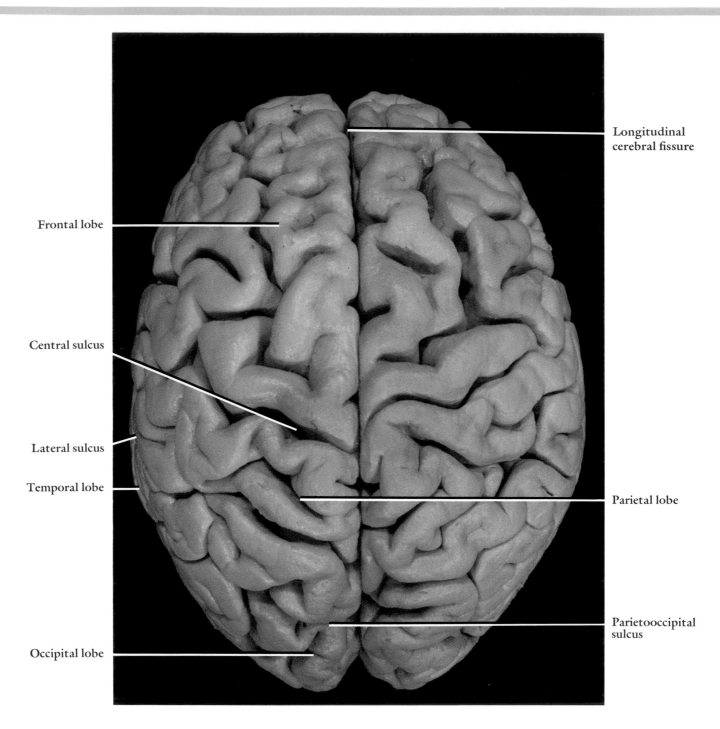

Longitudinal cerebral fissure

Frontal lobe

Central sulcus

Lateral sulcus

Temporal lobe

Parietal lobe

Parietooccipital sulcus

Occipital lobe

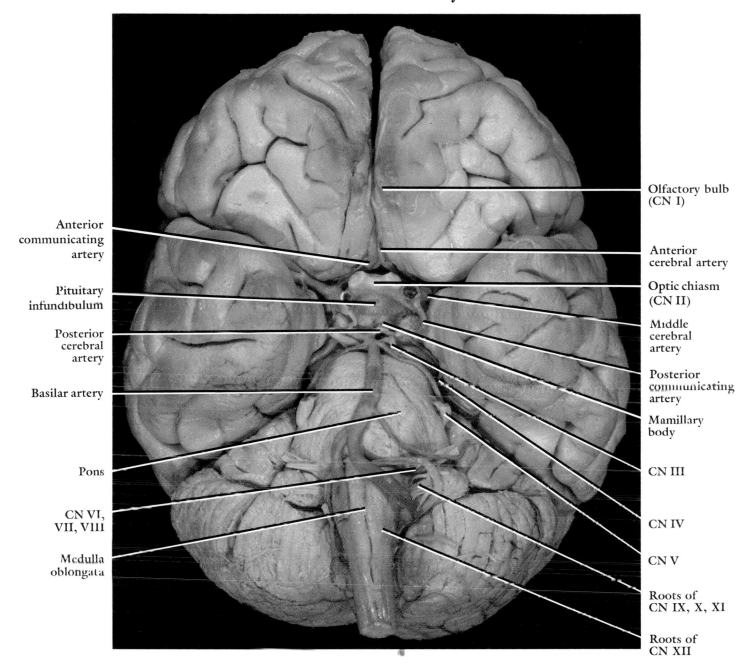

Olfactory bulb (CN I)

Anterior communicating artery

Anterior cerebral artery

Pituitary infundibulum

Optic chiasm (CN II)

Posterior cerebral artery

Middle cerebral artery

Basilar artery

Posterior communicating artery

Mamillary body

Pons

CN III

CN VI, VII, VIII

CN IV

Medulla oblongata

CN V

Roots of CN IX, X, XI

Roots of CN XII

Specific remarks: In this view all cranial nerves *(CN)* have been cut close to their respective points of exit from the cranial cavity, the *vertebral artery* at the *foramen magnum* and the *internal carotid artery* close to the *anterior clinoid process.* All separated structures were subsequently removed, together with the cranial division of the central nervous system, from the cranial cavity.

General remarks: The *internal carotid* and *vertebral arteries* are anastomosed to one another by way of the *basilar artery, cerebral arteries,* and *communicating arteries.* The arterial circle thus formed is an important formation for the blood supply and in the vascular pathology of the central nervous system.

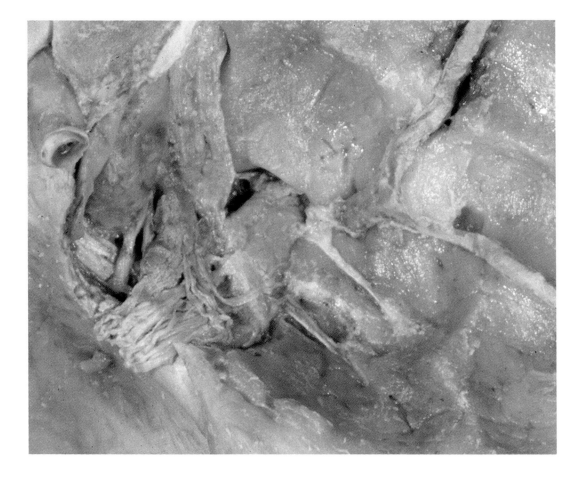

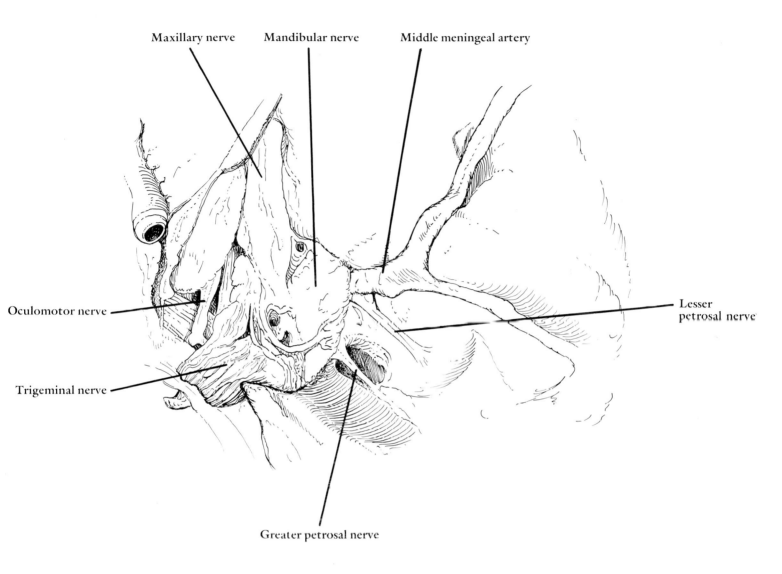

Maxillary nerve   Mandibular nerve   Middle meningeal artery

Oculomotor nerve

Lesser petrosal nerve

Trigeminal nerve

Greater petrosal nerve

Specific remarks: Although the *dura mater* in this view has been completely removed from the anterior surface of the petrous part of the temporal bone and the superior aspect of *trigeminal ganglion*, that part of dura mater which covers the floor of the *trigeminal impression* has been left intact. In the course of this procedure it was necessary to separate in situ the *petrosal nerves* and the *middle meningeal artery* from the meningeal layer. On the exposed surface of the petrous part the following structures are demonstrated: *arcuate eminence*, or projection of the *anterior semicircular canal*; *tegmen tympani*, or roof of the *tympanic cavity*; *hiatus for the greater petrosal nerve*; and *hiatus for the lesser petrosal nerve*.

General remarks: The *greater* and *lesser petrosal nerves*, which originate from the *facial* and *glossopharyngeal nerves*, respectively, represent preganglionic segments of the two parasympathetic pathways. The facial pathway is etiologically implicated in otogenic and rhinogenic headaches, conditions that are successfully treated by severance of the greater petrosal nerve on the anterior surface of the petrous part of the temporal bone.

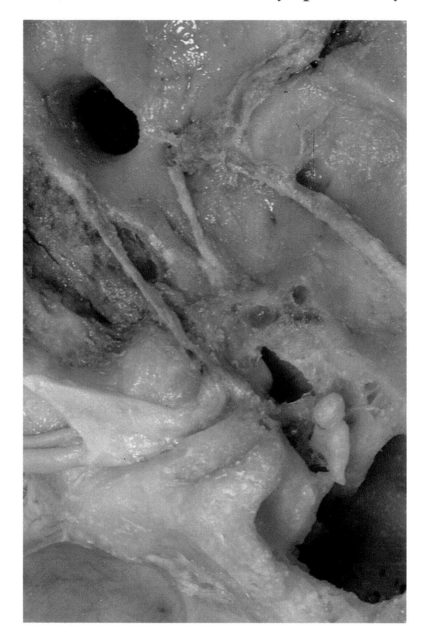

Superior aspect of the right inner ear, intraosseous segment of the facial nerve, and structures in the tympanic cavity

56

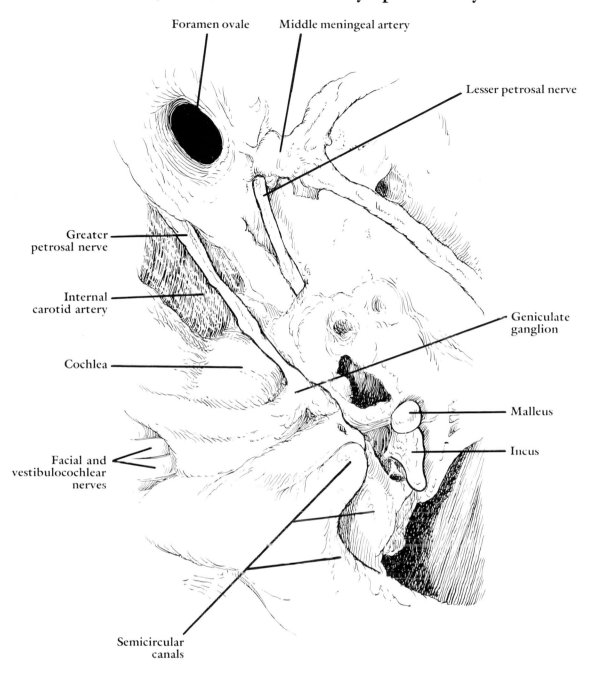

Foramen ovale   Middle meningeal artery

Lesser petrosal nerve

Greater petrosal nerve

Internal carotid artery

Cochlea

Facial and vestibulocochlear nerves

Geniculate ganglion

Malleus

Incus

Semicircular canals

Specific remarks: After removal of the bony roof (the *tegmen tympani*) from the middle ear cavity, the three *semicircular canals* and the *cochlea* have been dissected out of the bone. The first and second intraosseous segments of the *facial nerve,* the *geniculate ganglion,* and the initial intraosseous part of the *greater petrosal nerve* have been exposed at the same time. Inside the *tympanic cavity* two ossicles, the *malleus* and the *incus,* and the articulation between them, the *incudomalleolar joint,* are illustrated. At a deeper plane the tendon of the *tensor tympani muscle* is shown to cross the lumen of the tympanic cavity from the medial wall to the malleus, laterally. The *lesser petrosal nerve,* which ascends from the medial wall of the tympanic cavity, the

promontory, medial to the *tensor tympani muscle* is demonstrated as it courses toward the *foramen spinosum.*

General remarks: The incudomalleolar joint, together with the *head of malleus* and the *body* and *short crus of the incus,* is located in the *epitympanic recess of the tympanic cavity.* Because these structures are in a superior position to the *tympanic membrane,* they are not directly approachable by transtympanic exploration of the middle ear. The *epitympanic recess* communicates freely with the tympanic cavity, anteriorly and inferiorly, and with the *mastoid antrum,* posteriorly.

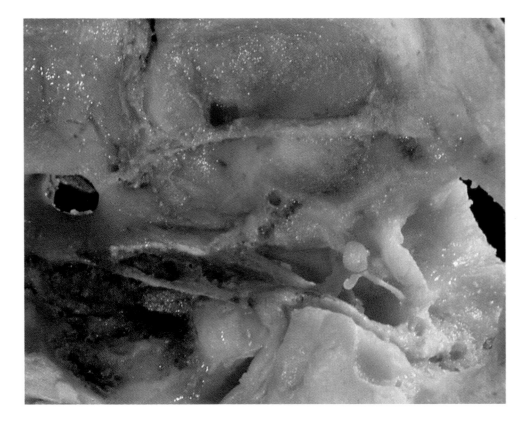

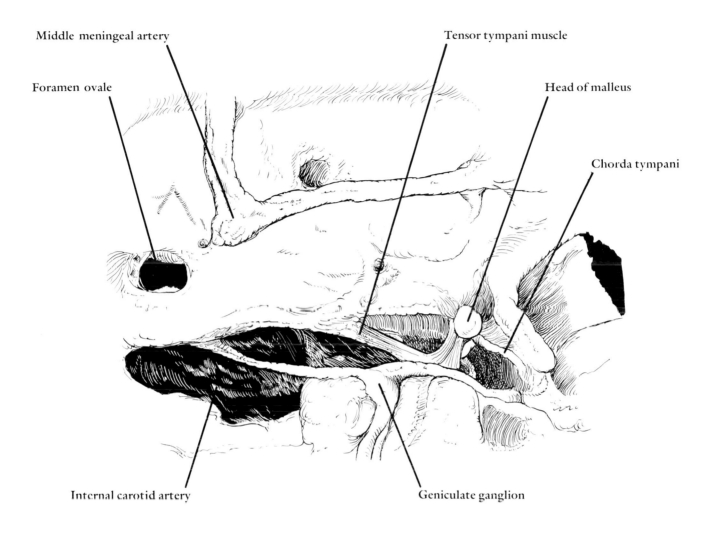

Middle meningeal artery

Foramen ovale

Tensor tympani muscle

Head of malleus

Chorda tympani

Internal carotid artery

Geniculate ganglion

Specific remarks: To demonstrate the two muscles of the middle ear, the *tensor tympani* and the *stapedius*, the *facial nerve*, *incus*, and the bony wall covering the superior aspect of these muscles have been dissected away. At this stage of dissection the lower, *hypotympanic recess* of the cavity and the *osseous part of auditory tube* can be observed. Because the superior half of the cochlear bony shell has been removed, the internal structure of the organ (i.e., *cochlear canal, spiral lamina, modiolus*) is exposed.

General remarks: The close relationship of the *internal carotid artery* in the *carotid canal* with the cochlear part of the inner ear is apparent in this dissection. Because of such anatomical proximity, the excessive pulsation in the artery may interfere with the normal recognition of sound waves by receptor cells in the *cochlea*.

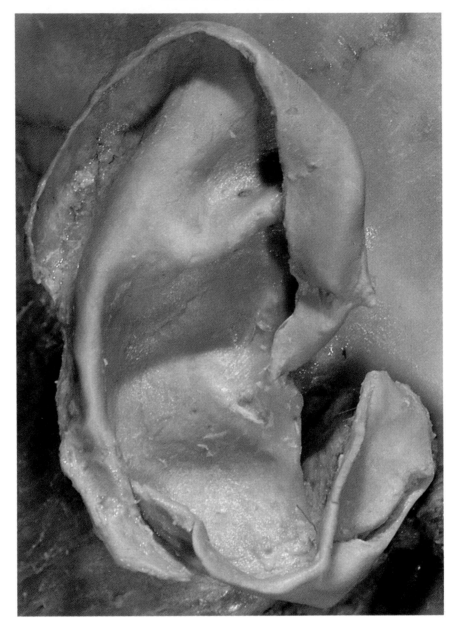

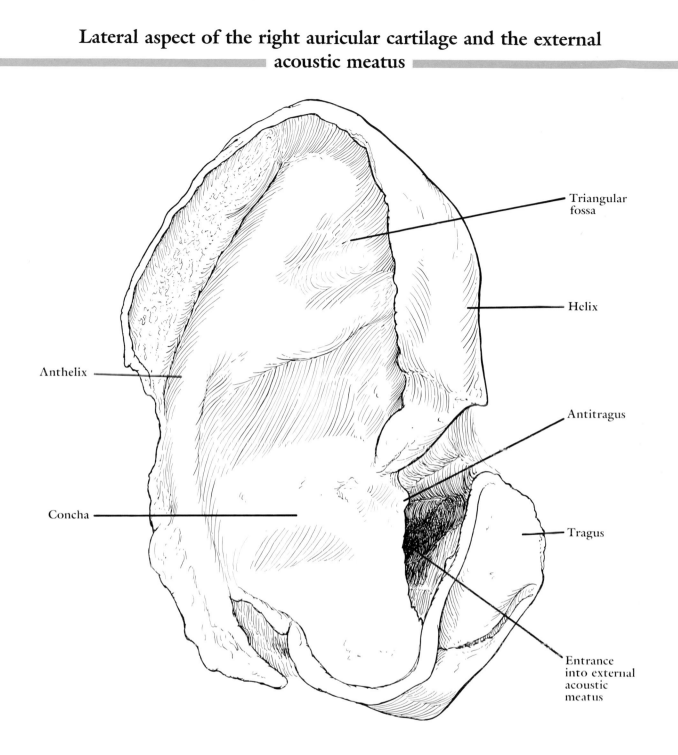

Triangular fossa

Helix

Antitragus

Anthelix

Concha

Tragus

Entrance into external acoustic meatus

Specific remarks: The *auricular cartilage* and the *cartilaginous external acoustic meatus* are demonstrated after the skin and a thin layer of subcutaneous tissue have been taken away. Because of uniformity in thickness of the skin and subcutaneous tissues that cover the cartilaginous skeleton, the auricular cartilage reflects, in general, the morphology of an intact *auricle,* except for the *auricular lobule,* which has no cartilaginous counterpart. The major subdivisions of the auricular cartilage are *tragus, antitragus, helix, anthelix, triangular fossa, scapha,* and *concha.* Depression of the concha continues into the cartilaginous external acoustic meatus.

General remarks: During the sixth week of prenatal differentiation three auricular primordia appear on the first pharyngeal arch and an additional three on the second pharyngeal arch. These six hillocks eventually fuse to form the definite auricule. However, congenital anomalies of the auricle, because of an irregular pattern or a lack of fusion among the primordial centers, are frequently observed. These include the fetal type of auricle, clefts, pits, fistulae, and synotia, fusion of both auricles. In view of the complex origin of this organ it is not surprising that several nerves *(cervical plexus, auriculotemporal, facial, vagus)* participate in the sensory perception of the auricle.

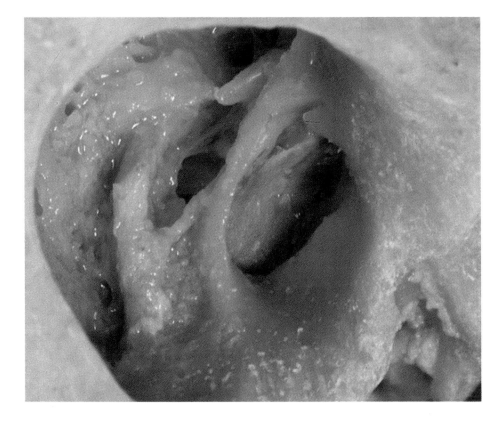

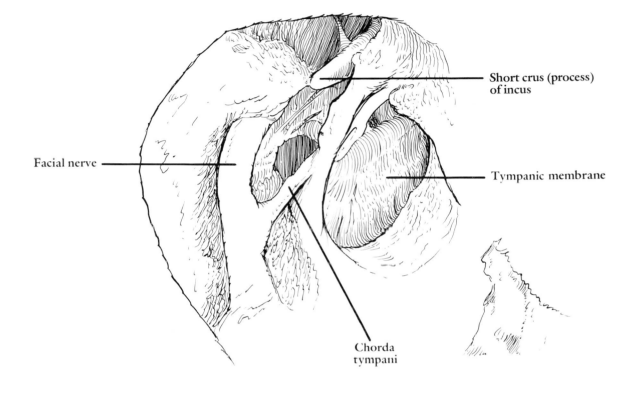

Short crus (process) of incus

Facial nerve

Tympanic membrane

Chorda tympani

Specific remarks: The third *vertical intraosseous segment of the facial nerve*, that which gives off the *nerve to the stapedius* and the *chorda tympani*, is embedded inside the bony mass of the *mastoid process*. In an approach to the nerve by piecemeal removal of the mastoid process and the *bony external acoustic meatus*, the *mastoid antrum* and the *epitympanic recess* have been perforated and the *tympanic membrane* exposed. Because the *handle of the malleus* is fused with and observable through the tympanic membrane, it is possible to determine membranous substructures (i.e. *umbo, flaccid part,* and *tense part*). From the epitympanic recess the *short crus of the incus* is pointed toward the mastoid antrum.

General remarks: The tympanic membrane represents a trilaminar layer that developmentally results from the opposing growths between the first pharyngeal cleft from the outside and the first pharyngeal pouch from the inside. Congenital deafness, although caused in most cases by abnormal development of the membranous or osseous labyrinths, might also be related to malformations of the ossicles and tympanic membrane.

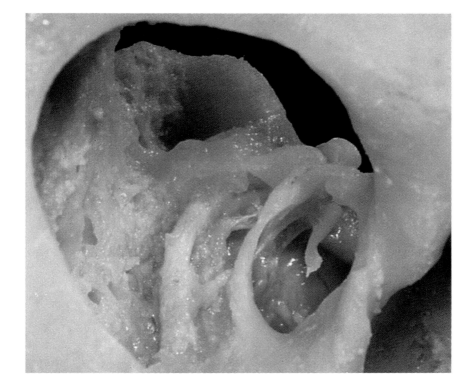

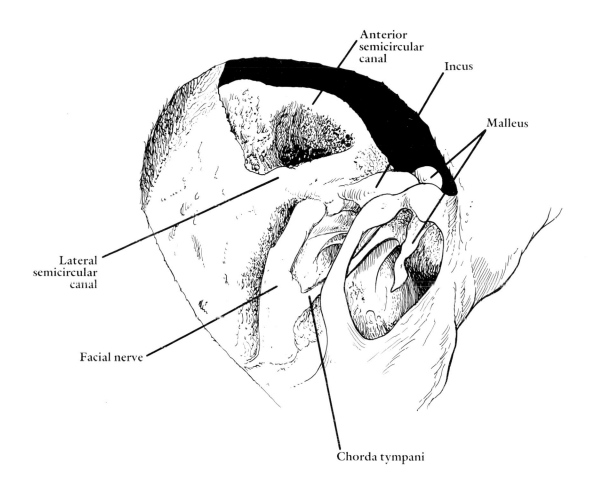

Anterior
semicircular
canal

Incus

Malleus

Lateral
semicircular
canal

Facial nerve

Chorda tympani

Specific remarks: After careful separation and subsequent removal of the *tympanic membrane* from around the bony ring and from the *handle of the malleus,* the *malleus* and the *incus* become exposed. Both segments of the *chorda tympani,* the intraosseous and the intratympanic, are now in evidence. This nerve passes immediately medial to the handle of the malleus and immediately lateral to the *long crus (process) of the incus* before it joins the *anterior ligament of the malleus* and exits the cavity at the *petrotympanic fissure.* Deep to the ossicles the following structures are also shown within the middle ear: *pyramid, promontory,* prominence of the *tensor tympani canal,* and *osseous auditory tube.*

General remarks: The *tympanic ring,* to which the membrane is attached, is laterally inclined at 55 degrees toward the floor of the meatus. This angle in the newborn, however, is much more acute because the membrane assumes an almost horizontal position. The depth of the *external acoustic meatus* is much shallower in neonates than in adults.

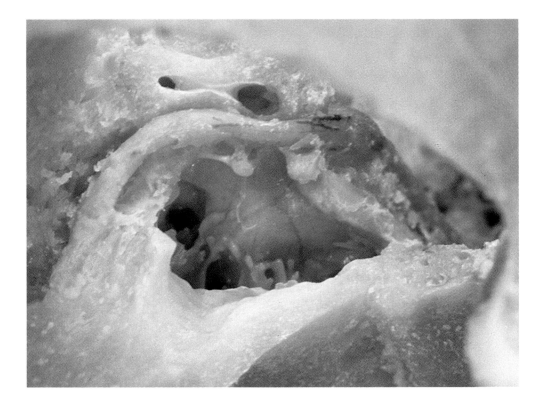

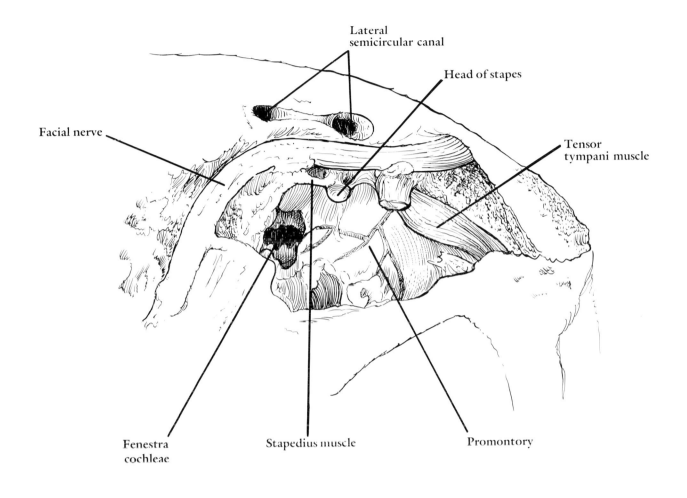

Lateral semicircular canal

Head of stapes

Facial nerve

Tensor tympani muscle

Fenestra cochleae

Stapedius muscle

Promontory

Specific remarks: With the *tympanic ring, malleus,* and *incus* removed, the *promontory* is brought into view. Ascending on the promontory from an inferior to a superior level are the *tympanic nerve, tympanic plexus,* and the *lesser petrosal nerve.* The *fenestra cochleae (round window)* and the *fenestra vestibuli (oval window)* with the *footplate of the stapes* in it are also identifiable. Both muscles of the middle ear, the *tensor tympani* and the *stapedius,* are exposed in their respective bony cavities. The latter muscle is attached to the *neck of the stapes.* The *third* and the *second horizontal intraosseous segments of the facial nerve, geniculate ganglion,* and the initial part of the *greater petrosal nerve* are also identified. To demonstrate the close relationship of the *lateral semicircular*

canal to the horizontal segment of the facial nerve, the canal has been perforated from one end to the other.

General remarks: The horizontal part of the facial nerve is contained in a bony canal that shows dehiscences in about 55% of instances. Because of such bony defects the nerve could become involved in pathological conditions that originated in an upper respiratory, tubal, or tympanic space.

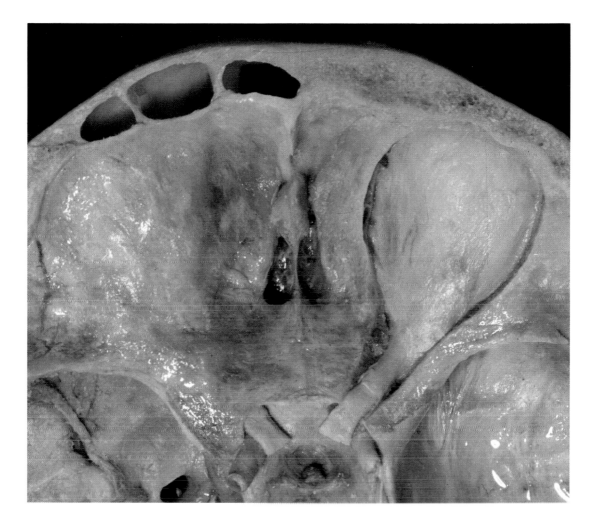

Specific remarks: The left half of this view is shown as a reference point for the dissection of the *orbit;* on the right the orbital roof has been removed to demonstrate the *periorbita,* the connective tissue sheath that envelops the contents of this space. Posteriorly the sheath becomes continuous with the *dura mater* along the *optic nerve,* but it ends anteriorly as the *orbital septum* within the eyelids, close to the corresponding *tarsal plates*.

General remarks: Although the orbital roof generally displays the typical structure of a flat bone (i.e., the superior and inferior compact tables separated by a thin spongy layer), sometimes it is pneumatized by *ethmoidal air cells* or a *frontal sinus* to the extent that the tables become dehiscent. This condition could contribute to the spread or complication of a sinus disease to either the orbital or the anterior cranial fossa contents.

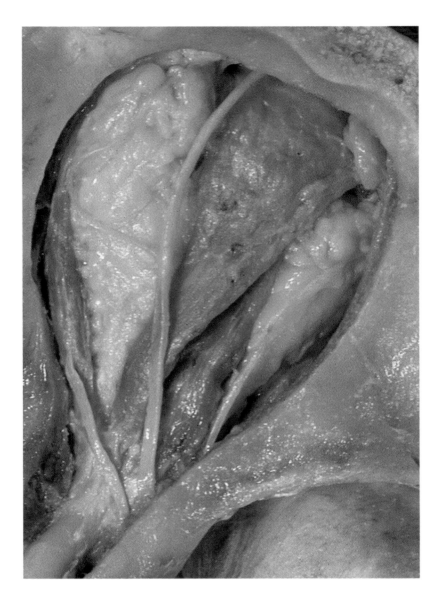

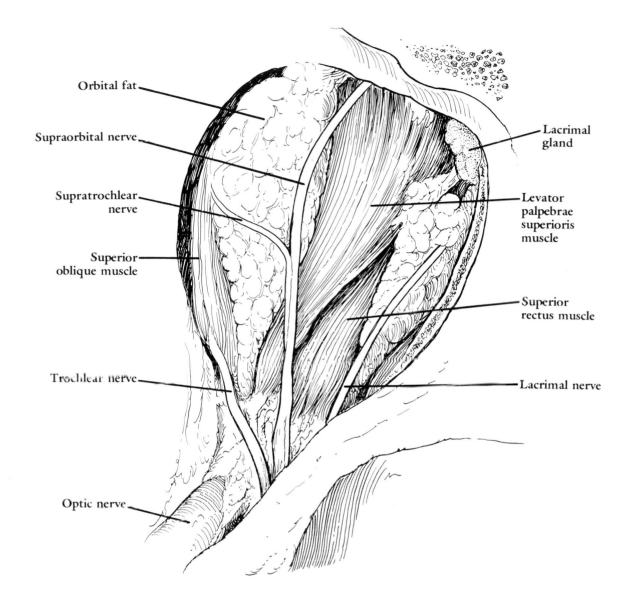

Orbital fat

Supraorbital nerve

Supratrochlear nerve

Superior oblique muscle

Trochlear nerve

Optic nerve

Lacrimal gland

Levator palpebrae superioris muscle

Superior rectus muscle

Lacrimal nerve

Specific remarks: Immediately deep to the *periorbita* three important nerves course in the most superior layer of the orbital space. Medially the *trochlear nerve* crosses above the *tendinous ring* to penetrate into the substance of the *superior oblique muscle.* In the middle the *frontal nerve* proceeds straight anteriorly, above the *superior rectus* and *levator palpebrae superioris muscles,* to divide into the *supratrochlear* and *supraorbital branches.* The divisions exit the orbital region through the respective notches and become distributed to the skin of the forehead and upper eyelids. Laterally the *lacrimal nerve* parallels the superior margin of the *lateral rectus muscle,* receives a *communicating branch from the zygomatic nerve* and continues through the substance of the *lacrimal gland* to the skin of the upper eyelid.

General remarks: A venous network also could be present in this orbital layer. Such veins would be representatives of the *superior ophthalmic system,* which connects the *facial veins* directly with the *cavernous venous sinus.* The fatty tissue lobules, which are interposed among the elements of the orbit, are essential as a support to muscular action and to movements of the eyeball.

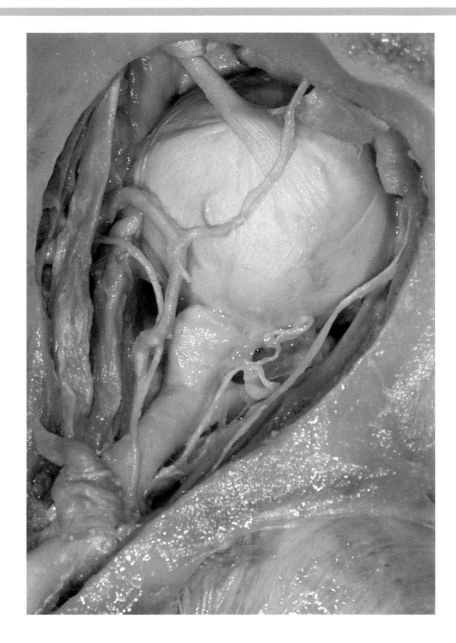

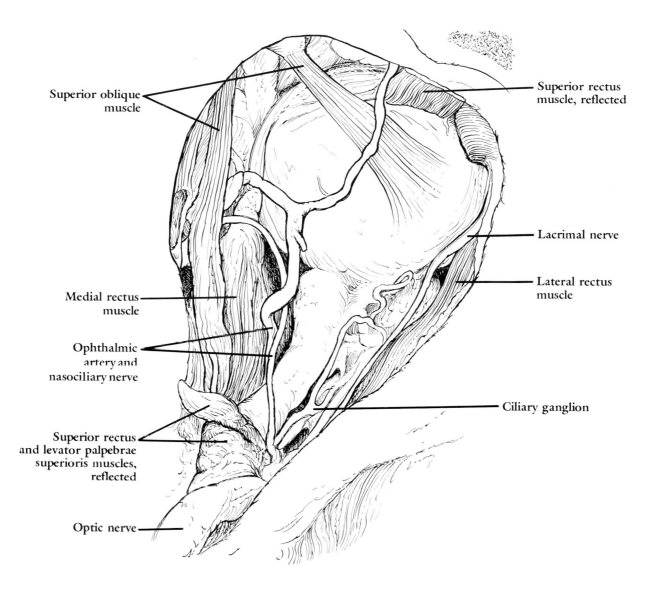

Superior oblique muscle

Superior rectus muscle, reflected

Lacrimal nerve

Lateral rectus muscle

Medial rectus muscle

Ophthalmic artery and nasociliary nerve

Ciliary ganglion

Superior rectus and levator palpebrae superioris muscles, reflected

Optic nerve

Specific remarks: The *levator palpebrae superioris* and *superior rectus muscles* have been cross-cut and the segments reflected anteriorly and posteriorly. Simultaneously the *frontal* and *trochlear nerves* have been completely removed. Consequently the attachment of the *superior rectus muscle* to the eyeball may now be appreciated and the *upper division of the oculomotor nerve* observed on the deep, reflected aspect of the posterior segment of superior rectus muscle. The fatty lobules also have been removed from the upper half of the orbital space to demonstrate the *trochlea* and reflected tendon of the *superior oblique muscle,* the *optic nerve, medial* and *lateral rectus muscles,* the *nasociliary nerve,* the *anterior ethmoidal nerve,* the *infratrochlear nerve,* the *ophthalmic artery,* the *ciliary ganglion, short ciliary nerves,* and the *lacrimal gland.*

General remarks: The ciliary ganglion is a parasympathetic ganglion that receives three roots: the sensory root from the nasociliary nerve, the preganglionic parasympathetic root from the *lower division of the oculomotor nerve,* and the postganglionic sympathetic root from the *internal carotid plexus* by way of the opthalmic artery. Because they are efferent branches of the ganglion, the short ciliary nerves carry the three types of axons to the intraocular structures.

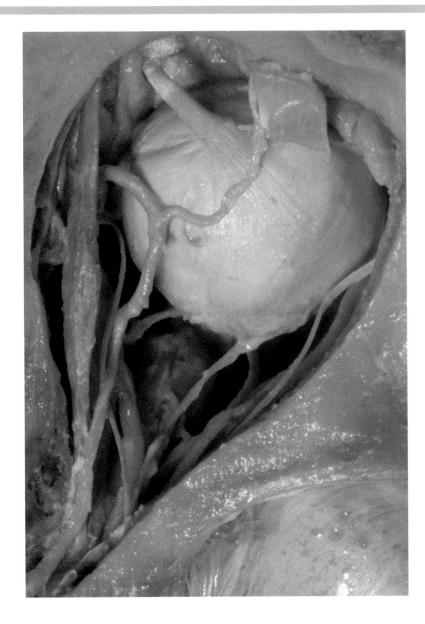

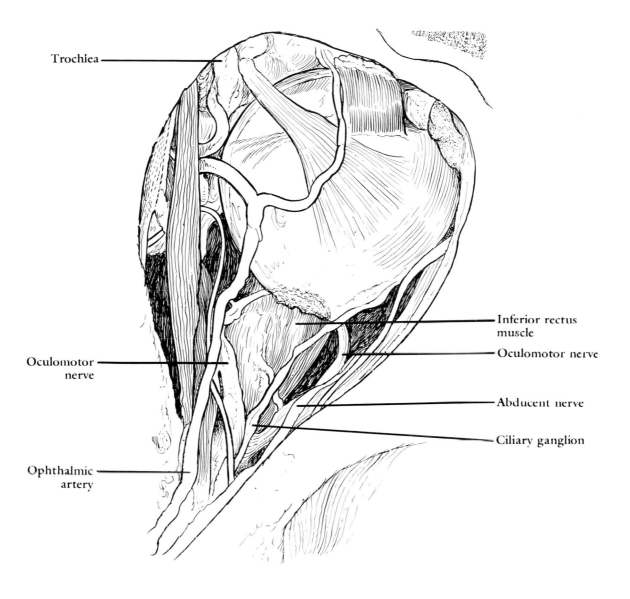

Trochlea

Oculomotor nerve

Ophthalmic artery

Inferior rectus muscle

Oculomotor nerve

Abducent nerve

Ciliary ganglion

Specific remarks: To allow exploration of the deeper, more inferior structures in the *orbit,* the *optic nerve* has been separated from the eyeball and completely reflected from the orbit and from the *optic canal.* Thus it is possible to follow the entire course of the *ophthalmic artery* in the optic canal and through the orbit and also to observe some of the branches—the *anterior ethmoidal,* the *infratrochlear,* and the *supraorbital.* The distribution of the *lower division of the oculomotor nerve* to the *medial rectus, inferior rectus, inferior oblique muscles,* and the *ciliary ganglion;* the *sensory root of the nasociliary nerve* to the ganglion; and the relationship of the *abducent nerve* to the medial aspect of the *lateral rectus muscle* are in the focus of this view.

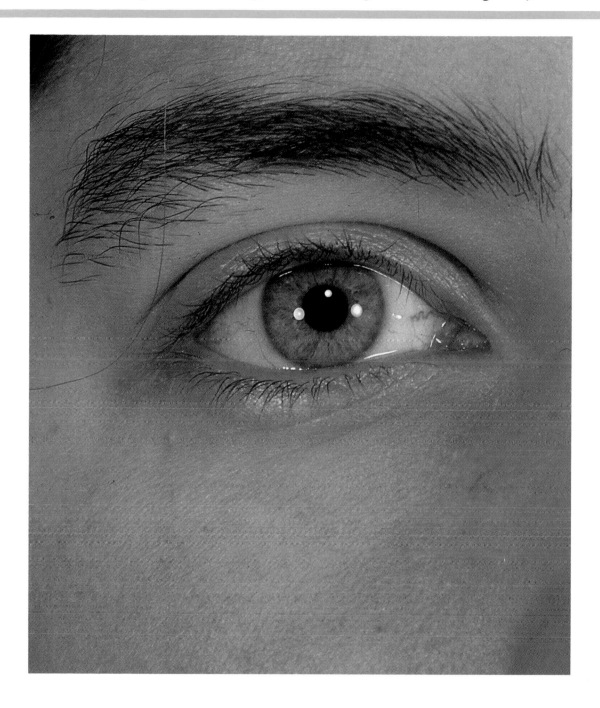

Specific remarks: The skin covering both eyelids is separated from the underlying *orbicularis oculi muscle* by an amount of loose connective tissue. The *superior* and *inferior tarsal plates,* which are located deep to the muscle, are visible as a slight prominences when the lids are moved. Both plates attach medially to the *medial palpebral ligament* and laterally to the *lateral palpebral ligament*. The former ligament could be demonstrated by gentle pulling of the lids in the lateral direction. In between the lids the *palpebral fissure* ends laterally at the *lateral angle,* or *canthus,* and medially at a triangular area, the *lacrimal lake*. The floor of the lake is represented by the *lacrimal caruncle,* which reflects the projection of the *lacrimal sac*. The elevations on the palpebral margins at the base of the lake, the *lacrimal pa-*

pillae, contain at their tips minute openings, the *lacrimal puncta,* from which the *lacrimal canaliculi* transport the lacrimal secretion first to the lacrimal sac and then to the *nasolacrimal duct*. With the palpebral fissure opened, structures of the eyeball that become visible are *cornea, sclera, iris,* and *pupil*.

General remarks: Small blood vessels that are readily observable on the sclera are at times used for diagnostic purposes. Some systemic diseases, e.g., renal failure, are accompanied by edema within the palpebral subcutaneous tissue.

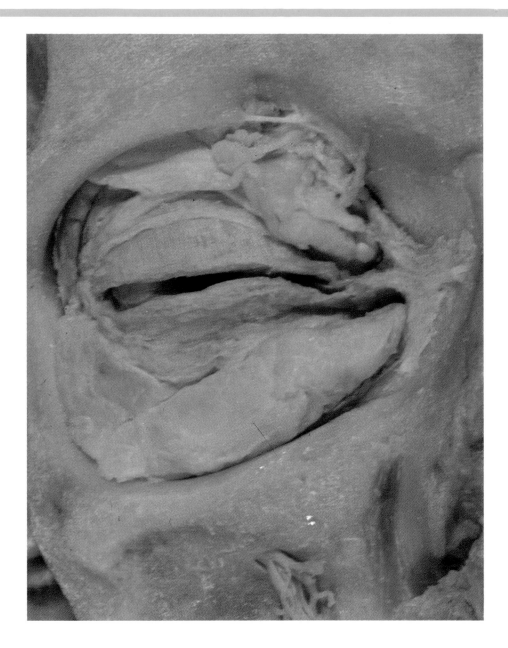

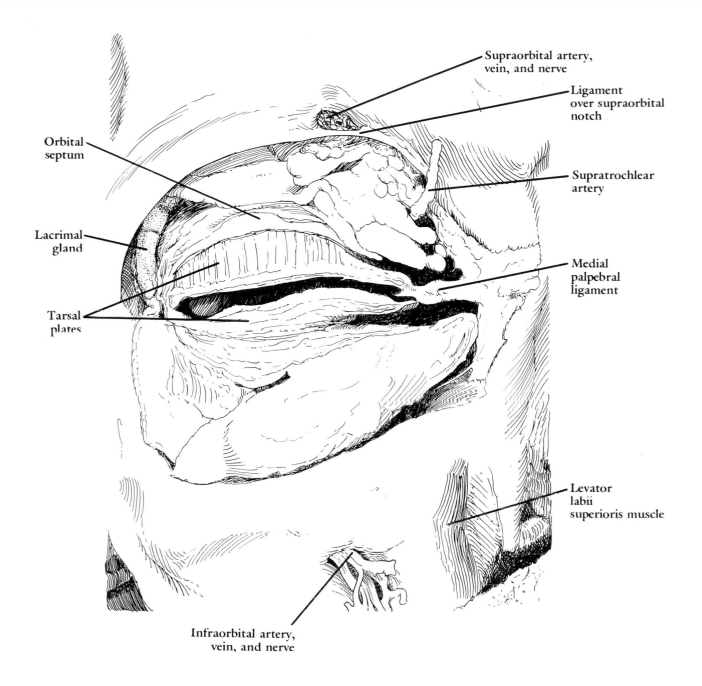

Supraorbital artery, vein, and nerve

Ligament over supraorbital notch

Orbital septum

Supratrochlear artery

Lacrimal gland

Medial palpebral ligament

Tarsal plates

Levator labii superioris muscle

Infraorbital artery, vein, and nerve

Specific remarks: Deep to the palpebral skin, loose subcutaneous tissue, and the *orbicularis oculi muscle,* all of which have been removed in this view, is the palpebral skeleton. It largely consists of the *tarsal plates* suspended within the palpebral substance by the *medial* and *lateral palpebral ligaments.* In addition, the *periorbita,* which fuses with the periosteum all around the orbital margins, extends into the palpebral substance, where it is named the *orbital septum.* As a septal layer of connective tissue it is more distinct peripherally, whereas it gradually disintegrates toward the convex margins of both tarsal plates. The orbital septum is perforated at several points by nerves and blood vessels that course from the *orbit* outward, or vice versa. These are *supraorbital, supratrochlear, infratrochlear, lacrimal,* and *angular-ophthalmic* venous and arterial anastomoses.

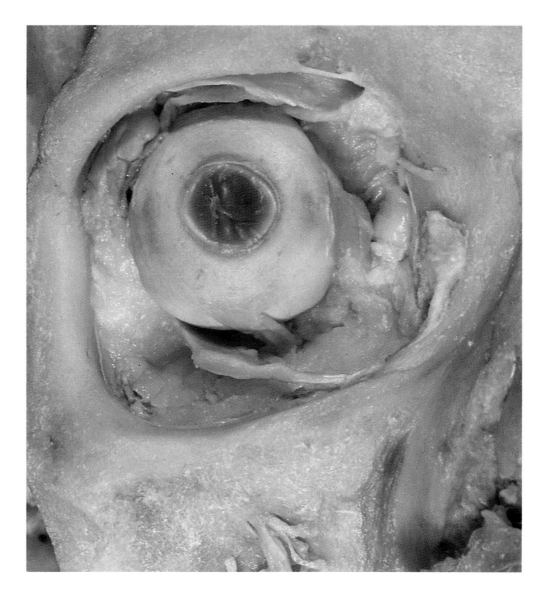

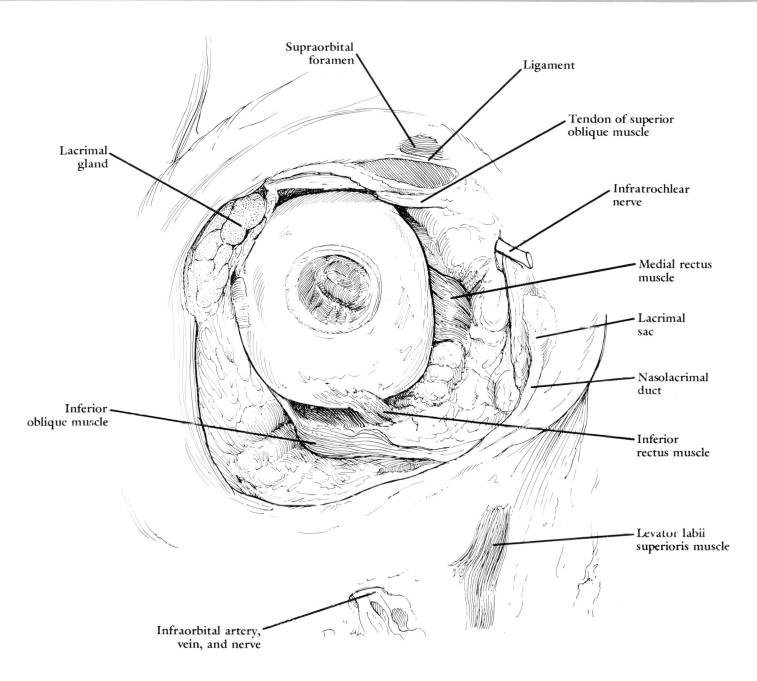

Supraorbital foramen

Ligament

Tendon of superior oblique muscle

Lacrimal gland

Infratrochlear nerve

Medial rectus muscle

Lacrimal sac

Nasolacrimal duct

Inferior oblique muscle

Inferior rectus muscle

Levator labii superioris muscle

Infraorbital artery, vein, and nerve

Specific remarks: The deep aspect of the eyelids, starting from the *palpebral fissure,* is lined by an epithelial layer, the *conjunctiva.* From all round the deep palpebral surface it reflects sharply onto the *sclera* to first form the *superior* and *inferior fornices* and then to attach to the eyeball in a circular fashion at the *sclerocorneal junction.* In this dissection all the palpebral layers, including the palpebral and ocular parts of conjunctiva, have been separated to expose the eyeball and the attachments on it of the *recti muscles.* Thus the *trochlea* and the *reflected tendon of superior oblique muscle,*

the *inferior oblique muscle,* the cut margin of the *levator palpebrae superioris muscle,* the *lacrimal gland,* the *supraorbital ligament* and the contents of the *supraorbital notch,* the *infratrochlear nerve,* and the *lacrimal sac* with the initial part of *nasolacrimal duct* are brought into this view.

General remarks: Once again, it is apparent in this view that the orbital lobules of fat are organized in a pattern that makes possible a great degree of movement of motor structures inside a relatively restricted space.

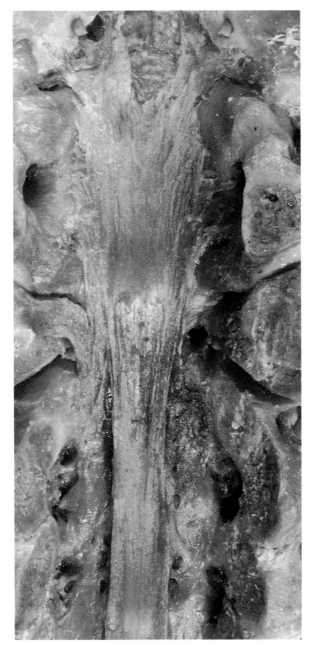

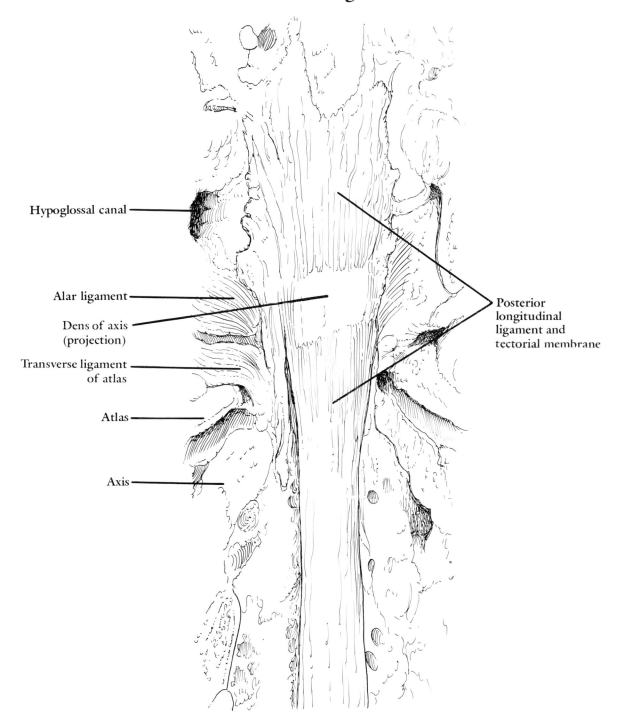

Hypoglossal canal

Alar ligament

Dens of axis
(projection)

Transverse ligament
of atlas

Atlas

Axis

Posterior
longitudinal
ligament and
tectorial membrane

Specific remarks: Following the removal of the *cervical spinal cord* and the cranial segment of the central nervous system, the posterior aspect of the *occipital base* and the upper *cervical vertebral bodies* come into view. The most prominent ligament on the posterior aspect of the vertebral bodies (i.e., on the anterior wall of the *vertebral canal*) is the *posterior longitudinal ligament*. It extends superiorly, beyond the prominence of the *dens of the axis,* to the occipital base. Deep to it and another ligamentous layer, the *tectorial membrane,* lies the *cruciform ligament of the atlas,* composed of weak longitudinal fascicles and the *strong transverse lig-*

ament of the atlas. The latter ligament attaches to the *lateral masses of the atlas,* whereas the *alar ligament* emerges from under the cover of the cruciform ligament to insert into the pericondylar bone.

General remarks: These ligaments are important in stabilizing the dens within the median *atlantoaxial joint.* Most of the rotatory movements are made possible at this joint and at the *lateral atlantoaxial joint.* Fracture of the dens diminishes greatly the stability at the atlantoaxial complex; the two vertebrae glide more freely over one another, thus endangering the integrity of the spinal cord.

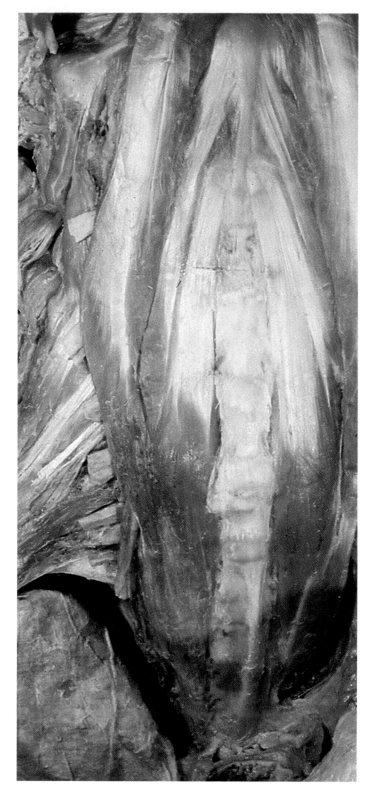

Anterior aspect of the right half of the cervical vertebral column and associated muscles

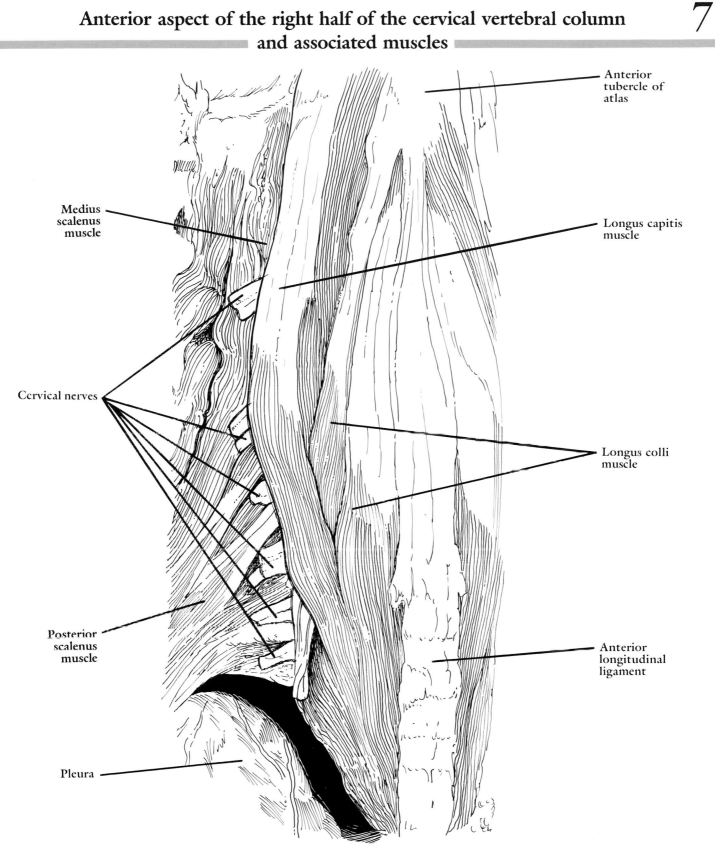

Medius scalenus muscle

Cervical nerves

Posterior scalenus muscle

Pleura

Anterior tubercle of atlas

Longus capitis muscle

Longus colli muscle

Anterior longitudinal ligament

Specific remarks: The *visceral compartment of the neck* has been removed to expose the *prevertebral muscles* of the neck, i.e., the *longus capitis* and the *longus colli*. Toward the midline, in between the left and right muscles, the *vertebral bodies* are covered by the *anterior longitudinal ligament*, which adheres at each intervertebral level to the corresponding *discs*. Lateral to the prevertebral muscles the cut *roots of the brachial plexus*, the attachment of the *scalene muscles*, and the *dome of the pleura* are also demonstrated.

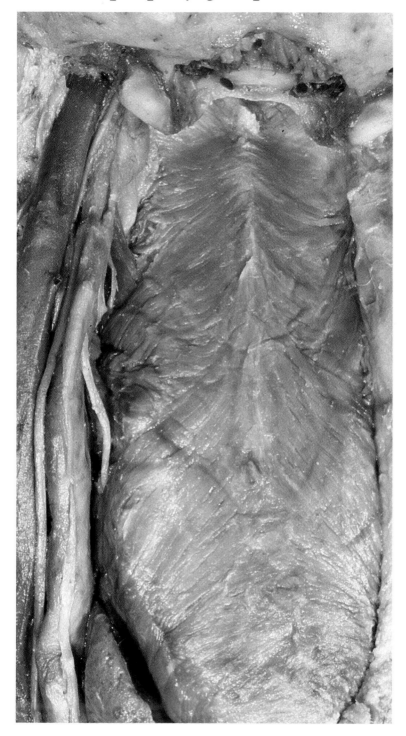

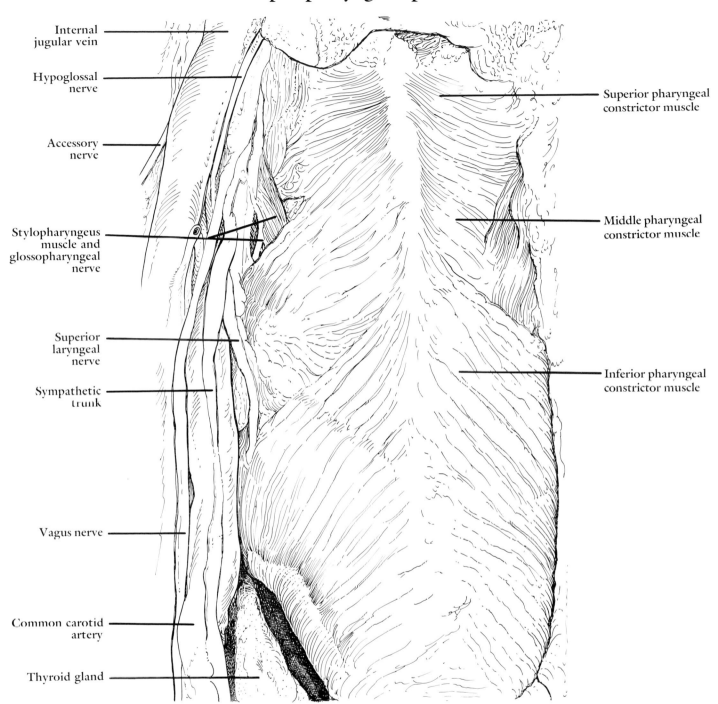

Internal jugular vein

Hypoglossal nerve

Accessory nerve

Stylopharyngeus muscle and glossopharyngeal nerve

Superior laryngeal nerve

Sympathetic trunk

Vagus nerve

Common carotid artery

Thyroid gland

Superior pharyngeal constrictor muscle

Middle pharyngeal constrictor muscle

Inferior pharyngeal constrictor muscle

Specific remarks: When the *vertebral column* is disarticulated at the *atlantooccipital joint* and removed together with the *prevertebral, scaleni,* and *levator scapulae muscles* from the *visceral compartment of the neck,* the three *pharyngeal constrictor muscles* are demonstrated. The following structures in the left *parapharyngeal space* are exposed from posterior to anterior: the *sympathetic trunk,* the *vagus nerve* and the *superior laryngeal branch,* the *hypoglossal nerve,* the *internal carotid artery,* the *internal jugular vein,* the *accessory nerve,* the *glossopharyngeal nerve,* and the *stylopharyngeal muscle.*

General remarks: The contents of parapharyngeal space are separated from those of the *parotid region* by the "styloid diaphragm," which is made of the *stylohyoid, styloglossus,* and *stylopharyngeus muscles.* The diaphragm is oriented from the deep aspect of the *sternocleidomastoid muscle* posterolaterally to the lateral pharyngeal wall anteromedially. During the radical exploration of the parotid space it is imperative to maintain the integrity of the diaphragm to preserve the important structures of the adjacent space.

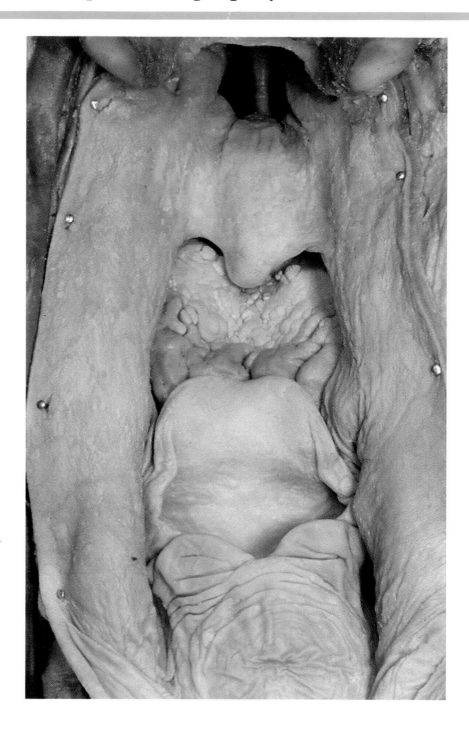

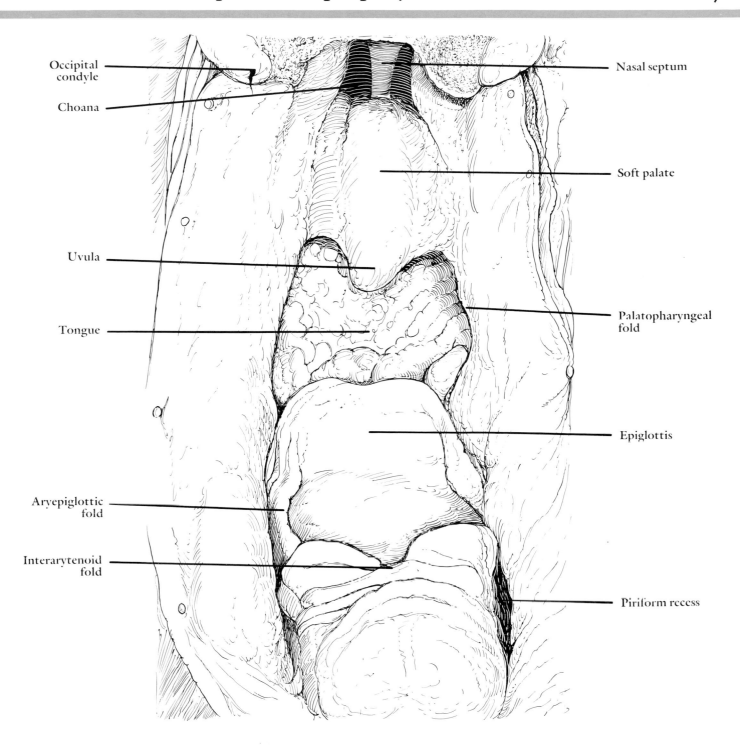

Occipital condyle

Choana

Uvula

Tongue

Aryepiglottic fold

Interarytenoid fold

Nasal septum

Soft palate

Palatopharyngeal fold

Epiglottis

Piriform recess

Specific remarks: The pharyngeal wall, which consists of muscular, membranous, and mucosal layers, has been cut longitudinally along the midline and horizontally along the attachment to the *occipital bone;* the two flaps subsequently were reflected to the corresponding sides. From the superior compartment of the *pharynx* inferiorly the following structures and spaces are demonstrated: the *torus tubarius, choanae,* the *salpingopharyngeal fold,* the *soft palate,* the *uvula,* the *palatopharyngeal fold,* the posterior aspect of the tongue with *papillae,* the *palatine tonsil,* the *isthmus faucium,* the *epiglottis,* the *aryepiglottic fold,* the *interarytenoid*

fold, the *aditus ad laryngis* (entrance to the larynx), the *piriform recess,* and the *prominence of the cricoid plate.*

General remarks: Deglutition is a composite musclear action that involves the *pharyngeal constrictors* and *levators,* muscles of the soft palate and tongue, laryngeal musculature, and several groups of extrinsic muscles, e.g., the *infrahyoids* and *suprahyoids.* This complexity extends to the nervous control of deglutition by the *cervical plexus* and the *trigeminal, facial, glossopharyngeal, vagus, accessory,* and *hypoglossal nerves.*

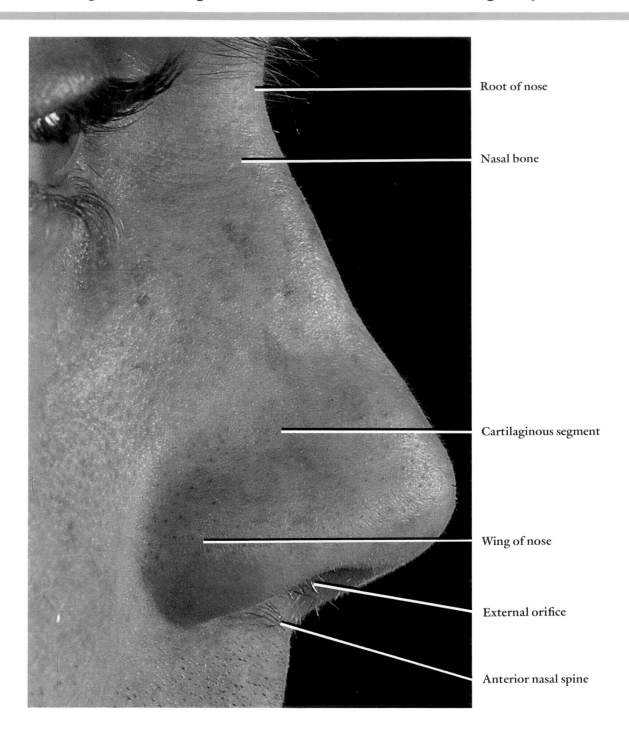

Root of nose

Nasal bone

Cartilaginous segment

Wing of nose

External orifice

Anterior nasal spine

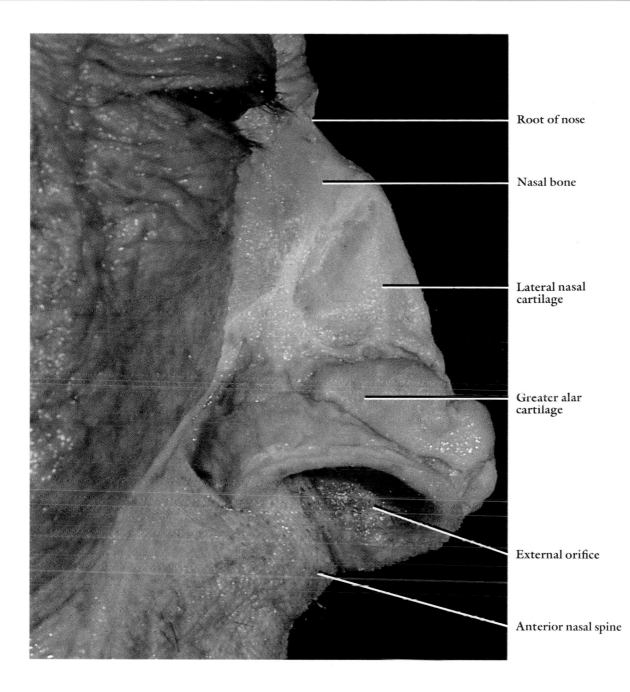

Root of nose

Nasal bone

Lateral nasal cartilage

Greater alar cartilage

External orifice

Anterior nasal spine

Specific remarks: The skin and subcutaneous tissue together with the periosteum and perichondrium have been removed to demonstrate two of the external nasal cartilages—the *lateral* and the *greater alar*.

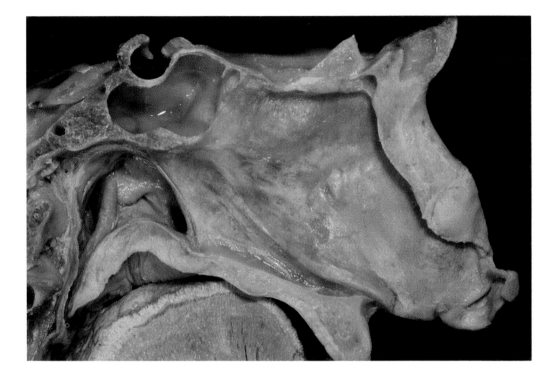

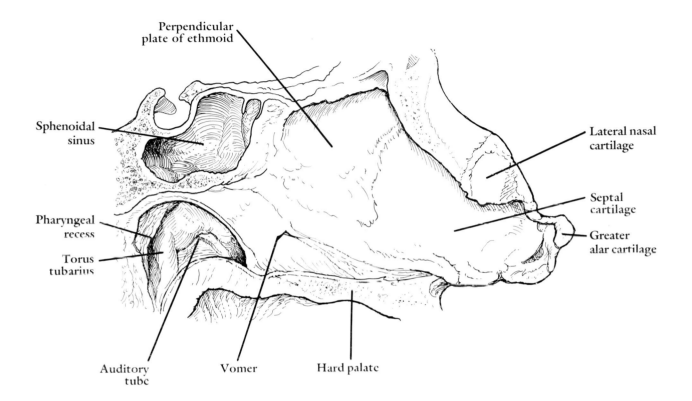

Perpendicular
plate of ethmoid

Sphenoidal
sinus

Lateral nasal
cartilage

Septal
cartilage

Greater
alar cartilage

Pharyngeal
recess

Torus
tubarius

Auditory
tube

Vomer

Hard palate

Specific remarks: To demonstrate the components of the *nasal septum* the head has been cut sagittally, immediately to the right of midline, and the mucosa has been removed from the septum. This procedure also exposes the roof and the floor of the right *nasal cavity*, the *sphenoidal sinus*, the *soft palate*, the lateral wall of the *nasopharynx*, the *pharyngeal opening of the auditory tube, torus tubarius,* and the *pharyngeal recess*. The three septal components—*septal cartilage, vomer,* and *perpendicular plate of the ethmoid*—are demonstrated.

General remarks: The vomer ossifies in membrane and the ethmoid plate in cartilage, whereas the septal cartilage persists throughout life. Because of developmental diversity among the three components, septal deformities are numerous, the most frequent of which is a deviated septum.

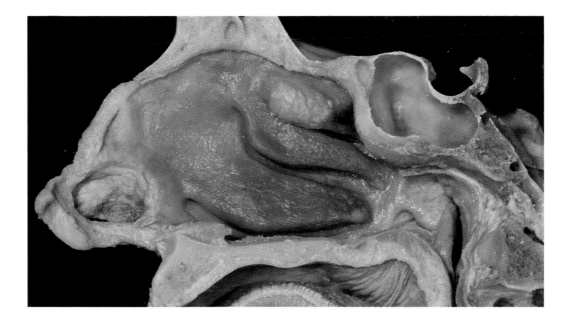

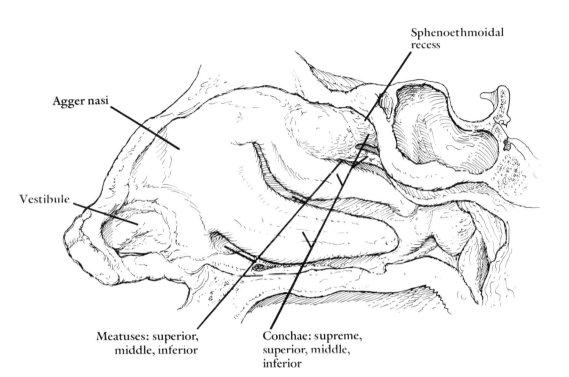

Sphenoethmoidal recess

Agger nasi

Vestibule

Meatuses: superior, middle, inferior

Conchae: supreme, superior, middle, inferior

Specific remarks: The *nasal septum,* which represents the *medial nasal wall,* has been removed from this view. The *lateral nasal wall* supports three *conchae,* which subdivide the nasal lumen into three subjacent *meatuses* and an upper space, the *sphenoethmoidal recess.* The *sphenoidal sinus* opens into the latter recess straight anteriorly.

General remarks: The *sphenopalatine foramen,* which transmits the sensory and visceromotor nerve impulses from the *pterygopalatine (sphenopalatine) ganglion* to the nasal mucosa, lies immediately posterior to the posterior end of the *middle concha.* This is an important landmark in local anesthesia of the nasal structures.

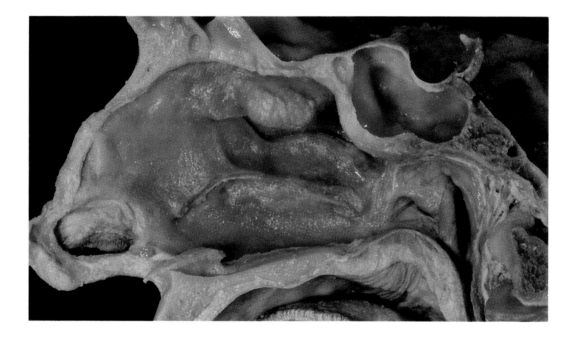

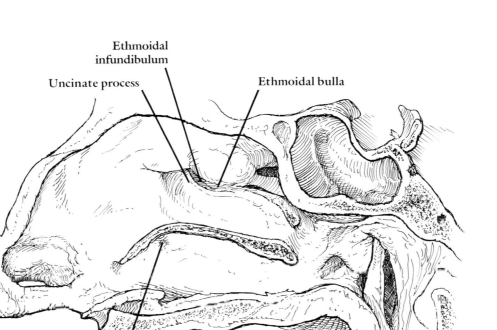

Ethmoidal
infundibulum

Uncinate process

Ethmoidal bulla

Opening of
nasolacrimal duct

Specific remarks: Once the *middle* and *inferior conchae* are separated from the *lateral nasal wall* and subsequently removed, the floors of the corresponding *meatuses* become exposed. Within the *middle meatus* the *ethmoidal bulla, uncinate process,* and the *ethmoid infundibulum* are demonstrated; within the *inferior meatus* the *nasal opening of the nasolacrimal duct* is shown.

General remarks: The *frontal sinus* opens in the anterior segment and the *maxillary sinus* in the posterior segment of the ethmoid infundibulum. In between these two openings there are numerous minute openings of the *anterior ethmoidal air cells.* Variations in the relative positions of any of these openings, however, are quite common.

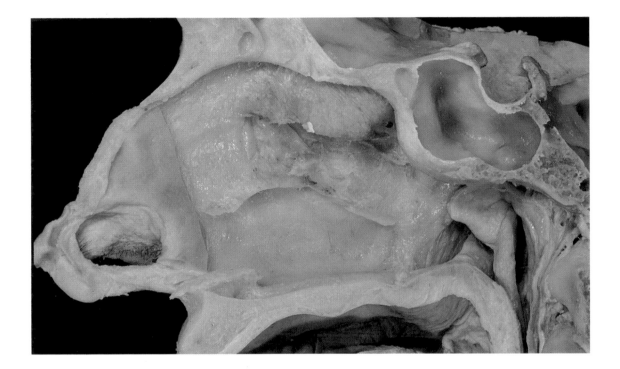

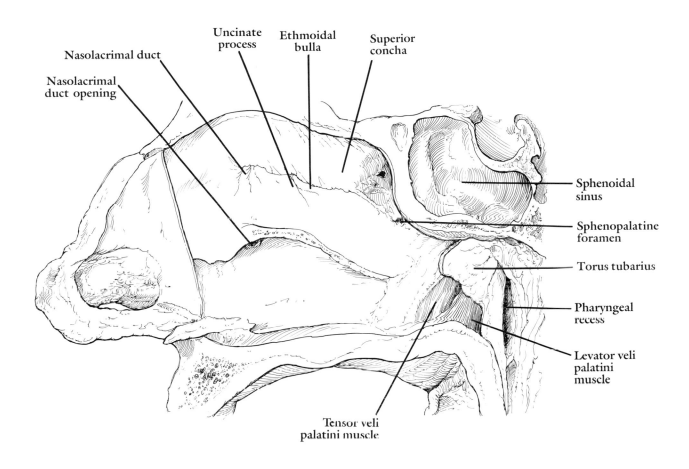

Nasolacrimal duct

Nasolacrimal
duct opening

Uncinate
process

Ethmoidal
bulla

Superior
concha

Sphenoidal
sinus

Sphenopalatine
foramen

Torus tubarius

Pharyngeal
recess

Levator veli
palatini
muscle

Tensor veli
palatini muscle

Specific remarks: The mucosa, submucosa, and periosteum have been dissected away from the most of the *lateral nasal wall*, but they have been kept in situ over the *nasal vestibule* and the *agger nasi*. In addition to the bony components of the wall, the *ethmoid labyrinth, superior concha, ethmoid bulla, uncinate process,* attachment of the *middle* and *inferior conchae, perpendicular plate of the palatine bone* with *orbital* and *sphenoid processes, nasolacrimal duct,* and *sphenopalatine foramen* are shown. Further posteriorly, within the *nasopharynx,* the *tensor* and *levator veli palatini muscles* are exposed. Because this view is a longitudinal section through the region, it is possible to ascertain the distribution of both muscular fibers inside the *soft palate.*

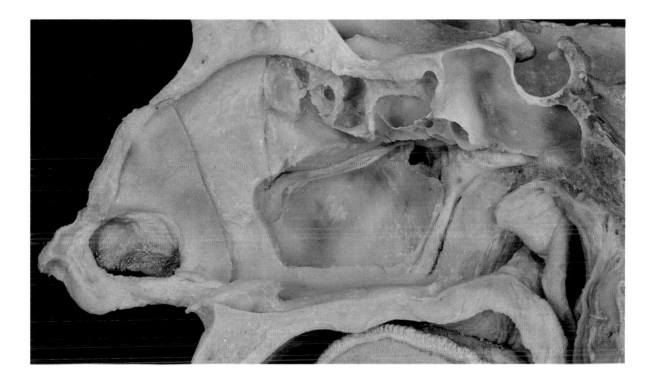

Specific remarks: In addition to the *maxillary* and *sphenoidal sinuses,* several *ethmoidal air cells* and the *frontal sinus* have been perforated and exposed from the *nasal cavity* for this view. The medial aspect of the *lacrimal sac* has also been exposed.

General remarks: The paranasal sinuses are variable to a great extent in size, general morphology, and relationships. Moreover, their functional importance in terms of resonance, maintainence of air temperature, olfaction, stability of the skull, and so on is not specifically determined.

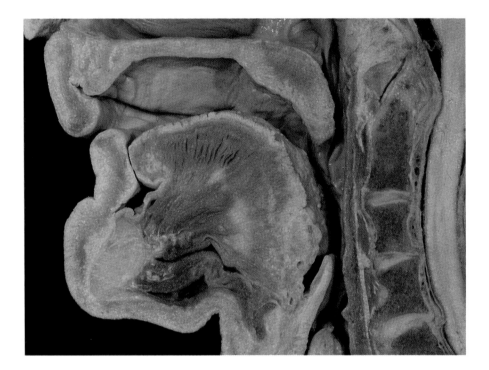

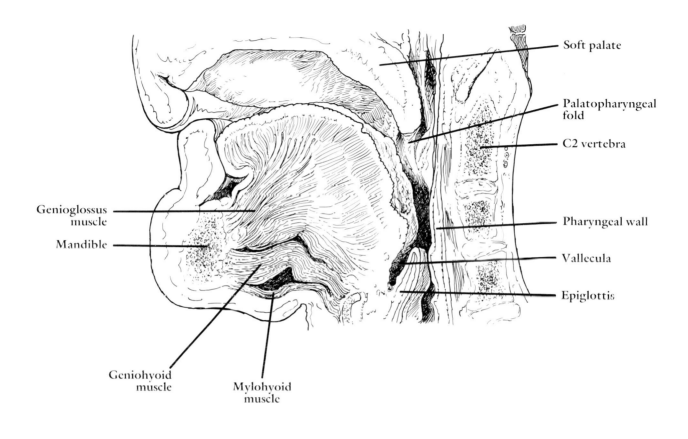

Soft palate

Palatopharyngeal fold

C2 vertebra

Pharyngeal wall

Vallecula

Epiglottis

Genioglossus muscle

Mandible

Geniohyoid muscle

Mylohyoid muscle

Specific remarks: The *oral cavity* is subdivided by the *maxillary* and *mandibular alveolar processes,* which in this subject are edentulous, together with corresponding teeth in the *vestibule* and the oral cavity proper. The vestibule is restricted by the alveolar processes on one side and the buccal and labial structures on the other side. The oral cavity proper expands within the concavities of the alveolar processes and opens posteriorly into the *oropharynx.* Musculomembranous layers of the floor of the mouth and the relationships of the *hyoid bone* to the tongue and to the *epiglottis* are clearly demonstrated in this view.

General remarks: The *parotid duct* opens on the buccal side of the oral vestibule, opposite the second maxillary molar.

Deep dissection of the right half of the hard palate and the tonsillar fossa

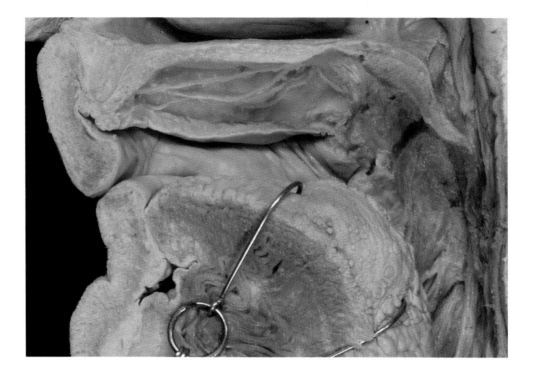

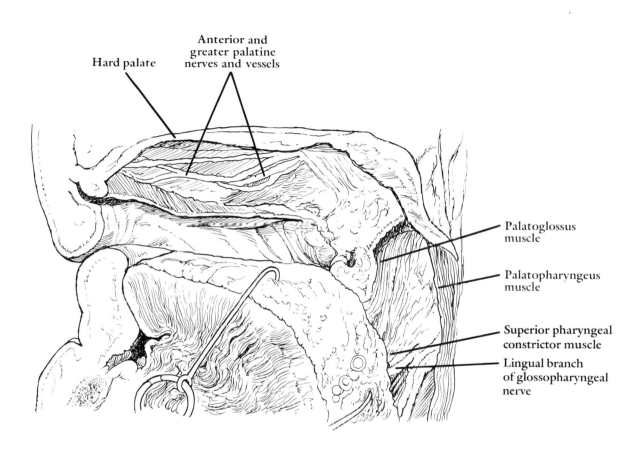

Hard palate

Anterior and greater palatine nerves and vessels

Palatoglossus muscle

Palatopharyngeus muscle

Superior pharyngeal constrictor muscle

Lingual branch of glossopharyngeal nerve

Specific remarks: By a careful separation of the palatal mucosa from the *hard palate* it is possible to expose the major nerves and blood vessels—*greater, lesser,* and *anterior palatine*—of that region. The mucosa and tonsillar tissues have been separated and removed from the tonsillar area and from the bordering folds. It is apparent from this view that the folds contain corresponding muscles—the *palato-glossus* and the *palatopharyngeus*. The floor of the fossa, on the other hand, is formed by the *superior pharyngeal con-strictor muscle* in relation to which the *lingual branch of glos-sopharyngeal nerve* approaches the substance of the tongue.

General remarks: Because of the proximity of major blood vessels on the outer aspect of the pharyngeal con-strictor muscle, it is important to respect this muscular layer during tonsillectomy.

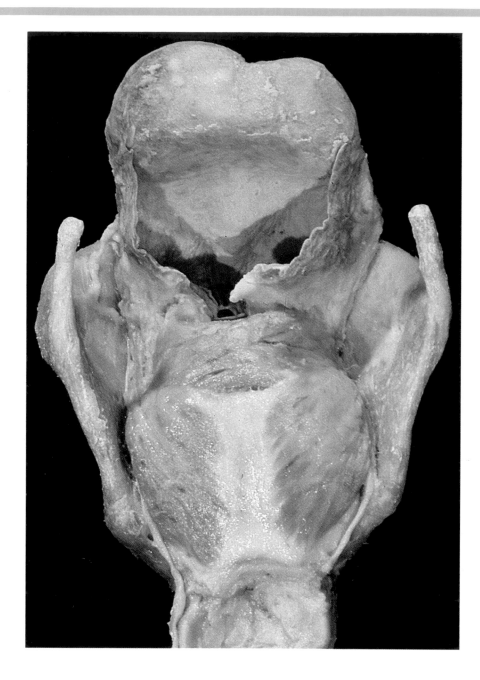

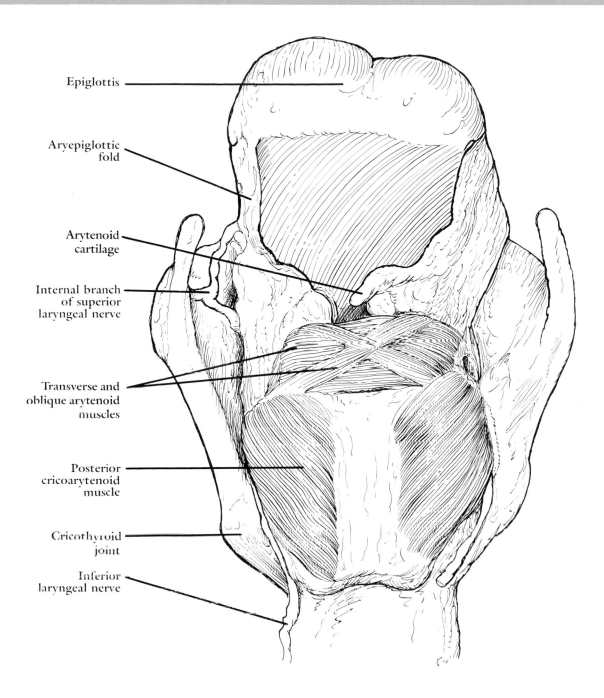

Epiglottis

Aryepiglottic fold

Arytenoid cartilage

Internal branch of superior laryngeal nerve

Transverse and oblique arytenoid muscles

Posterior cricoarytenoid muscle

Cricothyroid joint

Inferior laryngeal nerve

Specific remarks: The *larynx,* for this view, has been separated from *thyrohyoid membrane, hyoid bone, inferior pharyngeal constrictor,* and all other surrounding structures of the neck. In addition, the pharyngeal mucosal layer has been reflected completely from the posterior aspect of the organ. Consequently the following structures are brought into view: posterior margin of the *thyroid cartilage* with *superior* and *inferior horns,* submucosal layer of the *piriform recess* with the *internal branch of the superior laryngeal nerve* and the *inferior laryngeal nerve,* and the posterior group of intrinsic laryngeal muscles.

General remarks: The two laryngeal nerves exchange the *communicating rami* inside the deep layer of the piriform recess. This interaction makes a strict determination of terminal distribution of both nerves difficult. Some regional lymph nodes that control the outflow from the *vocal cords* are situated in the same recess.

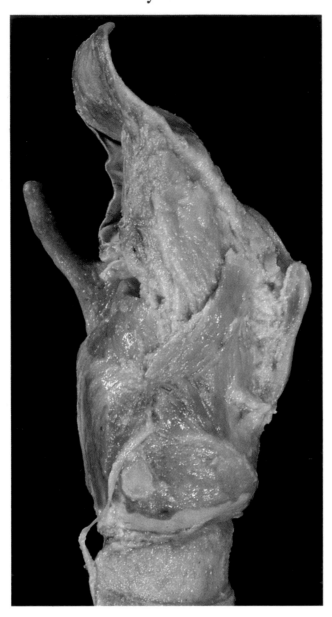

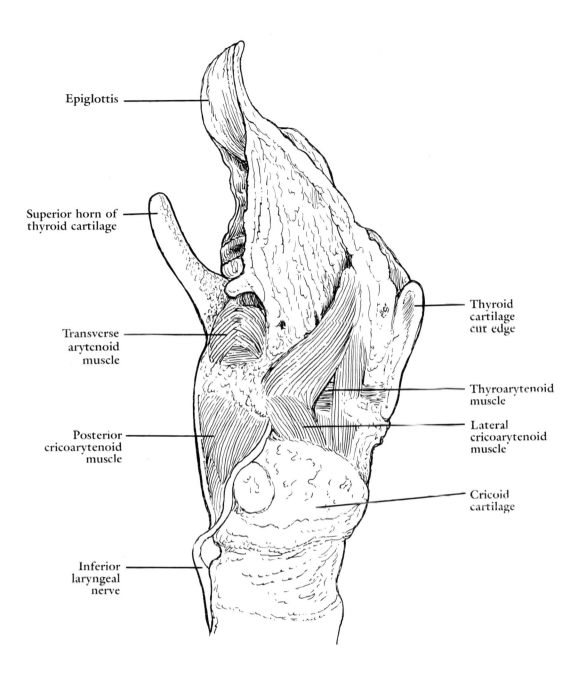

Epiglottis

Superior horn of
thyroid cartilage

Transverse
arytenoid
muscle

Posterior
cricoarytenoid
muscle

Inferior
laryngeal
nerve

Thyroid
cartilage
cut edge

Thyroarytenoid
muscle

Lateral
cricoarytenoid
muscle

Cricoid
cartilage

Specific remarks: To demonstrate deep laryngeal muscles on the medial wall of the *piriform recess,* the *thyroid lamina* has been vertically cut, just to the right of midline, and the *inferior horn* disarticulated at the *cricothyroid joint.* The cartilage, together with the *cricothyroid muscle,* has been sub- sequently removed to show the *arch of cricoid cartilage* and the *articular surface,* the *lateral cricoarytenoid muscle,* the *thyroarytenoid muscle,* the *superior thyroarytenoid muscle,* and the *thyroepiglottic muscle.*

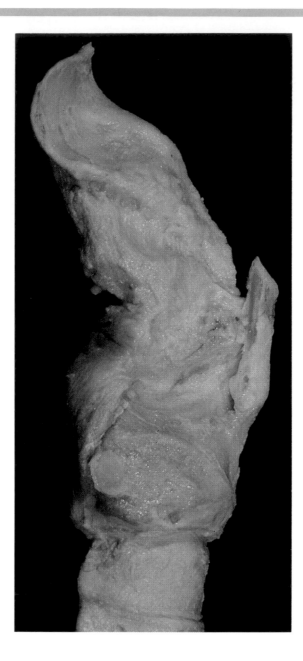

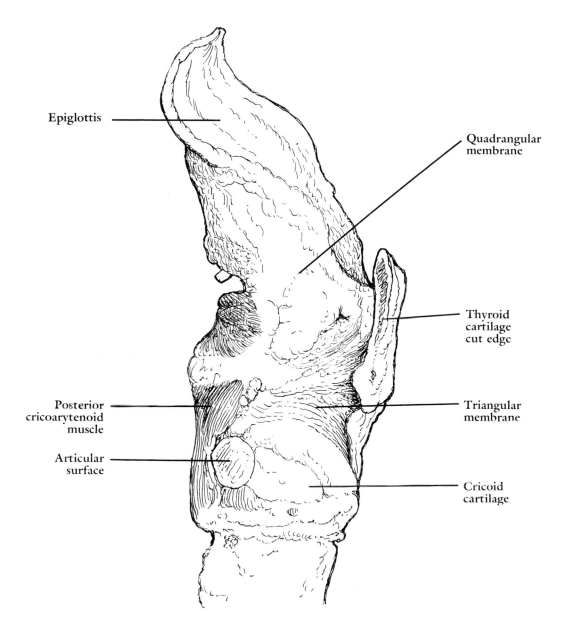

Epiglottis

Quadrangular
membrane

Thyroid
cartilage
cut edge

Posterior
cricoarytenoid
muscle

Triangular
membrane

Articular
surface

Cricoid
cartilage

Specific remarks: Following the removal of deep laryngeal muscles from the lateral aspect of the organ, the membranous layer becomes exposed. The *quadrangular membrane* is bordered by the *vestibular fold* inferiorly, the *thyroid* and *epiglottic cartilages* anteriorly, and the *arytenoid cartilage* posteriorly. The superior border of the membrane is freely contained within the *aryepiglottic fold*. The *triangular membrane*, or *conus elasticus,* attaches to the *vocal fold* superiorly, the *thyroid cartilage* and *cricothyroid ligament* anteriorly, and the superior margin of the *cricoid arch* and *lamina* and the *arytenoid cartilage* inferoposteriorly.

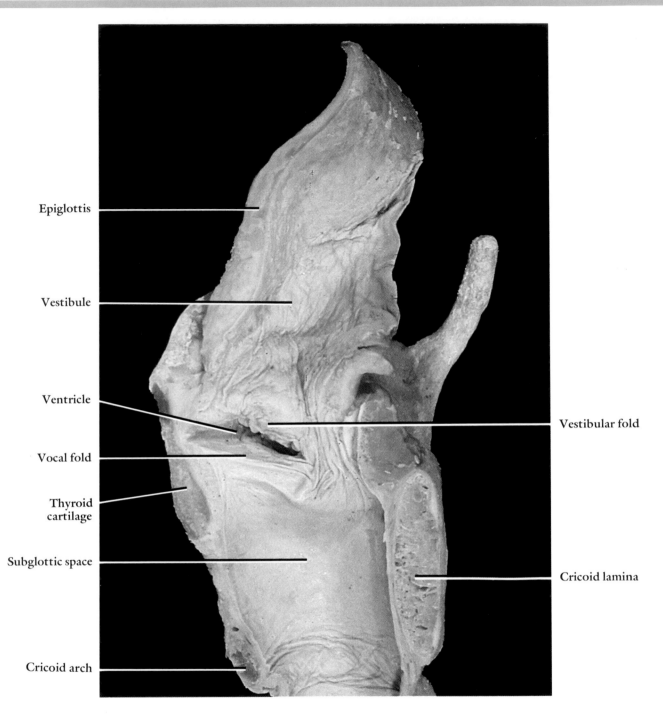

Epiglottis

Vestibule

Ventricle

Vocal fold

Thyroid cartilage

Subglottic space

Cricoid arch

Vestibular fold

Cricoid lamina

Specific remarks: The organ has been cut sagittally in the midline to demonstrate the structures of the lateral laryngeal wall.

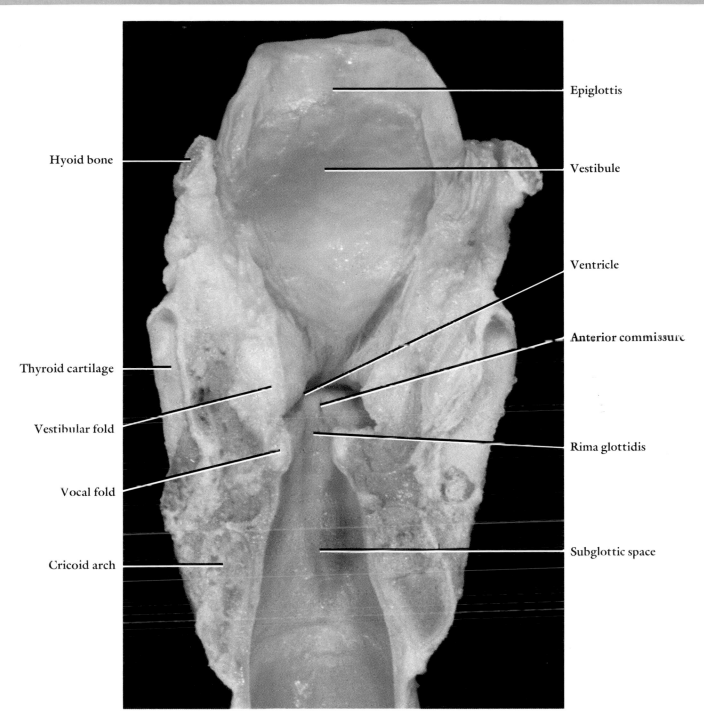

Hyoid bone

Thyroid cartilage

Vestibular fold

Vocal fold

Cricoid arch

Epiglottis

Vestibule

Ventricle

Anterior commissure

Rima glottidis

Subglottic space

Specific remarks: The organ has been cut frontally at about anteroposterior midline to demonstrate the structures at the anterior laryngeal wall.

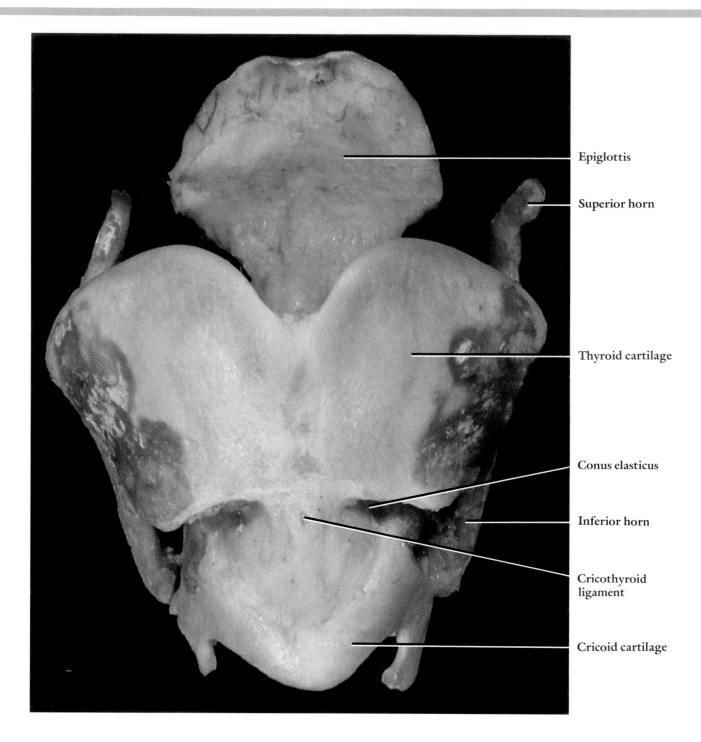

Epiglottis

Superior horn

Thyroid cartilage

Conus elasticus

Inferior horn

Cricothyroid ligament

Cricoid cartilage

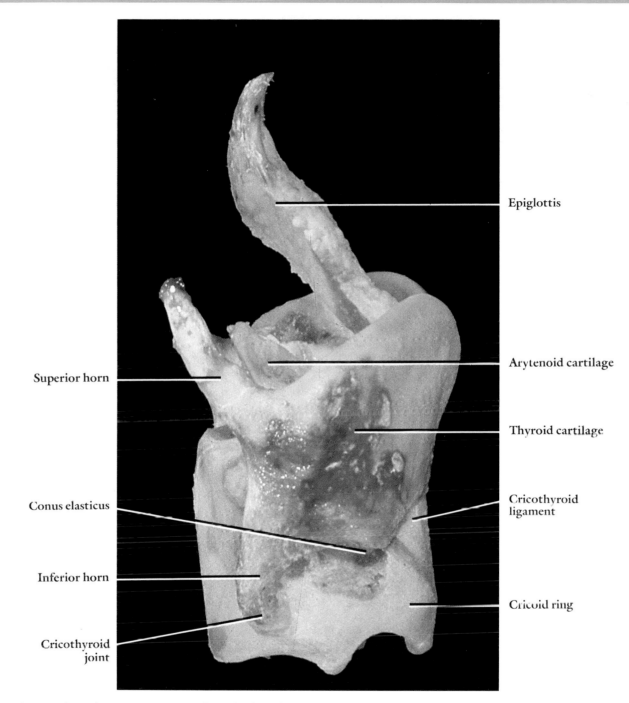

Epiglottis

Arytenoid cartilage

Thyroid cartilage

Cricothyroid ligament

Cricoid ring

Superior horn

Conus elasticus

Inferior horn

Cricothyroid joint

General remarks: The movements at the *cricothyroid joint* are around a transverse axis that passes through both joints. During the tension of *vocal cords* most of the movement is by the *cricoid cartilage* while the *thyroid cartilage* remains in situ.

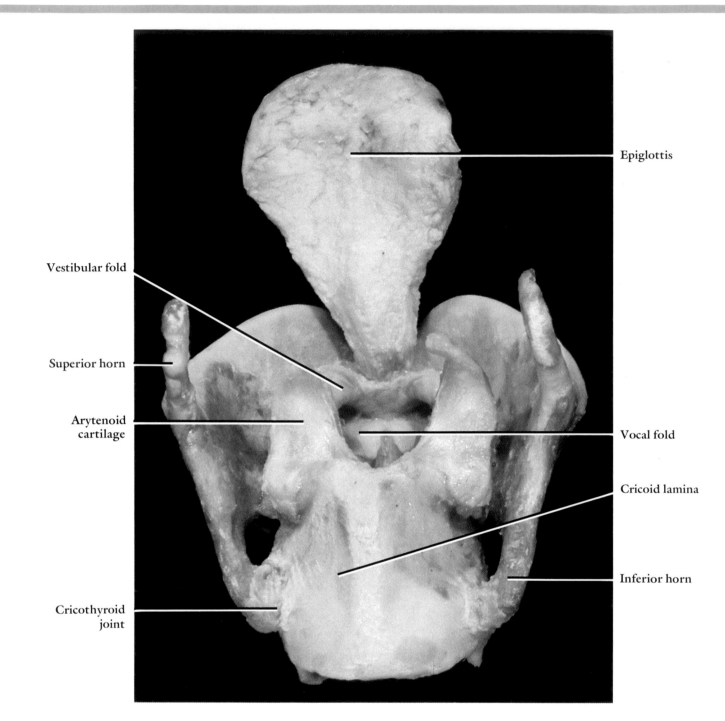

Epiglottis

Vestibular fold

Superior horn

Arytenoid
cartilage

Vocal fold

Cricoid lamina

Inferior horn

Cricothyroid
joint

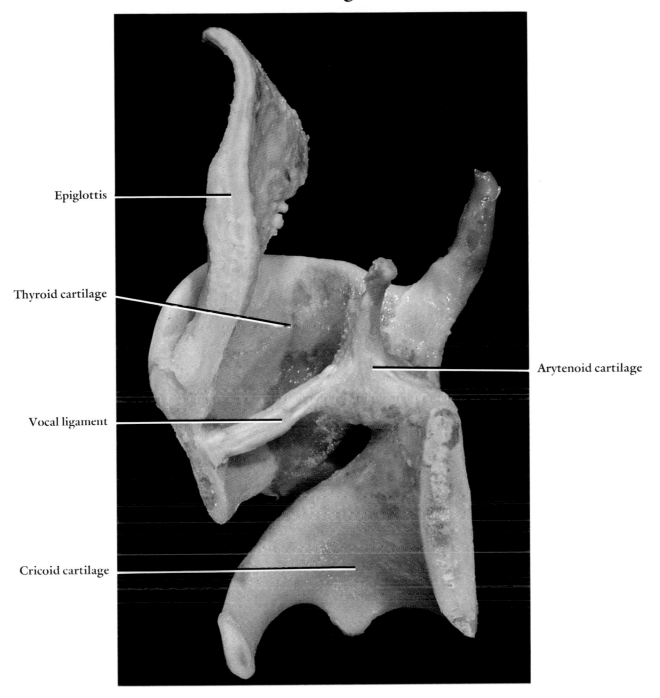

Epiglottis

Thyroid cartilage

Arytenoid cartilage

Vocal ligament

Cricoid cartilage

Specific remarks: For this view the laryngeal skeleton has been cut sagittally at the midline. The right *vocal ligament* has been preserved.

General remarks: During the abduction and adduction of vocal cords the *arytenoid cartilages* show two types of movement at the *cricoarytenoid joints*—rotation and gliding.

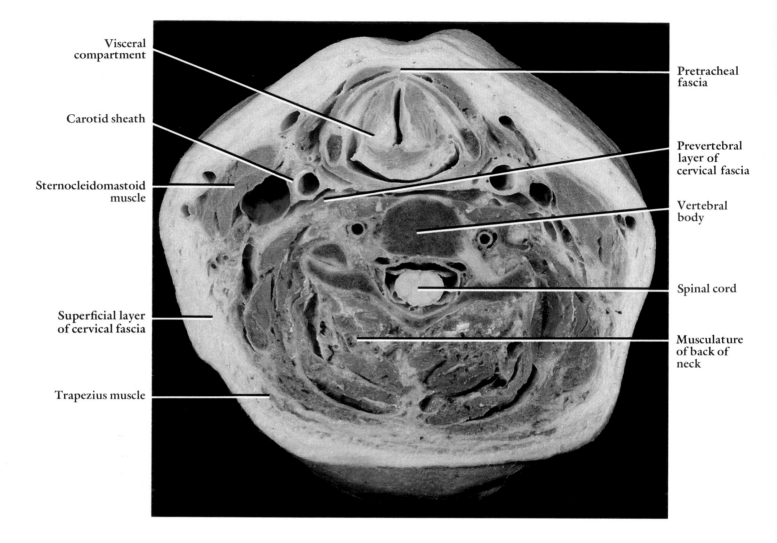

Visceral compartment

Carotid sheath

Sternocleidomastoid muscle

Superficial layer of cervical fascia

Trapezius muscle

Pretracheal fascia

Prevertebral layer of cervical fascia

Vertebral body

Spinal cord

Musculature of back of neck

Specific remarks: To show the overall organization of structures and fascial planes in the neck, this view is shown as a summary of individual anatomical demonstrations presented in the previous illustrations.

References

1

Berry, A.C., and Berry, R.J.: Epigenetic variation in the human cranium, J. Anat. **101**:361, 1967.

Enlow, D.H.: Textbook of facial growth, Philadelphia, 1975, W.B. Saunders Co.

Ford, E.H.R.: The growth of the foetal skull, J. Anat. **90**:63, 1956.

Keen, J.A.: Study of differences between male and female skulls, Am. J. Phys. Anthrop. **8**:65, 1950.

Todd, J.T., and Mark, L.S.: Issues related to the prediction of craniofacial growth, Am. J. Orthod. **79**:63, 1981.

2

Enlow, D.H., and Harris, D.B.: A study of the postnatal growth of the human mandible, Am. J. Orthod. **50**:25, 1964.

Erickson, G.E., and Waite, D.E.: Mandibular asymmetry, J. Am. Dent. Assoc. **89**:1369, 1974.

Meikle M.C.: The role of the condyle in the postnatal growth of the mandible, Am. J. Orthod. **64**:50, 1973.

Moss, M.L., and Salentijn, L.: The logarithmic growth of the human mandible, Acta Anat. **77**:341, 1970.

Ricketts, R.M.: A principle of arcial growth of the mandible, Angle Orthod. **42**:368, 1972.

3

Pierce, R.H., Mainc, M.W., and Bosma, J.F.: The cranium of the newborn infant: an atlas of tomogoraphy and anatomical sections, DHEW Pub. No. (NIH)78-788, Bethesda, Md., 1978.

Scott J.H.: Dento-facial development and growth, Oxford, England, 1967, Pergamon Press.

4

Webber, R.L.: Angular invariants in developing human mandible, Science **206**:689, 1979.

5

Inman, V.T., and Saunders, J.B. de C.M.: The ossification of the human frontal bone, with special reference to its presumed pre- and post-frontal elements, J. Anat. **71**:383, 1937.

Montagu, M.F.A.: Wallbrook frontal bone, Am. J. Phys. Anthrop. **9**:5, 1951.

Pritchard, J.J., Scott, J.H., and Girgis, F.G.: The structure and development of cranial and facial sutures, J. Anat. **90**:73, 1956.

6

Ford, E.H.: Growth of the human cranial base, Am. J. Orthod. **44**:498, 1958.

Latham, R.A.: Observations on the growth of the cranial base in the human skull. J. Anat. **100**:435P, 1966.

Latham, R.A.: The sella point and postnatal growth of the human cranial base, Am. J. Orthod. **61**:156, 1972.

7

Burdi, A.R., and Faist, K.: Morphogenesis of the palate in normal human embryos with special emphasis on the mechanisms involved, Am. J. Anat. **120**:149, 1967.

Vidić, B.: The structure of the palatum osseum and its toral overgrowth, Acta Anat. **71**:94, 1968.

Vidić, B.: The variations in height of the palatum osseum as a function of the variations of some other vertical dimensions and angles of the skull, J. Dent. Res. **50**:14, 1971.

8

Durst, J.H., and Snow, J.E.: Multiple mandibular canals: oddities or fairly common anomalies? Oral Surg. **49**:272, 1980.

Gabriel, A.C.: Some anatomical features on the mandible, J. Anat. **92**:580, 1958.

Vidić, B.: The variations in length of the pterygoid process as a function of the variations of the sphenoid angle, Anat. Rec. **160**:527, 1968.

10

Enlow, D.H.: Growth and remodeling of the human maxilla, Am. J. Orthod. **51**:446, 1965.

Noback, C.R., and Moss, M.L.: The topology of the human premaxillary bone, Am. J. Phys. Anthrop. **11**:181, 1953.

Woo, J.K.: Ossification and growth of the human maxilla, premaxilla, and palatine bones, Anat. Rec. **105**:737, 1949.

Wood, N.K., et al.: Osteogenesis of the human upper jaw: proof of the nonexistence of a separate premaxillary centre, Arch. Oral Biol. **14**:1331, 1969.

18

Best, T.H., and Anson, B.J.: The temporal bone and the ear, Springfield, Ill., 1949, Charles C Thomas, Publisher.

20

Singh, S.: Variations of the superior articular facets of atlas vertebrae, J. Anat. **99**:565, 1965.

Töndury, G.: Zur Anatomie der Halswirbelsäule. Gibt es Uncovertebralgelenke? Z. Anat. Entwgesch. **112**:448, 1943.

25

Davis, R.A., et al.: Surgical anatomy of the facial nerve and parotid gland based upon a study of 350 cervicofacial halves, Surg. Gynecol. Obstet. **102**:384, 1956.

Génis-Gálvez, J.M., et al.: On the double innervation of the parotid gland: an experimental study, Acta Anat. **63**:398, 1966.

Podvinec, M., and Pfaltz, C.P.: Studies on the anatomy of the facial nerve, Acta Otolaryngol. **81**:173, 1976.

26

Einstein, R.A., and Katz, A.D.: Parotid area swelling caused by a prominent transverse process of atlas, Arch. Otolaryngol. **101**:558, 1975.

Guffarth, A., and Graumann, W.: Über die Lagebeziehung der Arteria carotis externa zur Glandula parotis, Arch. Oto-Rhino-Laryngol. **211**:17, 1975.

Vidić, B.: The anatomy and development of the facial nerve, Ear Nose Throat J. **57**:236, 1978.

27

Burkitt, A.N., and Lightoller, G.S.: The facial musculature of the Australian aboriginal, J. Anat. **61**:14; **62**:33, 1926.

Lightoller, G.H.S.: Facial muscles: the modiolus and muscles surrounding the rima oris with some remarks about the panniculus adiposus, J. Anat. **60**:1, 1925.

28

Fishel, D., et al.: Roentgenologic study of the mental foramen, Oral Surg. Med. Pathol. **41**:682, 1976.

Kadanoff, D.: Die sensiblen Nervenendigungen in der mimischen Musculatur des Menschen, Z. Mikrosk. Anat. Forsch. **62**:1, 1956.

29

MacDougall, J.D.B.: The attachments of the masseter muscle, Br. Dent. J. **98**:193, 1955.

Perkins, R.E., et al.: Electromyographic analysis of the "buccinator mechanism" in human beings, J. Dent. Res. **56**:783, 1977.

Rees, L.A.: The structure and function of the mandibular joint, Br. Dent. J. **96**:125, 1954.

30

Blackwood, H.J.J.: The development, growth, and pathology of the mandibular condyle, Queen's U. thesis, Belfast, 1959.

Harpman, J.A., and Woollard, H.H.: The tendon of the lateral pterygoid muscle, J. Anat. **73**:112, 1938.

Jones, D.L., and Blanton, P.L.: Electromyographic analysis of the separated heads of the lateral pterygoid muscle in man, Anat. Rec. **205**:93A, 1983.

Lacouture, C., et al.: The anatomy of the maxillary artery in the infratemporal fossa in relationship to oral infections, Anat. Rec. **205**:104A, 1983.

31

Carter, R.B., and Keen, E.N.: The intramandibular course of the inferior alveolar nerve, J. Anat. **108**:433, 1971.

Koritzer, R.T., and Suarez, F.R.: Accessory medial pterygoid muscle, Acta Anat. **107**:467, 1980.

Suarez, F.R., et al.: A preliminary study of computerized tomographs of the temporomandibular joint, Compendium Cont. Ed. **1**:217, 1980.

33

de Sousa, O.M.: Estudo electromiogràfico do m. platysma, Folia Clin. Biol. **33**:42, 1964.

34

Gaughran, G.R.L.: Mylohyoid boutonnière and sublingual bouton, J. Anat. **97**:565, 1963.

Moyers, R.E.: Electromyographic analysis of certain muscles involved in temporomandibular movement, Am. J. Orthod. **36**:481, 1950.

35

Harris, W.: The morphology of the brachial plexus, London, England, 1939, Oxford University Press.

Raveau, F.: Note sur les variations de la morphologie externe de l'encéphale de macaque rhésus, Arch. Anat. Pathol. **16**:A220, 1968.

36

Campbell, E.J.M.: The role of the scalene and sternomastoid muscles in breathing in normal subjects: an electromyographic study, J. Anat. **89**:378, 1955.

Curto, F.S., Suarez, F., and Kornblut, A.D.: The extracranial hypoglossal nerve: 112 cadaver dissections, Ear Nose Throat J. **59**:94, 1980.

Werner, S.: The thyroid, ed. 3, New York, 1969, Harper & Row, Publishers.

37

Lazorthes, G.: Le système neurovasculaire, Paris, 1949, Masson.

Pick, J., and Sheehan, D.: Sympathetic rami in man, J. Anat. **80**:12, 1946.

Sunderland, S., and Bedbrook, G.M.: Relative sympathetic contribution to individual roots of the brachial plexus in man, Brain **72**:297, 1949.

39

Bearn, J.G.: An electromyographic study of the trapezius, deltoid, pectoralis major, biceps and triceps muscles, during static loading of the upper limb, Anat. Rec. **140**:103, 1961.

44

Hoffmann, E., and Thiel, W.: Untersuchungen vermeintlicher und wirkincher Abflusswege aus dem Subdural- und Subarachnoidealraum, Z. Anat. Entwgesch. **119**:283, 1956.

Kimmel, D.L.: Innervation of spinal dura mater and dura mater of the posterior cranial fossa, Neurology **11**:800, 1961.

45

Davson, H.: Physiology of the cerebrospinal fluid, London, England, 1970, Churchill, Livingstone.

Turnbull, I.M., Brieg, A., and Hassler, D.: Blood supply of cervical spinal cord in man: a microangiographic cadaver study, J. Neurosurg. **24**:951, 1966.

46

Baumel, J.J., and Beard, D.J.: The accessory mcningeal artery of man, J. Anat. **95**:386, 1961.

Kimmel, D.L.: The nerves of the cranial dura mater and their significance in dural headache and referred pain, Chicago Med. School Quart. **22**:16, 1961.

48

Baló, J.: The dural venous sinuses, Anat. Rec. **106**:319, 1950.

49

Butler, H.: The development of certain human dural venous sinuses, J. Anat. **91**:510, 1957.

Klintworth, G.K.: The comparative anatomy and phylogeny of the tentorium cerebelli, Anat. Rec. **160**:635, 1968.

51

Schaltenbrand, G., and Woolsey, C.N., editors: Cerebral localization and organization, Madison, Wisc., 1964, University of Wisconsin Press.

53

Gluhbegović, N., and Williams, T.H.: The human brain: a photographic guide, Hagerstown, Md., 1980, Harper & Row, Publishers.

54

Rhoton, A.L., Kobayashi, S., and Hollinshead, W.H.: Nervus intermedius, J. Neurosurg. **29**:609, 1968.

Samarasinghe, D.D.: The innervation of the cerebral arteries in the rat: an electron microscope study, J. Anat. **99**:815, 1965.

Zaki, W.: The trochlear nerve in man: study relative to its origin, its intracerebral traject, and its structure, Arch. Anat. Histol. Embryol. **43**:105, 1960.

55

Krmpotić, J., and Sunarić, R.: Shirurgische Behandlung otogener und rhinogener Kopfschmerzen, Z. Laryng. Rhinol. Otol. **42**:260, 1963.

Vidić, B., and Young, P.A.: Gross and microscopic observations on the communicating branch of the facial nerve to the lesser petrosal nerve, Anat. Rec. **158**:257, 1967.

56

Vidić, B., and O'Rahilly, R.: An atlas of the anatomy of the ear, Philadelphia, 1971, W.B. Saunders Co.

57

Proctor, B.: The development of middle ear spaces and their surgical significance, J. Laryngol. **78**:631, 1964.

58

Smith, D.W.: Recognizable patterns of human malformation: genetic, embryologic, and clinical aspects, Philadelphia, 1970, W.B. Saunders Co.

59

Altmann, F.: Malformations, anomalies and vestigial structures of the inner ear, A.M.A. Arch. Otolaryng. **57**:591, 1953.

Johnson, F.R., McMinn, R.M.H., and Atfield, G.N.: Ultrastructural and biochemical observations on the tympanic membrane, J. Anat. **103**:297, 1968.

60

Vidić, B.: Anatomical variations in pediatric otorhinolaryngology. In Jazbi, B., editor: Pediatric otorhinolaryngology, Amsterdam, Holland, 1979, Excerpta Medica.

61

Arslan, M.: The innervation of the middle ear, Proc. R. Soc. Med. **53**:1068, 1960.

Baxter, A.: Dehiscence of fallopian canal: an anatomical study J. Laryngol. Otol. **85**:587, 1971.

Blevins, C.E.: Innervation patterns of the human stapedius muscle, Arch. Otolaryngol. **86**:136, 1967.

Candiollo, L., and Levi, A.C.: Study on the morphogenesis of the middle ear muscles in man, Arch. Ohr-Nas-Kelkheilk **195**:55, 1969.

62

Vidić, B.: Extreme development of the paranasal sinuses: report of a case, Ann. Otol. Rhinol. Laryngol. **78**:1291, 1969.

63

Ruskell, G.L.: The distribution of autonomic postganglionic nerve fibers in the lacrimal gland in the rat, J. Anat. **109**:229, 1971.

64

Hayrek, S.S.: Arteries of the orbit in the human being, Br. J. Surg. **50**:938, 1963.

65

Cogan, D.G.: Neurology of ocular muscles, Springfield, Ill., 1956, Charles C Thomas, Publishers.

66

McEven, W.K., and Goodner, E.T.: Secretion of tears and blinking. In Davson, H., editor: The eye, New York, 1962, Academic Press, Inc.

69

Ganguly, D.N., and Roy, K.K.: A study on the cranio-vertebral joint in man, Anat. Anz. **114**:433, 1964.

70

Andreassi, G.: Sur la topographie de l'apex pulmonaire chez l'homme, C.R. Assoc. Anat. **137**:141, 1967.

Fountain, F.P., Minear, W.L., and Allison, R.D.: Function of longus colli and longissimus cervicis muscles in man, Arch. Phys. Med. **47**:665, 1966.

71

Ebbesson, S.O.E.: Quantitative studies of superior cervical sympathetic ganglia in a variety of primates, including man. II. Neuronal packing density, J. Morphol. **124**:181, 1968.

Jamieson, R.W., Smith, D.B., and Anson, B.J.: The cervical sympathetic ganglia: an anatomical study of 100 cervicothoracic dissections, Quart. Bull. Northwestern U. Med. School **26**:219, 1952.

72

Bosma, J.F.: Sensorimotor examination of the mouth and pharynx, Front. Oral Physiol. **2**:78, 1976.

Khoo, F.Y., Kanagasuntheram, R., and Chia, K.B.: Variations of the lateral recesses of the nasopharynx, Arch. Otolaryngol. **88**:456, 1969.

74

Warbrick, J.C.: The early development of the nasal cavity and upper lip in the human embryo, J. Anat. **94**:351, 1960.

77

Van Alyea, O.E.:The ostium maxillare, Arch. Otolaryngol. **24**:553, 1936.

78

Körner, F.: Die Musculi Tensor und Levator Veli palatini. Z. Anat. Entwgesch. **111**:508, 1942.

Vidić, B.: L'innervation du muscle releveur du voile du palais chez l'homme et chez certain mammifères, Arch. Anat. Histol. Embryol. **47**:339, 1964.

79

Ruskell, G.L.: The distribution of autonomic postganglionic nerve fibres in the lacrimal gland in the rat, J. Anat. **109**:229, 1971.

Scit, S., and Dellon, A.L.: Autonomic relationships between the human levator and tensor veli palatini and the eustachian tube, Cleft Palate J. **15**:329, 1978.

80

Blanton, P.L., and Biggs, N.L.: Eighteen hundred years of controversy: the paranasal sinuses, Am. J. Anat. **124**:135, 1969.

Vidić, B.: Paranasal sinuses: past and present, Ear Nose Throat J. **55**:305, 1976.

82

Sherif, M.F., Al-Zuhair, A.G., and Albert, E.N.: Proprioceptive innervation of the rat lingual musculature, Anat. Rec. **205**:182, 1983.

Sicher, H., and DuBrul, E.L.: Oral anatomy, St. Louis, 1970, The C.V. Mosby Co.

86

Garrett, J.R.: The innervation of salivary glands. II. The ultrastructure of nerves in normal glands of the cat, J.R. Microscop. Soc. **85**:149, 1966.

87

Harris, W.: Fifth and seventh cranial nerves in relation to nervous mechanism of taste sensation: new approach, Br. Med. J. **1**:831, 1952.

Hrycyshyn, A.W., and Basmajian, J.V.: Electromyography of the oral stage of swallowing in man, Am. J. Anat. **133**:333, 1972.

Weiffenbach, J.M., editor: Taste and development: the genesis of sweet preference, DHEW Publication No. (NIH) 77-1068, 1977.

88

Bowden, R.E.M.: Surgical anatomy of the recurrent laryngeal nerve, Br. J. Surg. **43**:153, 1955.

English, D.T., and Blevins, C.E.: Motor units of laryngeal muscles, Arch. Otolaryngol. **89**:778, 1969.

89

Rueger, R.S.: The superior laryngeal nerve and the interarytenoid muscle in humans: an anatomical study, Laryngoscope **82**:2008, 1972.

Yeager, V.L., and Archer, C.R.: Calcification and ossification of the larynx as it affects interpretation of computed tomography scans, Anat. Rec. **196**:211A, 1980.

90

Tautz, C., and Rohen, J.W.: Über den konstruktiven Bau des M. vocalis beim Menschen, Ana. Anz. **120**:409, 1967.

91

Terracol, J., et al.: L'anatomie functionelle du larynx, Biol. Méd. **54**:180, 1965.

93

Pressman, J.J.: Physiology of vocal cords in phonation and respiration, Arch. Otolaryngol. **35**:355, 1942.

Tucker, J.A., et al.: Survey of the development of laryngeal epithelium, Ann. Otol. Rhinol. Laryngol. **85**(suppl. 30):3, 1976.

97

Frable, M.A.: Computation of motion at the cricoarytenoid joint, Arch. Otolaryngol. **73**:551, 1961.

Part Two
UPPER LIMB

Skeleton of upper limb, thorax, abdomen, and pelvis

Claviscapular skeleton

Costovertebral skeleton

Skeleton of elbow

Skeleton of wrist and hand

Pectoral, mammary, axillary, and anterior brachial regions

Anterior antebrachial and hand regions

Scapular and posterior brachial regions

Posterior antebrachial and hand regions

Shoulder joint

Elbow joint

Wrist and hand joints

Costovertebral joints

Intervertebral joints

Anterior aspect of the right half of the thoracic, upper limb, abdominal, and pelvic skeleton

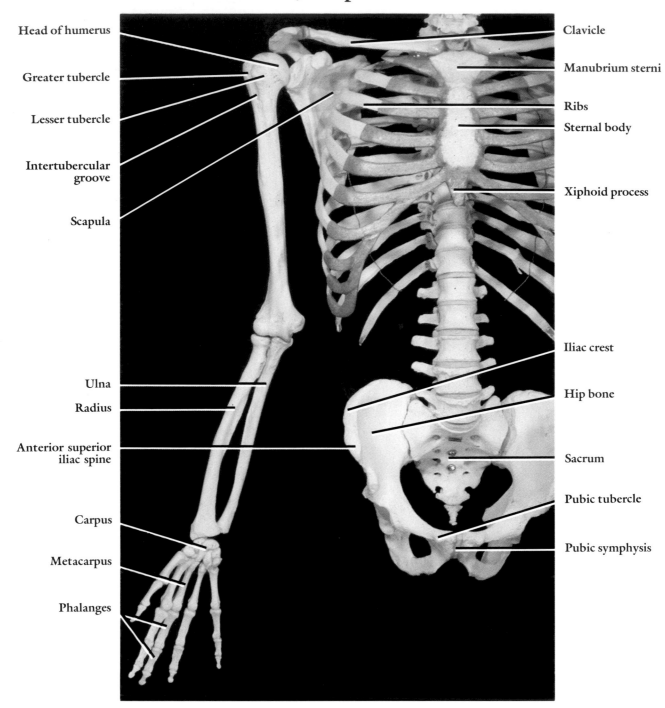

Head of humerus

Greater tubercle

Lesser tubercle

Intertubercular groove

Scapula

Ulna

Radius

Anterior superior iliac spine

Carpus

Metacarpus

Phalanges

Clavicle

Manubrium sterni

Ribs

Sternal body

Xiphoid process

Iliac crest

Hip bone

Sacrum

Pubic tubercle

Pubic symphysis

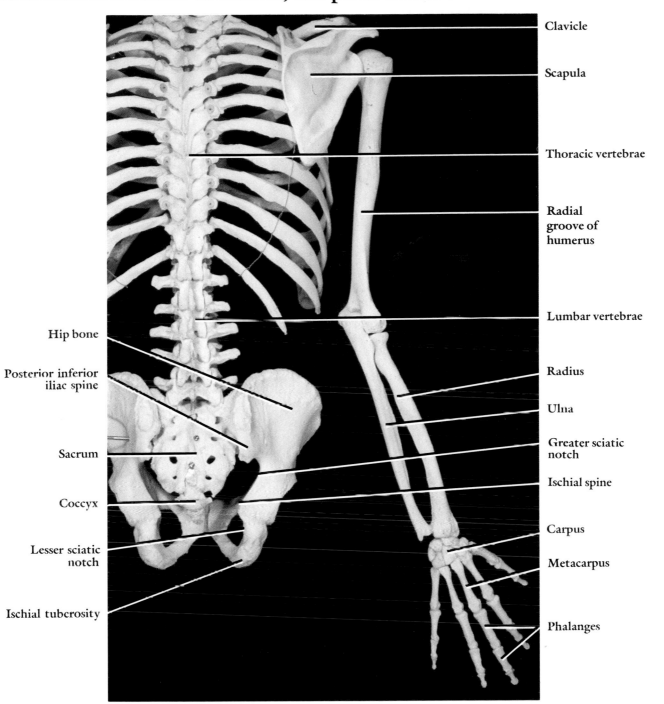

Clavicle

Scapula

Thoracic vertebrae

Radial groove of humerus

Lumbar vertebrae

Hip bone

Posterior inferior iliac spine

Radius

Ulna

Greater sciatic notch

Ischial spine

Sacrum

Coccyx

Carpus

Metacarpus

Lesser sciatic notch

Ischial tuberosity

Phalanges

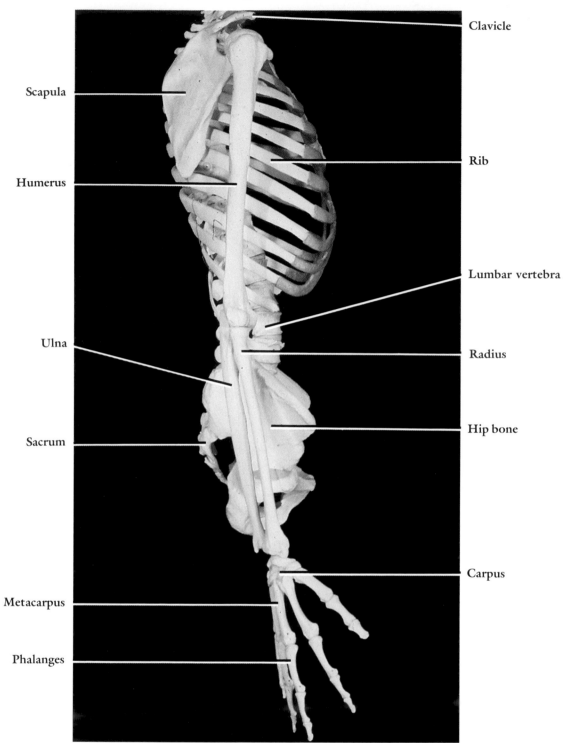

Clavicle

Scapula

Humerus

Rib

Lumbar vertebra

Ulna

Radius

Sacrum

Hip bone

Carpus

Metacarpus

Phalanges

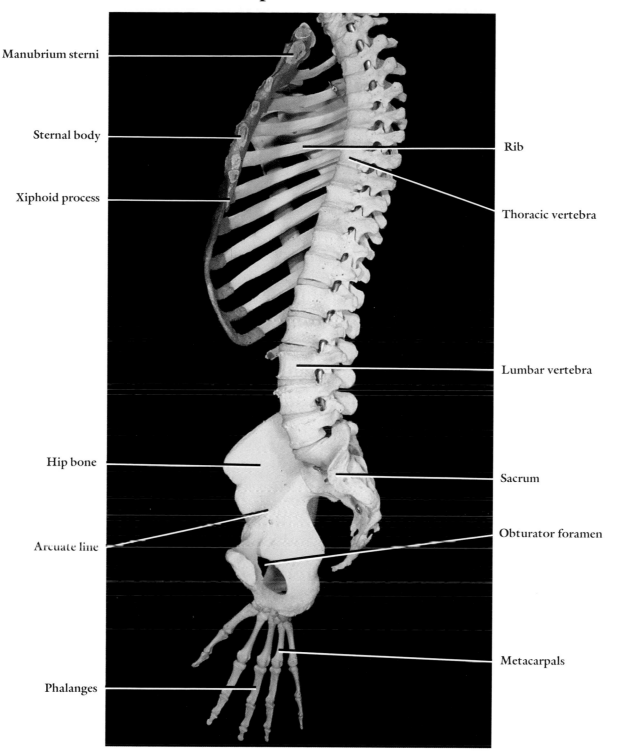

Manubrium sterni

Sternal body

Xiphoid process

Rib

Thoracic vertebra

Lumbar vertebra

Hip bone

Sacrum

Arcuate line

Obturator foramen

Metacarpals

Phalanges

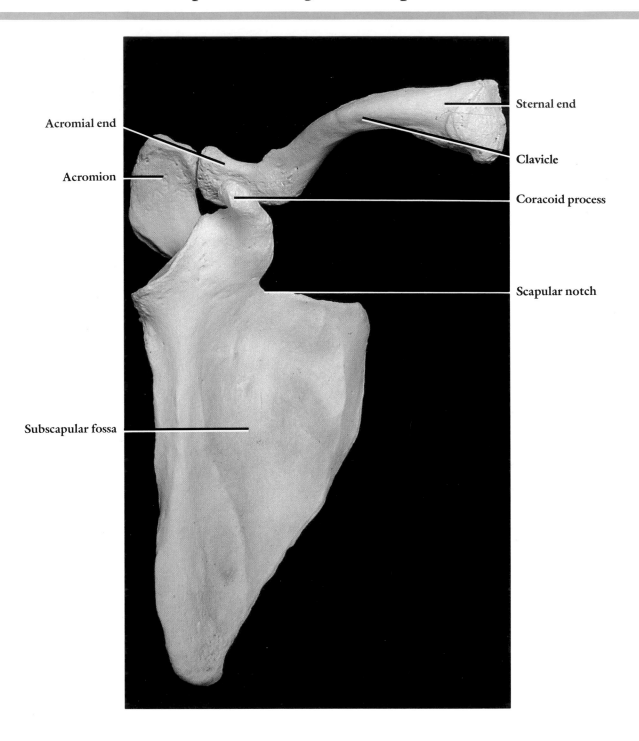

Acromial end

Acromion

Sternal end

Clavicle

Coracoid process

Scapular notch

Subscapular fossa

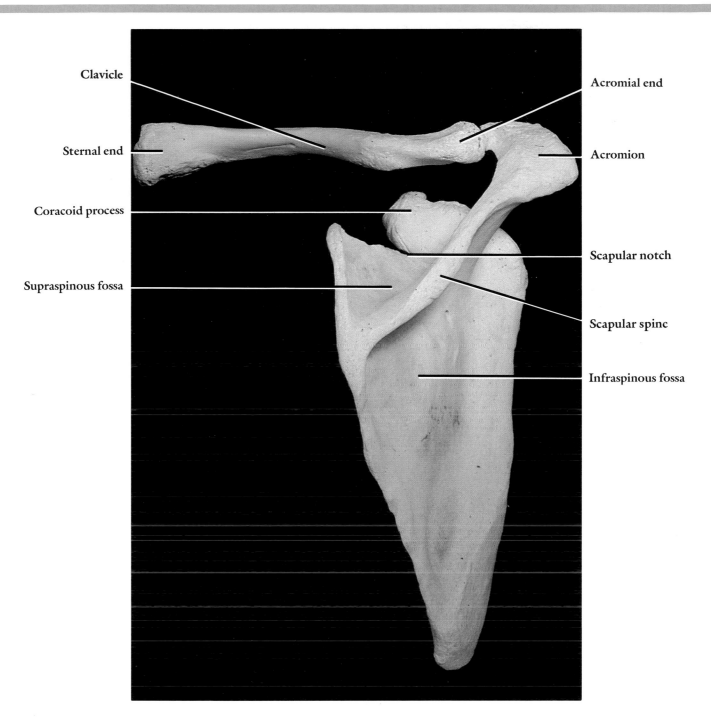

Clavicle

Sternal end

Coracoid process

Supraspinous fossa

Acromial end

Acromion

Scapular notch

Scapular spinc

Infraspinous fossa

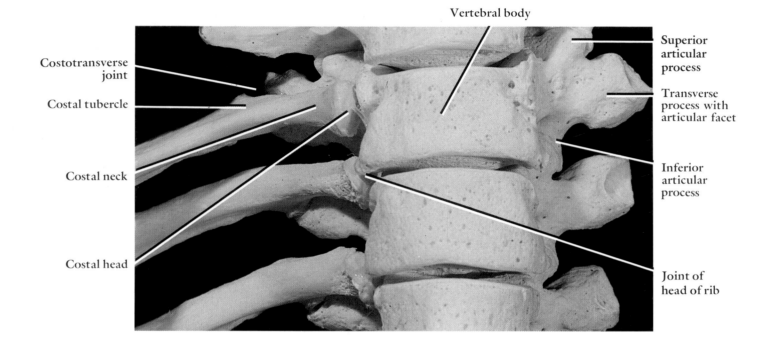

Vertebral body

Costotransverse joint

Costal tubercle

Costal neck

Costal head

Superior articular process

Transverse process with articular facet

Inferior articular process

Joint of head of rib

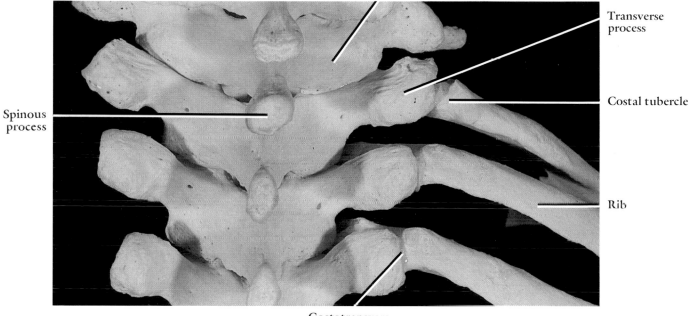

Vertebral lamina

Transverse process

Spinous process

Costal tubercle

Rib

Costotransverse joint

General remarks: A *vertebrosternal rib* moves during respiration about two axes: (1) passing from just lateral to the *costal tubercle* to the sternal midline and (2) passing from the costal tubercle to the *costal head*.

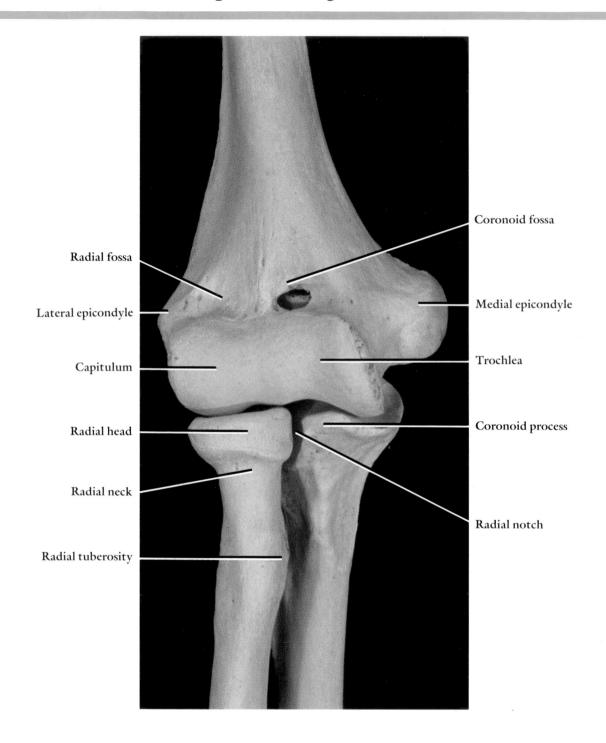

Radial fossa

Coronoid fossa

Lateral epicondyle

Medial epicondyle

Capitulum

Trochlea

Radial head

Coronoid process

Radial neck

Radial notch

Radial tuberosity

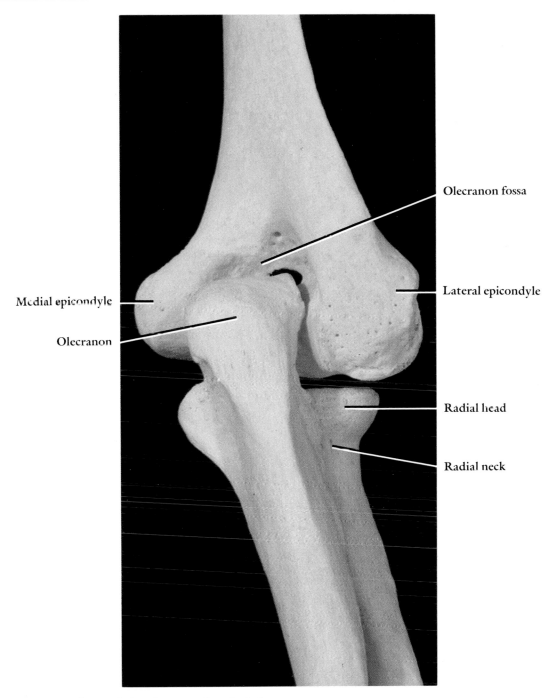

Olecranon fossa

Lateral epicondyle

Medial epicondyle

Olecranon

Radial head

Radial neck

General remarks: Bony floor of the *olecranon fossa* is deficient in this instance and hence is opened anteriorly into the *coronoid fossa*. Most frequently, however, the two fossae are separated by a thin bony lamina.

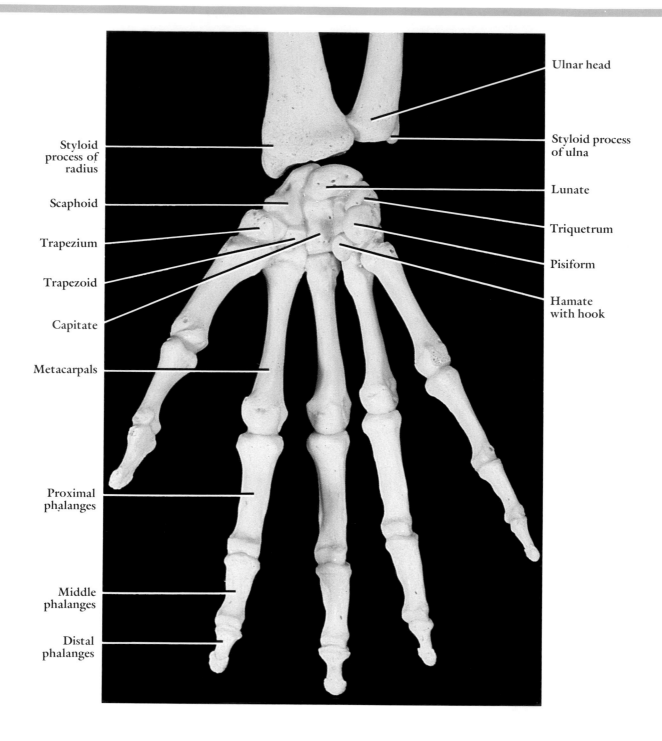

Styloid process of radius

Scaphoid

Trapezium

Trapezoid

Capitate

Metacarpals

Proximal phalanges

Middle phalanges

Distal phalanges

Ulnar head

Styloid process of ulna

Lunate

Triquetrum

Pisiform

Hamate with hook

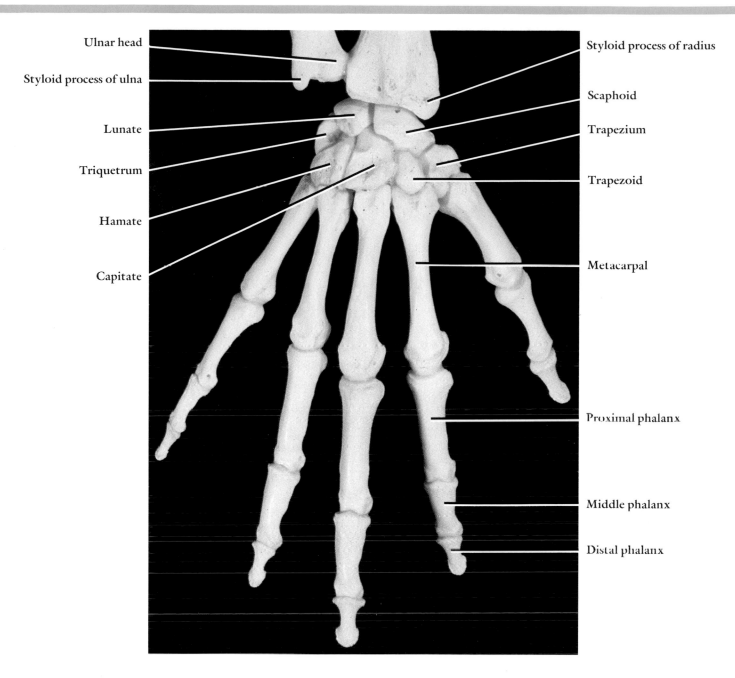

Ulnar head

Styloid process of ulna

Lunate

Triquetrum

Hamate

Capitate

Styloid process of radius

Scaphoid

Trapezium

Trapezoid

Metacarpal

Proximal phalanx

Middle phalanx

Distal phalanx

Anterior aspect of the arm, thorax, and abdomen
in a living male subject

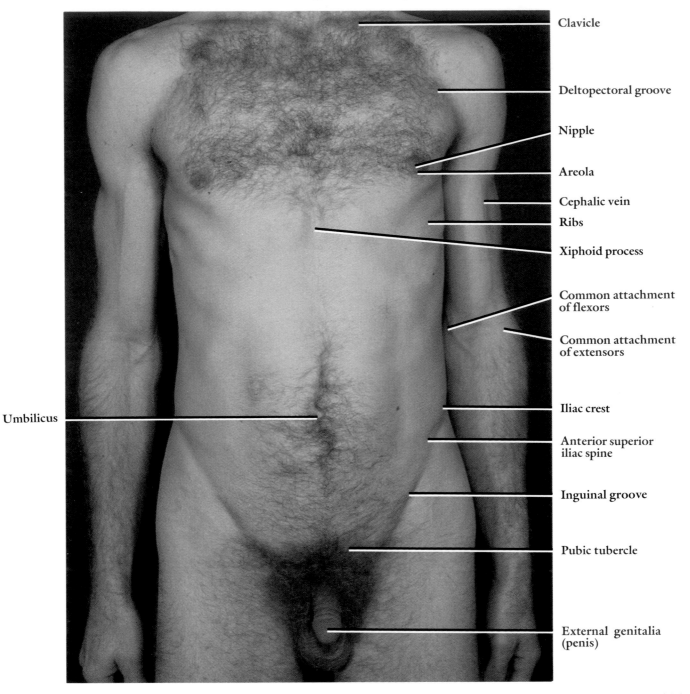

Clavicle

Deltopectoral groove

Nipple

Areola

Cephalic vein

Ribs

Xiphoid process

Common attachment of flexors

Common attachment of extensors

Iliac crest

Anterior superior iliac spine

Inguinal groove

Pubic tubercle

External genitalia (penis)

Umbilicus

General remarks: Ribs and *intercostal spaces* are routinely used as topographical landmarks during physical examination or in planning a radical exploration of the thoracic contents. The anterior and lateral abdominal walls, which are composed of several muscular layers, on the other hand, give a free access to internal structures by palpation.

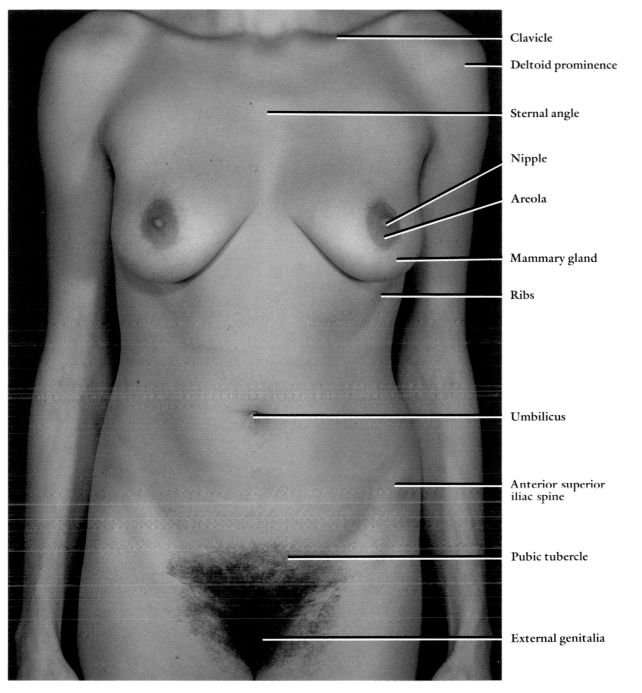

Clavicle

Deltoid prominence

Sternal angle

Nipple

Areola

Mammary gland

Ribs

Umbilicus

Anterior superior iliac spine

Pubic tubercle

External genitalia

General remarks: The *mammary gland* consists in prepubertal individuals mainly of *lactiferous ducts*. At the time of puberty these further develop under the influence of estrogen hormones to form precursors of *glandular alveoli*. The secreting tissue, however, differentiates only during pregnancy as a result of placental estrogen and progesterone stimuli.

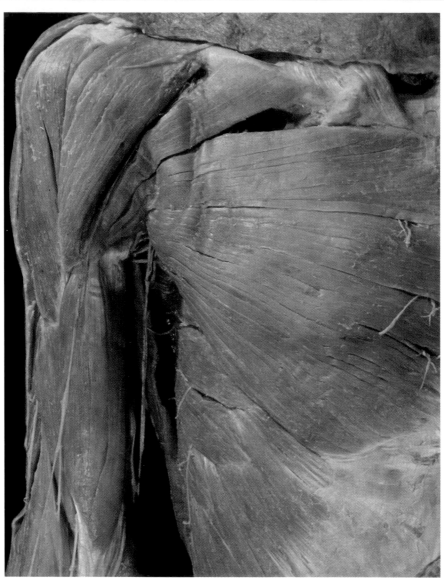

114
Anterior aspect of the mammary tissue

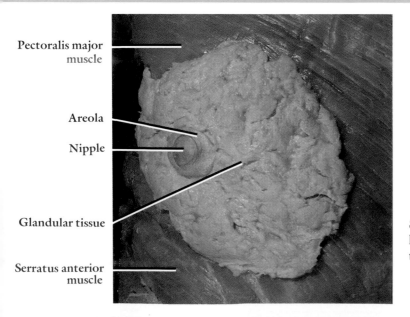

Pectoralis major
muscle

Areola

Nipple

Glandular tissue

Serratus anterior
muscle

Specific remarks: The skin, subcutaneous tissue, and fascia have been removed from this region, but the mammary tissue has been maintained in situ in this female subject.

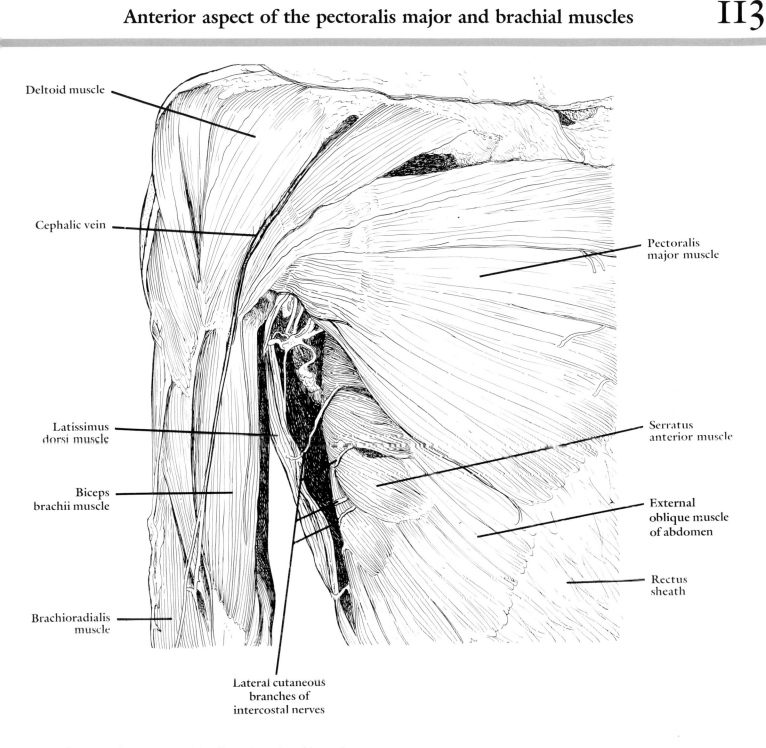

Deltoid muscle

Cephalic vein

Latissimus dorsi muscle

Biceps brachii muscle

Brachioradialis muscle

Lateral cutaneous branches of intercostal nerves

Pectoralis major muscle

Serratus anterior muscle

External oblique muscle of abdomen

Rectus sheath

Specific remarks: During this dissection the skin, subcutaneous tissue, and regional fascia have been removed to demonstrate the *pectoralis major muscle,* the *deltoid muscle,* the *biceps brachii muscle,* and the *cephalic vein.*

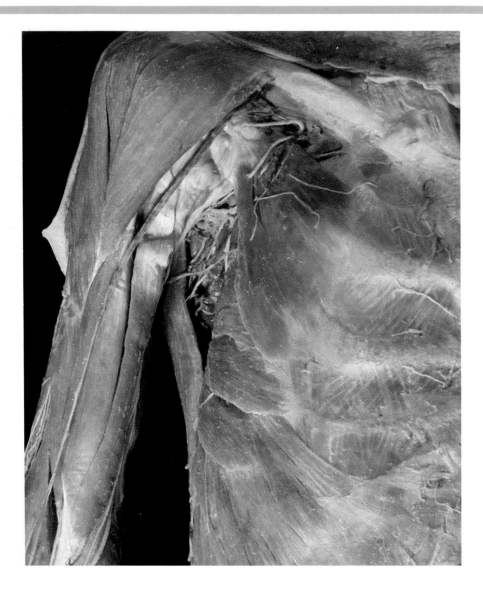

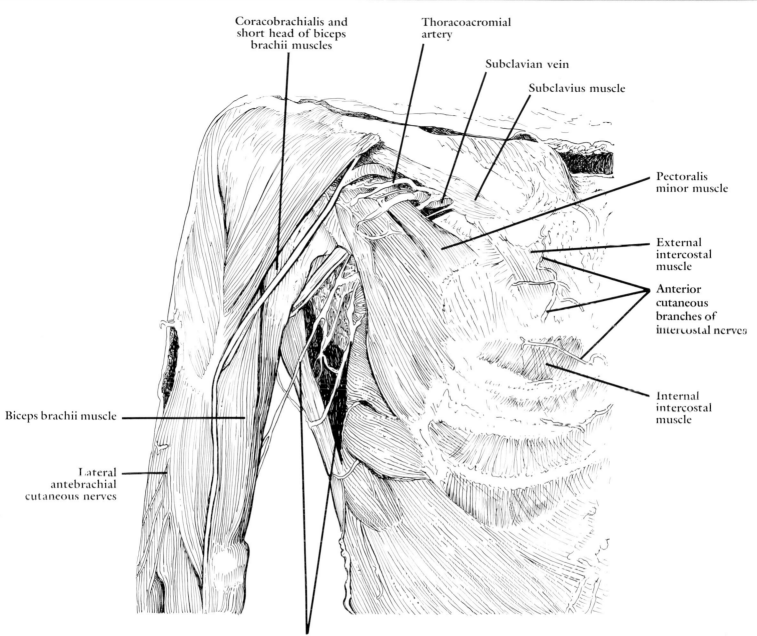

Coracobrachialis and short head of biceps brachii muscles

Thoracoacromial artery

Subclavian vein

Subclavius muscle

Pectoralis minor muscle

External intercostal muscle

Anterior cutaneous branches of intercostal nerves

Biceps brachii muscle

Internal intercostal muscle

Lateral antebrachial cutaneous nerves

Medial brachial cutaneous and intercostobrachial nerves

Specific remarks: For the approach to the axillary content the *pectoralis major muscle* has been removed. Now the *subclavius, pectoralis minor, coracobrachialis,* and the *short head of the biceps brachii muscles* are demonstrated, in addition to those structures that are partially exposed in the *axilla*.

General remarks: Pectoralis major and minor muscles, together with their investing fascia, represent the anterior wall of the *axillary fossa*.

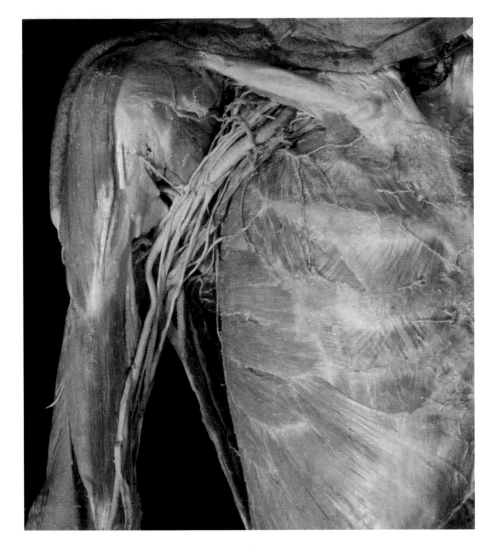

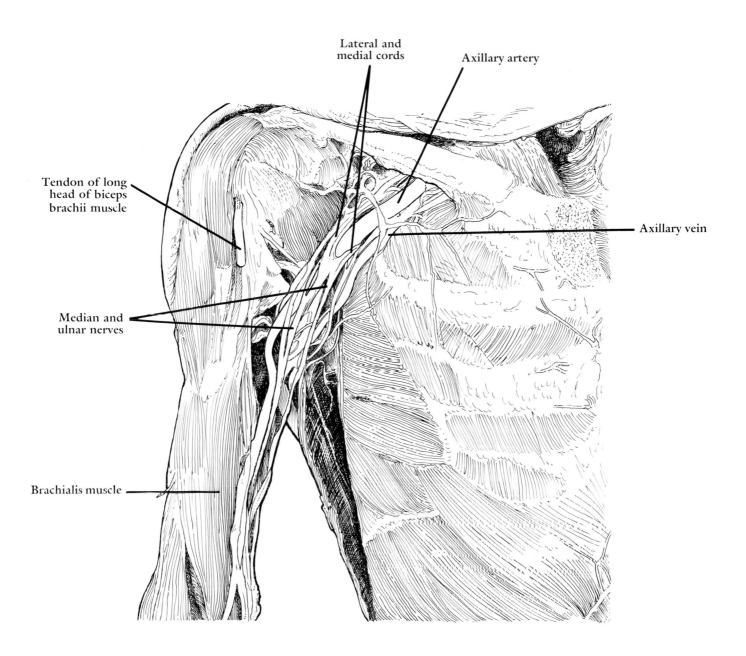

Lateral and
medial cords

Axillary artery

Tendon of long
head of biceps
brachii muscle

Axillary vein

Median and
ulnar nerves

Brachialis muscle

Specific remarks: Following the removal of *pectoralis minor, biceps brachii,* and *deltoid muscles* the content of the *axillary fossa* becomes exposed. In addition to *cords of the brachial plexus* and their collateral and terminal branches, the *axillary artery* and its continuation, the *brachial artery,* and their respective branches are shown. The attachment of *serratus anterior* and *intercostal muscles* on the thoracic wall are also demonstrated.

General remarks: The serratus anterior muscle forms the medial wall of the *axilla.* The *coracobrachialis muscle, short head of biceps brachii muscle,* and the *humeral shaft* contribute to the lateral axillary wall. *Axillary lymph nodes* are usually divided into several groups: lateral, anterior, posterior, central, and apical. They drain, in addition to upper limb, the axillary walls, mammary gland, and the skin from thoracic and abdominal walls above the *umbilicus.*

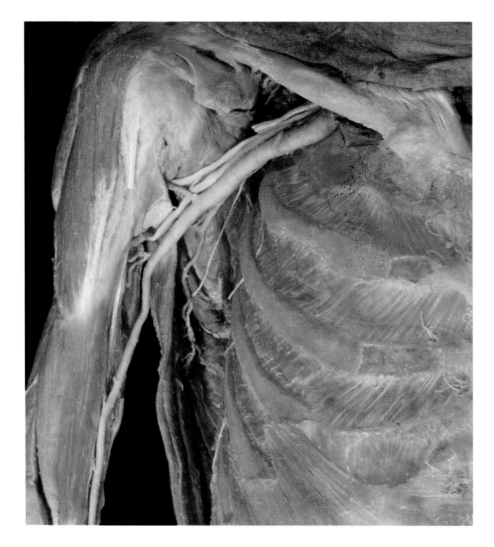

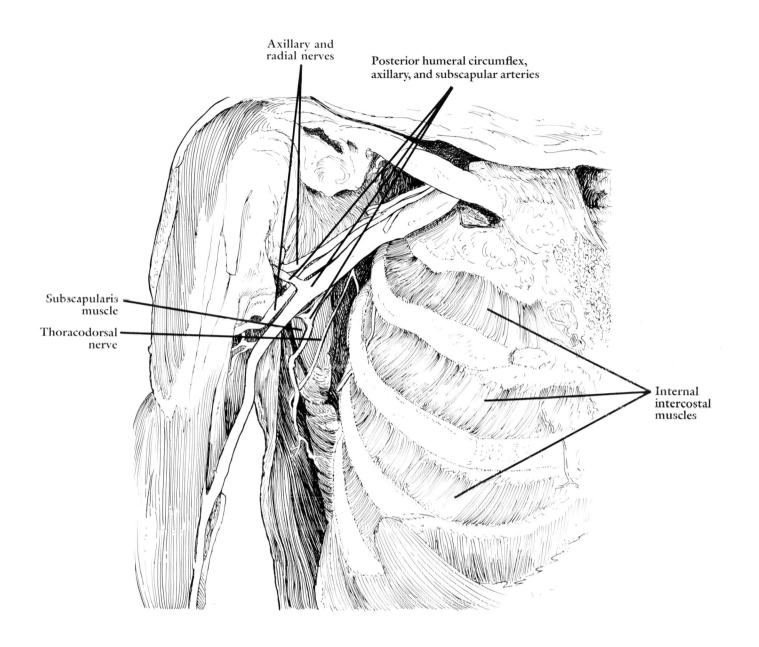

Axillary and
radial nerves

Posterior humeral circumflex,
axillary, and subscapular arteries

Subscapularis
muscle

Thoracodorsal
nerve

Internal
intercostal
muscles

Specific remarks: Because more superficial elements have been removed from the *axillary fossa*, it is possible to bring into evidence the *posterior cord of the brachial plexus* and its branches and accompanying blood vessels. Besides the two collateral branches of the plexus, the *upper* and *lower subscapular nerves*, the *axillary* and *radial nerves* are also exposed. The axillary nerve, together with the *posterior humeral circumflex artery*, penetrates into the *quadrangular space* to become distributed to the *deltoid* and *teres minor muscles* and to the skin over the posterior aspect of the arm. The radial nerve, which is accompanied with the *profunda brachii artery*, continues into the posterior brachial compartment and further inferiorly into the posterior compartment of the forearm and hand.

General remarks: The quadrangular space is bordered by the teres minor muscle superiorly, the *teres major muscle* inferiorly, the *long head of the triceps brachii muscle* medially, and by the *humeral shaft* laterally.

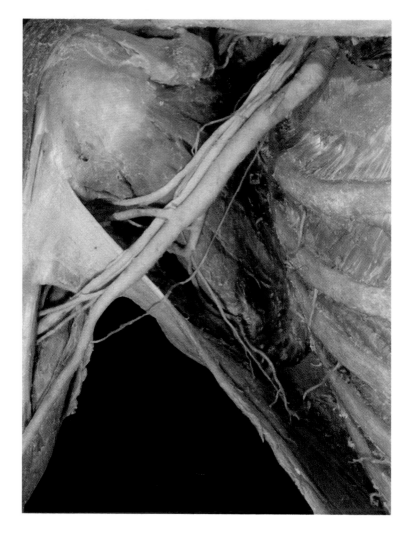

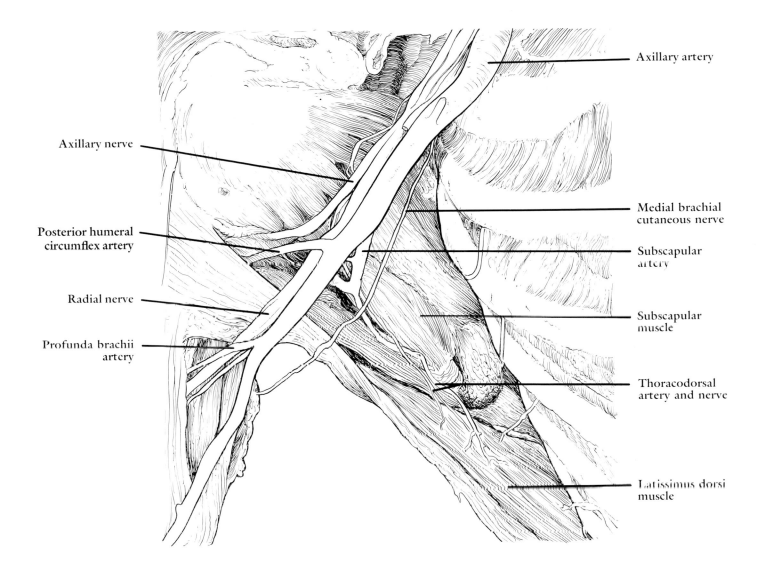

Axillary artery

Axillary nerve

Medial brachial cutaneous nerve

Posterior humeral circumflex artery

Subscapular artery

Radial nerve

Subscapular muscle

Profunda brachii artery

Thoracodorsal artery and nerve

Latissimus dorsi muscle

Specific remarks: Most of the posterior axillary wall is formed by the *subscapular muscle*. The muscle extends from the anterior aspect of the *scapula*—the *subscapular fossa*—medially to the *lesser tubercle of the humerus* laterally. Because it is directly related to the *glenohumeral joint* posteriorly, the muscle is protected by the *subscapular bursa*, the cavity of which is continuous with that of the joint by an opening between the *superior* and *middle glenohumeral ligaments*.

General remarks: The *intercostal muscles* are arranged within *intercostal spaces* in three layers: external, internal, and innermost. They are important in moving ribs during respiration to increase or decrease the anteroposterior and transverse diameters of the thoracic cage.

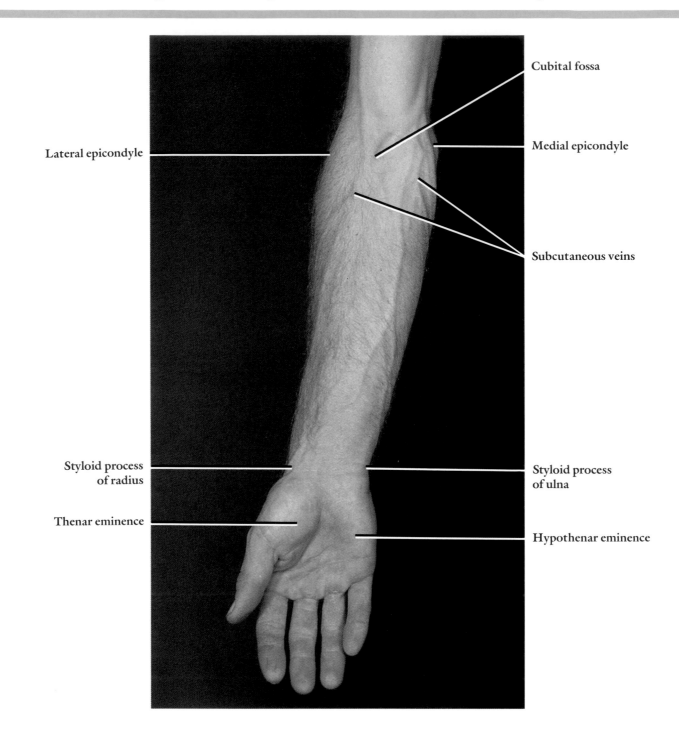

Cubital fossa

Medial epicondyle

Lateral epicondyle

Subcutaneous veins

Styloid process of radius

Styloid process of ulna

Thenar eminence

Hypothenar eminence

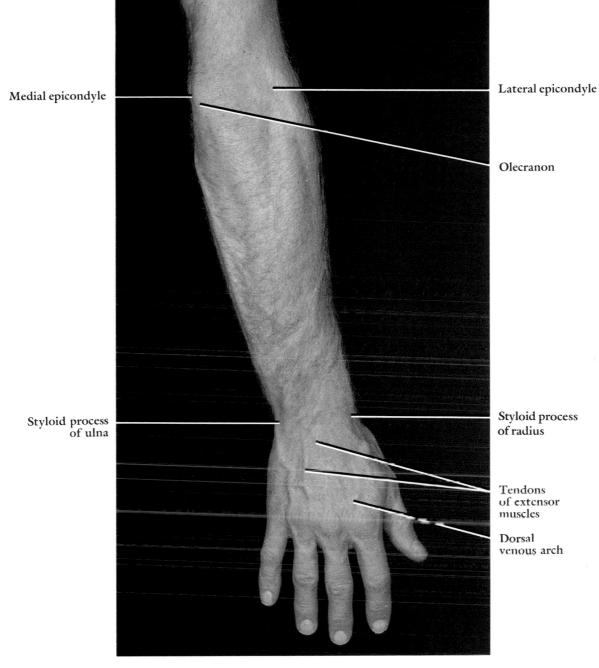

Medial epicondyle

Lateral epicondyle

Olecranon

Styloid process
of ulna

Styloid process
of radius

Tendons
of extensor
muscles

Dorsal
venous arch

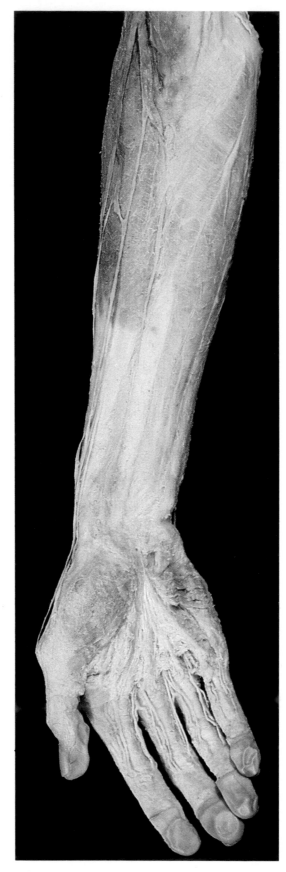

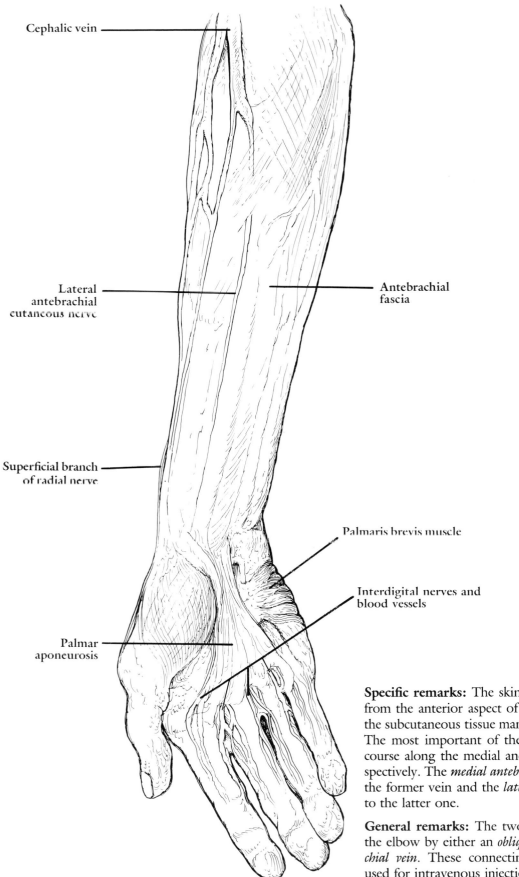

Cephalic vein

Lateral antebrachial cutaneous nerve

Antebrachial fascia

Superficial branch of radial nerve

Palmaris brevis muscle

Interdigital nerves and blood vessels

Palmar aponeurosis

Specific remarks: The skin has been completely removed from the anterior aspect of the forearm and hand. Within the subcutaneous tissue many *antebrachial veins* are present. The most important of these, the *basilic* and the *cephalic,* course along the medial and lateral sides of the region respectively. The *medial antebrachial cutaneous nerve* relates to the former vein and the *lateral antebrachial cutaneous nerve* to the latter one.

General remarks: The two major veins are connected at the elbow by either an *oblique cubital* or a *median antebrachial vein.* These connecting vessels are most frequently used for intravenous injection and withdrawal of blood.

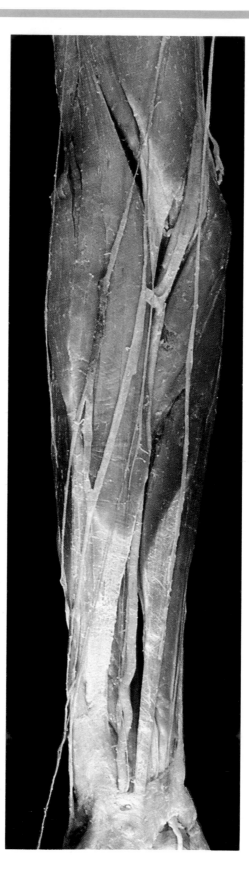

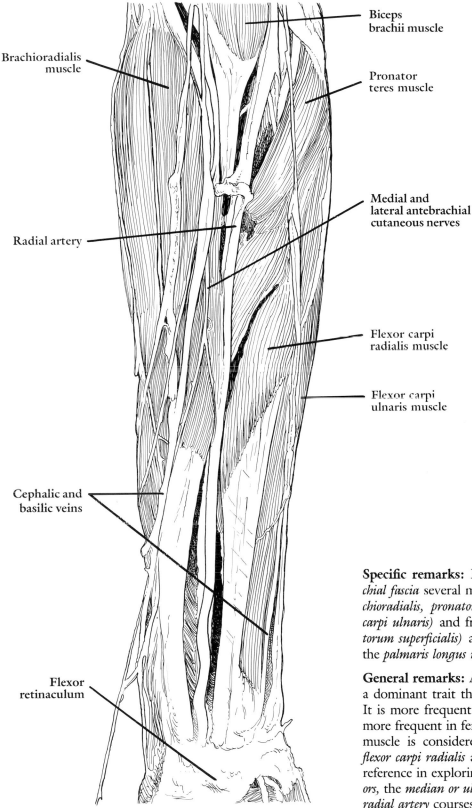

Brachioradialis
muscle

Radial artery

Cephalic and
basilic veins

Flexor
retinaculum

Biceps
brachii muscle

Pronator
teres muscle

Medial and
lateral antebrachial
cutaneous nerves

Flexor carpi
radialis muscle

Flexor carpi
ulnaris muscle

Specific remarks: Following the removal of the *antebrachial fascia* several muscles from the superficial group *(brachioradialis, pronator teres, flexor carpi radialis, and flexor carpi ulnaris)* and from the next deeper group *(flexor digitorum superficialis)* are shown. In this particular individual the *palmaris longus muscle* is absent.

General remarks: Agenesis of the *palmaris longus muscle* is a dominant trait that occurs in 12.9% of the population. It is more frequent on the left side than on the right and more frequent in females than in males. The tendon of this muscle is considered, together with the tendons of the *flexor carpi radialis* and *ulnaris muscles*, as a point of initial reference in exploring either the tendons of the *digital flexors*, the *median or ulnar nerve*, or the *ulnar blood vessels*. The *radial artery* courses medial to the tendon of *brachioradialis muscle* and lateral to that of the *flexor carpi radialis muscle*. Because of the relatively superficial position of the artery in this location and its close relationship with the underlying *radius*, this artery is most commonly used for taking the pulse.

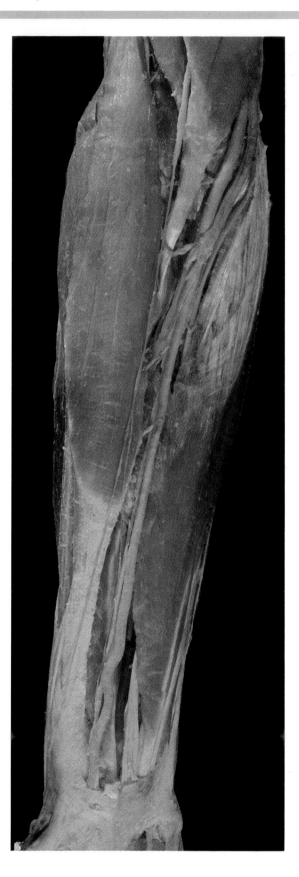

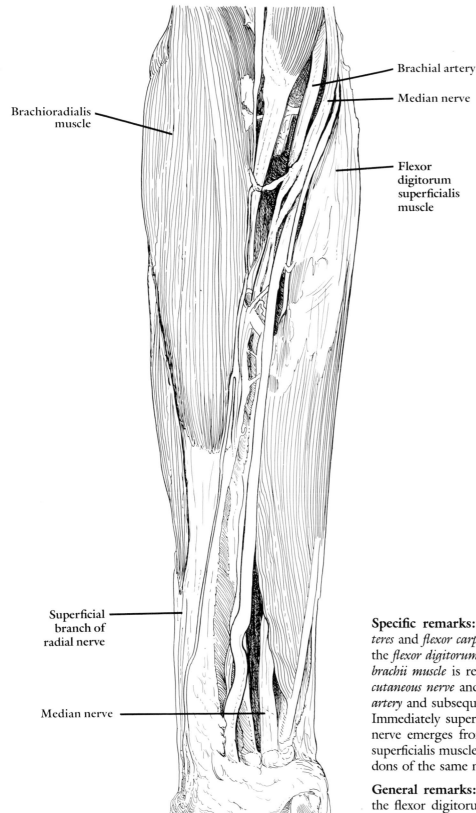

Brachioradialis muscle

Brachial artery

Median nerve

Flexor digitorum superficialis muscle

Superficial branch of radial nerve

Median nerve

Specific remarks: Two superficial muscles, the *pronator teres* and *flexor carpi radialis*, were removed to demonstrate the *flexor digitorum superficialis muscle*. The tendon of *biceps brachii muscle* is related laterally to the *lateral antebrachial cutaneous nerve* and medially to the still undivided *brachial artery* and subsequently the *radial artery* and *median nerve*. Immediately superior to the *flexor retinaculum* the median nerve emerges from under the cover of flexor digitorum superficialis muscle to become placed just lateral to the tendons of the same muscle.

General remarks: Although the anatomical variations in the flexor digitorum superficialis muscle are encountered, the topographical relation between the median nerve and the muscle is constant. The muscular variations most frequently include absence of the radial head, prevalent action on the *index,* and absence of the muscular part or tendon of the fifth digit.

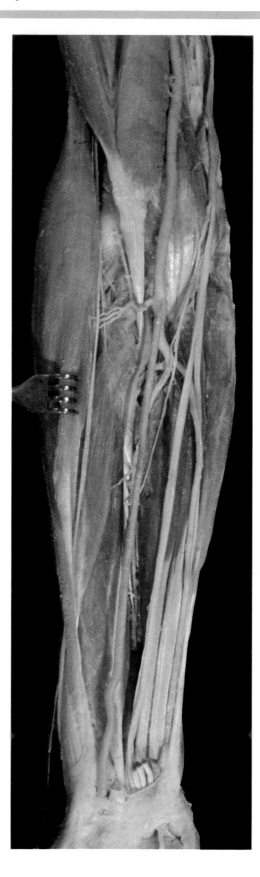

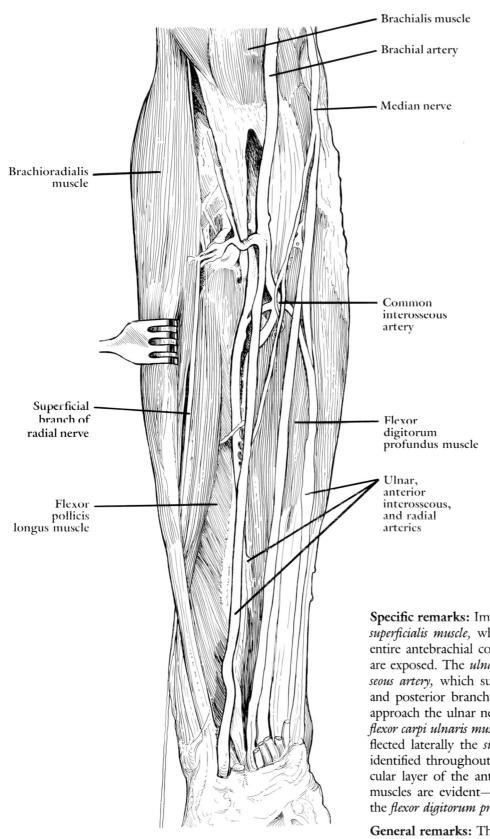

Brachialis muscle

Brachial artery

Median nerve

Brachioradialis
muscle

Common
interosseous
artery

Superficial
branch of
radial nerve

Flexor
digitorum
profundus muscle

Ulnar,
anterior
interosseous,
and radial
arteries

Flexor
pollicis
longus muscle

Specific remarks: Immediately deep to the *flexor digitorum superficialis muscle,* which was removed for this view, the entire antebrachial courses of the *median* and *ulnar nerves* are exposed. The *ulnar artery* gives off the *common interosseous artery,* which subsequently divides into the anterior and posterior branches, and continues medioinferiorly to approach the ulnar nerve along the anterior margin of the *flexor carpi ulnaris muscle.* With the *brachioradialis muscle* reflected laterally the *superficial branch of the radial nerve* is identified throughout the forearm. Within the third muscular layer of the anterior antebrachial compartment two muscles are evident—the *flexor pollicis longus* laterally and the *flexor digitorum profundus* medially.

General remarks: The flexor digitorum profundus muscle is innervated by two branches of the *brachial plexus.* The median nerve supplies the lateral half and the ulnar nerve the medial half of the muscle. Such a dual innervation is important in differential diagnosis of neurological conditions related to either of the two nerves.

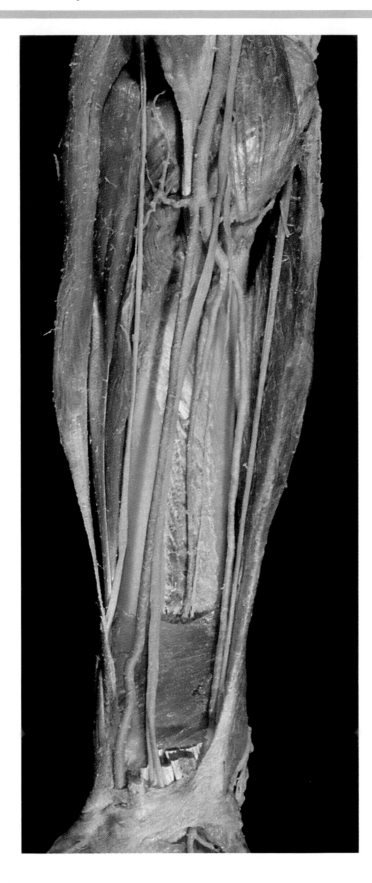

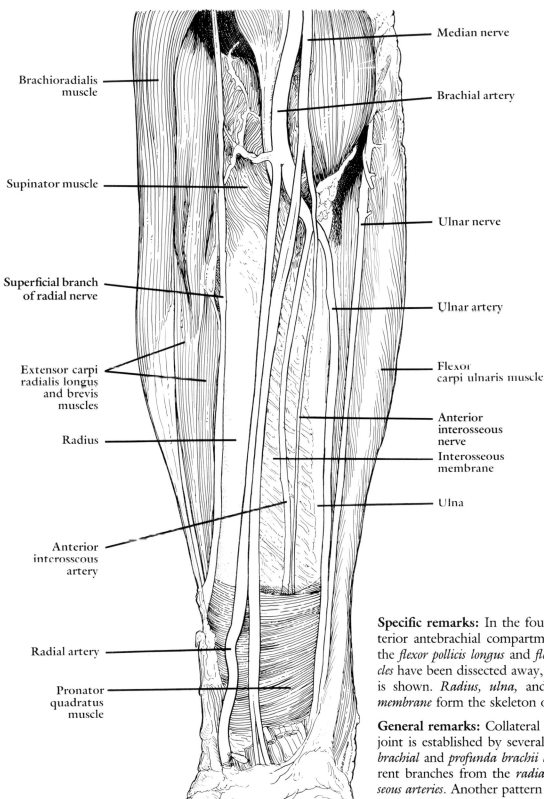

Brachioradialis muscle

Supinator muscle

Superficial branch of radial nerve

Extensor carpi radialis longus and brevis muscles

Radius

Anterior interosseous artery

Radial artery

Pronator quadratus muscle

Median nerve

Brachial artery

Ulnar nerve

Ulnar artery

Flexor carpi ulnaris muscle

Anterior interosseous nerve

Interosseous membrane

Ulna

Specific remarks: In the fourth muscular layer of the anterior antebrachial compartment, demonstrated here after the *flexor pollicis longus* and *flexor digitorum profundus muscles* have been dissected away, the *pronator quadratus muscle* is shown. *Radius, ulna,* and the intervening *interosseous membrane* form the skeleton of the forearm.

General remarks: Collateral circulation around the elbow joint is established by several collateral branches from the *brachial* and *profunda brachii arteries* and by a set of recurrent branches from the *radial, ulnar,* and *common interosseous arteries.* Another pattern is developed between the *anterior* and *posterior interosseous arteries,* which exchange numerous anastomosing twigs through the interosseous membrane. These collateral bridges between the major arteries, similar to ones established around the *scapula,* in the arm, or in the hand, enable blood to be distributed even to those parts of the upper limb in which the regional arteries may have been physically or otherwise disrupted.

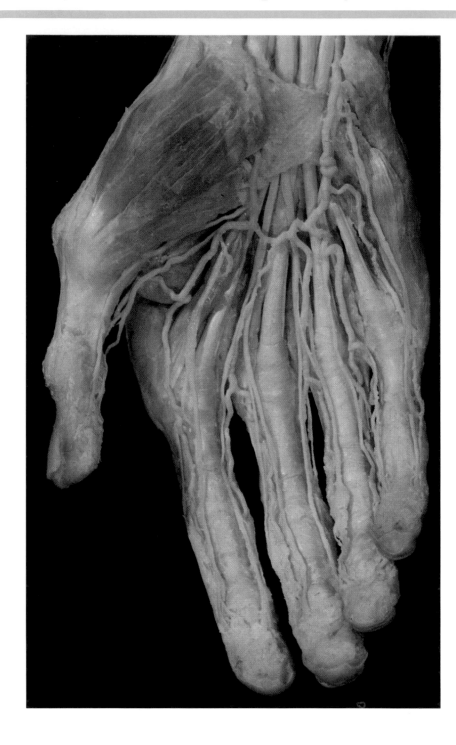

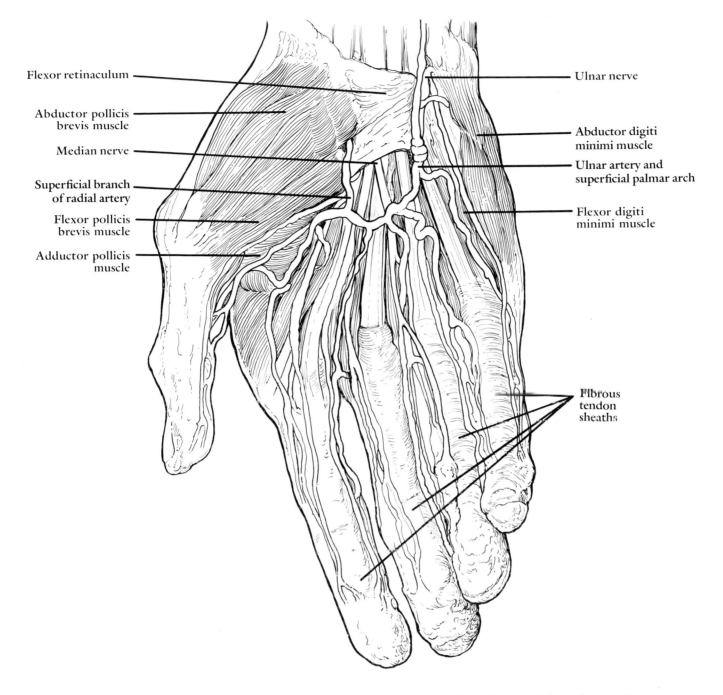

Flexor retinaculum

Abductor pollicis
brevis muscle

Median nerve

Superficial branch
of radial artery

Flexor pollicis
brevis muscle

Adductor pollicis
muscle

Ulnar nerve

Abductor digiti
minimi muscle

Ulnar artery and
superficial palmar arch

Flexor digiti
minimi muscle

Fibrous
tendon
sheaths

Specific remarks: Immediately deep to the *palmar aponeurosis* are the *superficial palmar arch,* its branches, and the *digital branches of the median* and *ulnar nerves.* These elements overlap directly tendons of the *flexor digitorum superficialis muscle,* which, from the metacarpophalangeal level distally, are enclosed in their respective *synovial sheaths.* Muscles of the *thenar* and *hypothenar eminences* are shown as they extend from the *flexor retinaculum* to the first and fifth digits respectively.

General remarks: The superficial palmar arch is an important anastomosis between the *ulnar artery* medially and the *radial artery* laterally. Because of its superficial position immediately deep to the aponeurosis, the arch is frequently damaged in hand injuries.

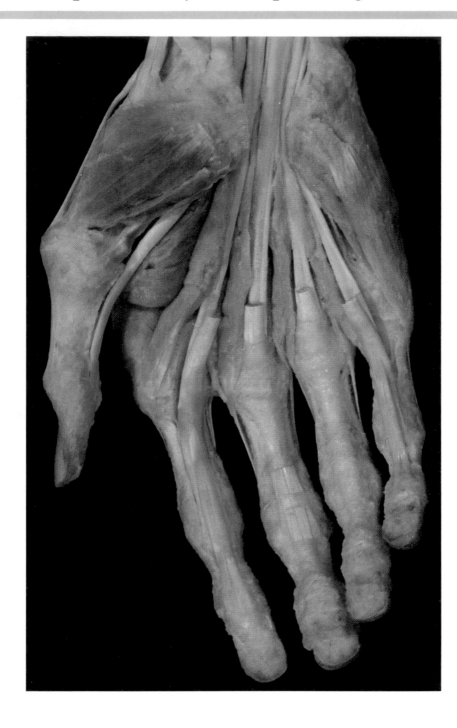

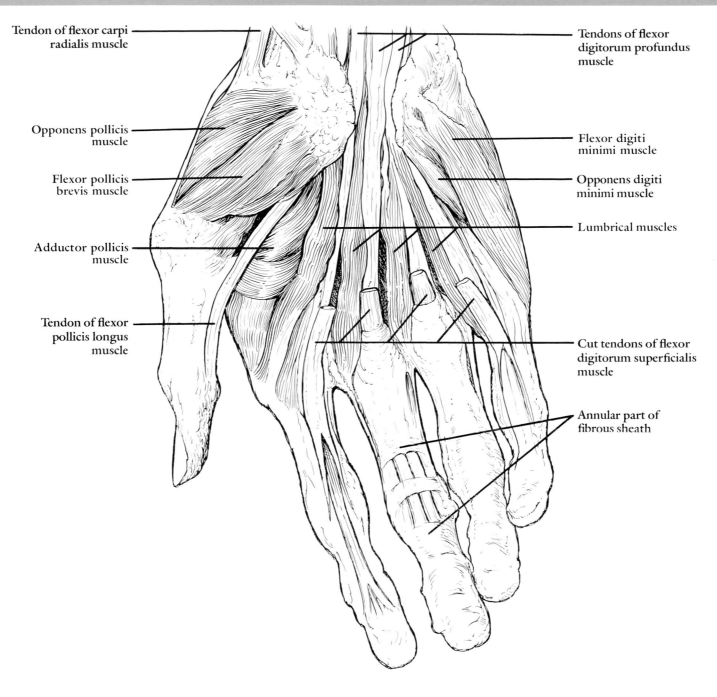

Tendon of flexor carpi radialis muscle

Opponens pollicis muscle

Flexor pollicis brevis muscle

Adductor pollicis muscle

Tendon of flexor pollicis longus muscle

Tendons of flexor digitorum profundus muscle

Flexor digiti minimi muscle

Opponens digiti minimi muscle

Lumbrical muscles

Cut tendons of flexor digitorum superficialis muscle

Annular part of fibrous sheath

Specific remarks: For this view the *superficial palmar arch* and branches and the *digital branches of the median* and *ulnar nerves* have been completely removed, and tendons of the *flexor digitorum superficialis muscle* have been cut close to the metacarpophalangeal level and also removed. In addition, the *abductor pollicis brevis muscle* has been dissected away from the *thenar eminence* and the *flexor retinaculum* from the *carpal canal (tunnel)*. The relationship of the *lumbrical muscles* to tendons of the *flexor digitorum profundus muscle*, as well as their digital extension, are evident. Tendons of the superficial and deep digital flexors are completely exposed in the second and fifth digits, but they are only partially shown in the third digit as maintained in situ by the *annular part* of the digital sheath. Those in the fourth digit are completely enclosed in both the *fibrous* and *synovial sheaths*.

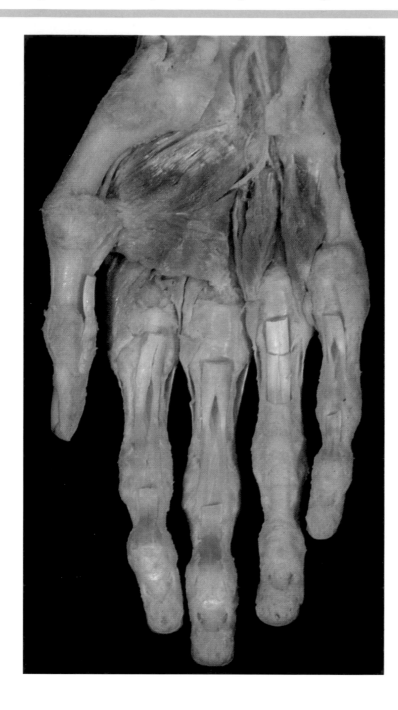

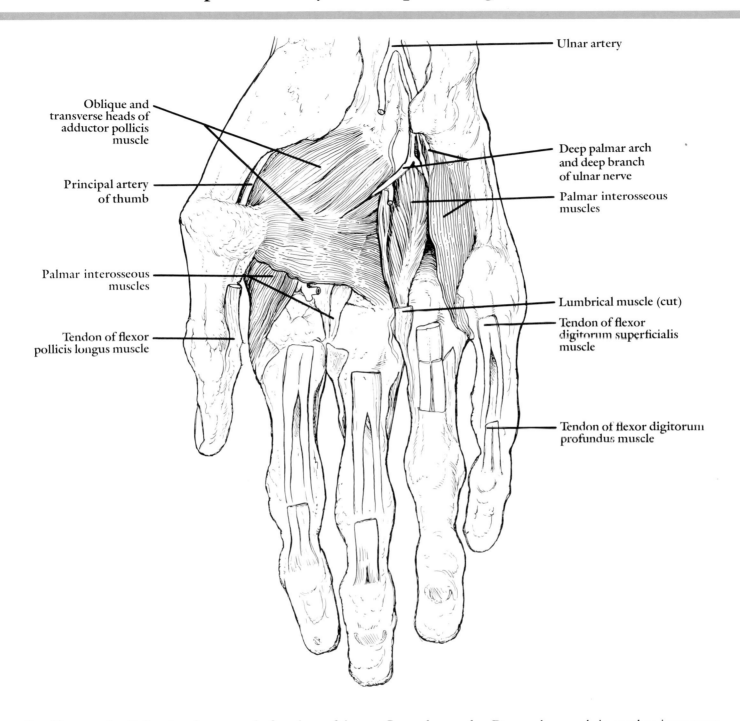

Ulnar artery

Oblique and transverse heads of adductor pollicis muscle

Deep palmar arch and deep branch of ulnar nerve

Principal artery of thumb

Palmar interosseous muscles

Palmar interosseous muscles

Lumbrical muscle (cut)

Tendon of flexor digitorum superficialis muscle

Tendon of flexor pollicis longus muscle

Tendon of flexor digitorum profundus muscle

Specific remarks: Following the removal of tendons of the *flexor digitorum superficialis* and *profundus muscles* and of the *flexor pollicis longus muscle* and muscles of the *thenar* and *hypothenar eminences* the deep structures of the region could be demonstrated: 1. *adductor pollicis muscle*; 2. *palmar interossei*; 3. *dorsal interossei*; and 4. *deep palmar arch*.

General remarks: Deep palmar arch is another important anastomosis between the *radial artery* laterally and the *ulnar artery* medially. It is accompanied by the *deep branch of the ulnar nerve* which supplies the interossei, two medial *lumbricals*, hypothenar muscles, adductor pollicis muscle, and most frequently the *flexor pollicis brevis muscle*.

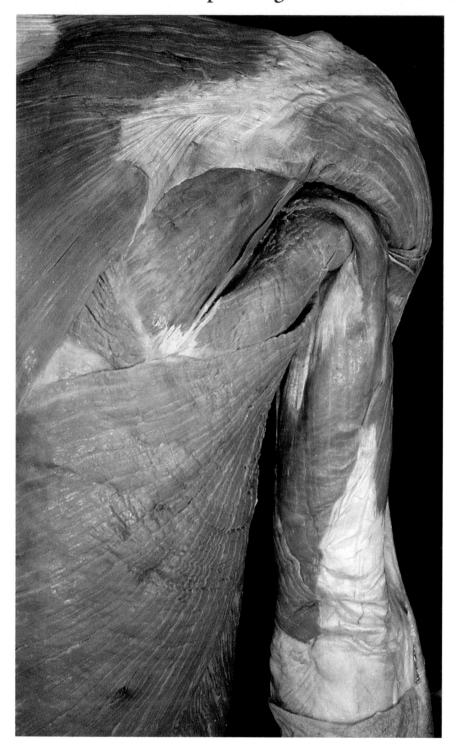

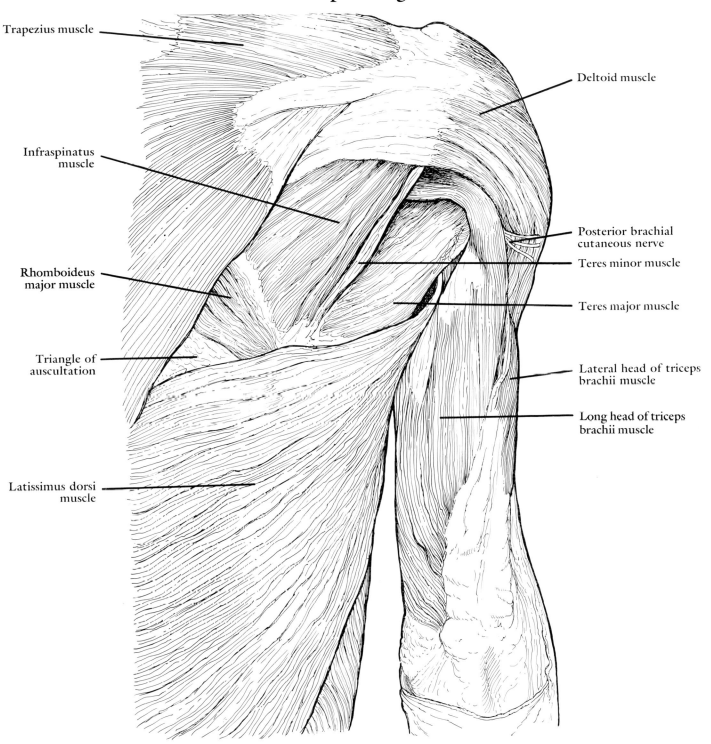

Trapezius muscle

Deltoid muscle

Infraspinatus muscle

Posterior brachial cutaneous nerve

Teres minor muscle

Rhomboideus major muscle

Teres major muscle

Triangle of auscultation

Lateral head of triceps brachii muscle

Long head of triceps brachii muscle

Latissimus dorsi muscle

Specific remarks: The most superficial muscles of these two regions are shown in this view, after the skin, subcutaneous tissue, and the regional fascia have been removed.

General remarks: The *triangular space,* which transmits *circumflex scapular blood vessels,* is bordered superiorly by the *teres minor muscle,* inferiorly by the *teres major muscle,* and laterally by the *long head of the triceps brachii muscle.* Another triangular space of this region, the *triangle of auscultation,* is also shown between the *latissimus dorsi muscle* inferiorly, the *rhomboideus major muscle* superolaterally, and the *trapezius muscle* superomedially.

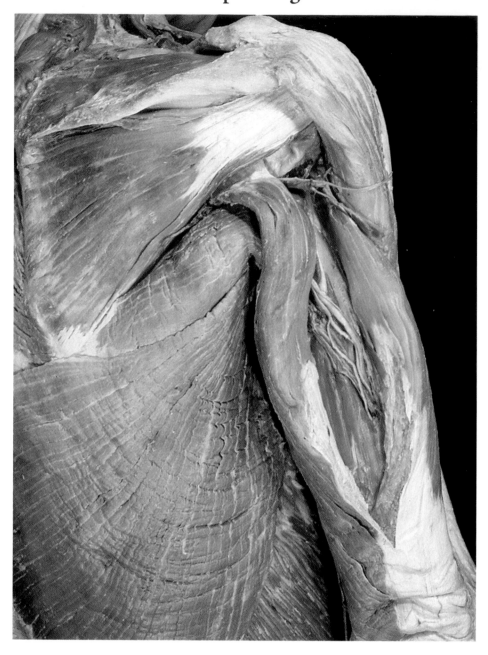

Supraspinatus muscle

Scapular spine

Axillary nerve

Teres minor muscle

Circumflex scapular vessels

Long head of triceps brachii muscle

Teres major muscle

Radial nerve and profunda brachii vessels

Lateral head of triceps brachii muscle

Medial head of triceps brachii muscle

External oblique muscle of abdomen

Specific remarks: With the *trapezius muscle* removed, the *supraspinatus* and *infraspinatus muscles* come into view. In this dissection the *long* and *lateral heads of the triceps brachii muscle* have been separated from one another and reflected medially and laterally respectively. Between these two heads a part of the *medial head* of the same muscle and the *radial nerve* and *profunda brachii vessels* are shown.

General remarks: Because the most posterior part of the *deltoid muscle* has been separated and removed, boundaries of the *quadrangular space* and a part of the *subdeltoid bursa* can be demonstrated. The boundaries of the quadrangular space are the *teres minor muscle* superiorly, the *teres major muscle* inferiorly, the *long head of the triceps brachii muscle* medially, and the *humeral shaft* laterally. The space transmits the *axillary nerve* and *posterior humeral circumflex vessels*.

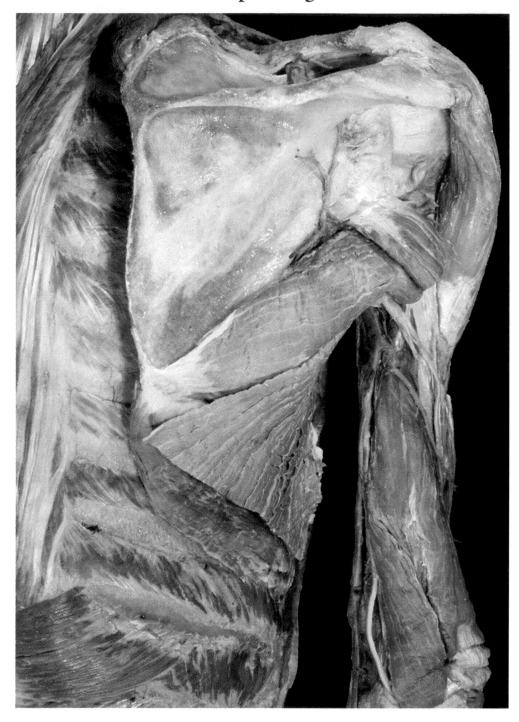

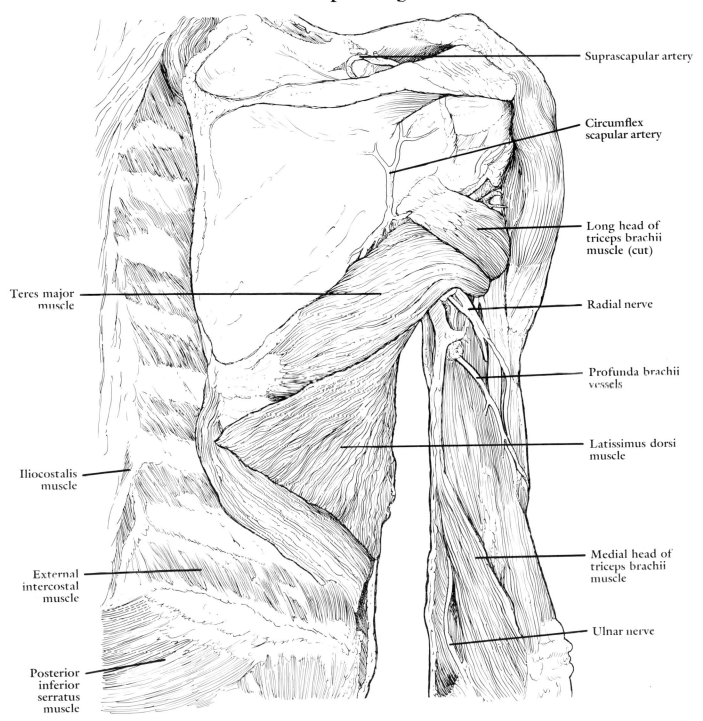

Suprascapular artery

Circumflex scapular artery

Long head of triceps brachii muscle (cut)

Radial nerve

Profunda brachii vessels

Teres major muscle

Latissimus dorsi muscle

Iliocostalis muscle

Medial head of triceps brachii muscle

External intercostal muscle

Ulnar nerve

Posterior inferior serratus muscle

Specific remarks: The posterior scapular aspect is demonstrated in this dissection after removal of the *supraspinatus, infraspinatus, rhomboid,* and *teres minor muscles*. The *long head,* except the segment still attached to the *infraglenoid tubercle,* and the *lateral head of triceps brachii muscle* have been completely removed to better demonstrate the *radial nerve, profunda brachii vessels, medial head,* and the *ulnar nerve* at the elbow.

General remarks: Three major arteries supply the scapular region: the *suprascapular* of the *thyrocervical trunk,* the *circumflex scapular* of the *subscapular,* and the *dorsal scapular* of the *transverse cervical*. They are interconnected by large anastomotic branches that circulate blood steadily throughout the region, even when some muscular groups are in action.

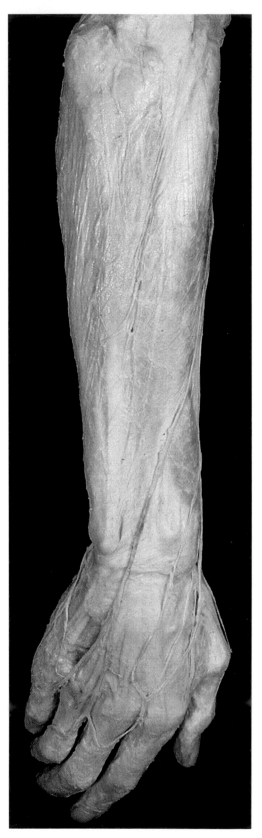

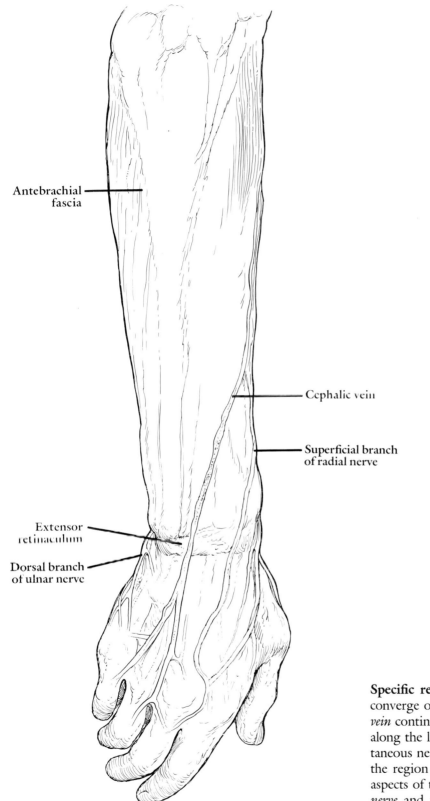

Antebrachial fascia

Cephalic vein

Superficial branch of radial nerve

Extensor retinaculum

Dorsal branch of ulnar nerve

Specific remarks: *Digital veins* are demonstrated as they converge onto the *dorsal venous arch*. From here the *basilic vein* continues along the medial aspect and the *cephalic vein* along the lateral aspect of the forearm. The two major cutaneous nerves of the dorsum of the hand and digits enter the region from the forearm along the medial and lateral aspects of the wrist. They are the *dorsal branch of the ulnar nerve* and the *superficial branch of the radial nerve* respectively.

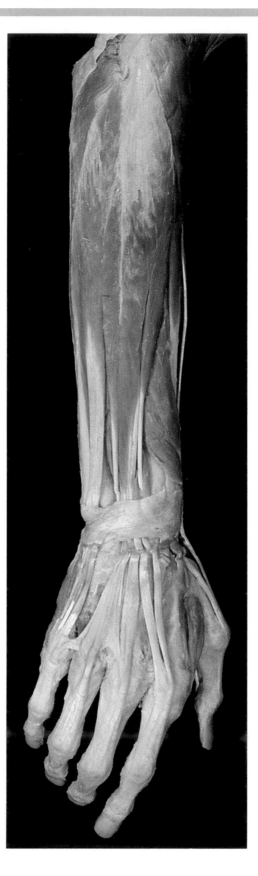

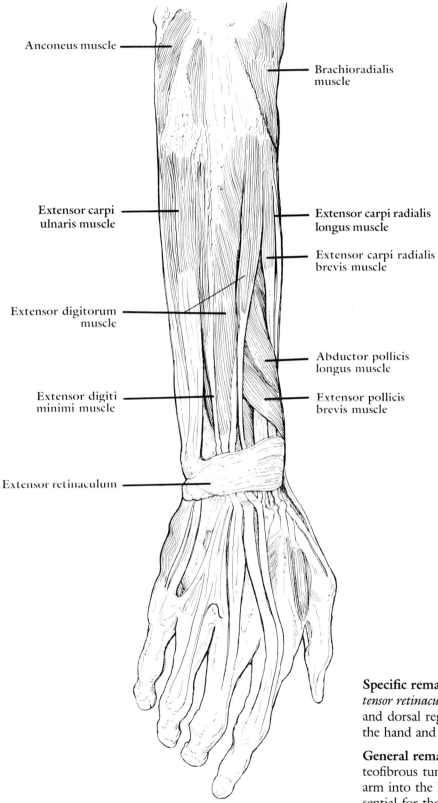

Anconeus muscle

Brachioradialis muscle

Extensor carpi ulnaris muscle

Extensor carpi radialis longus muscle

Extensor carpi radialis brevis muscle

Extensor digitorum muscle

Abductor pollicis longus muscle

Extensor digiti minimi muscle

Extensor pollicis brevis muscle

Extensor retinaculum

Specific remarks: The fascia, with the exception of the *extensor retinaculum,* has been removed from the antebrachial and dorsal region of the hand. Distribution of tendons in the hand and their digital expansions are demonstrated.

General remarks: The extensor retinaculum covers six osteofibrous tunnels, which transmit tendons from the forearm into the hand. The integrity of this retinaculum is essential for the proper functioning of the extensor muscles. Tendons, while in their respective tunnels, are protected by *synovial sheaths.*

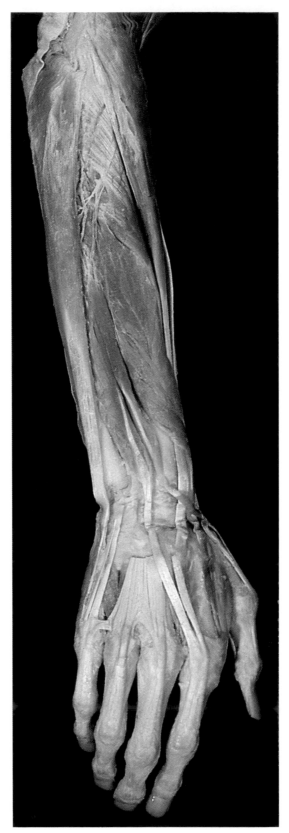

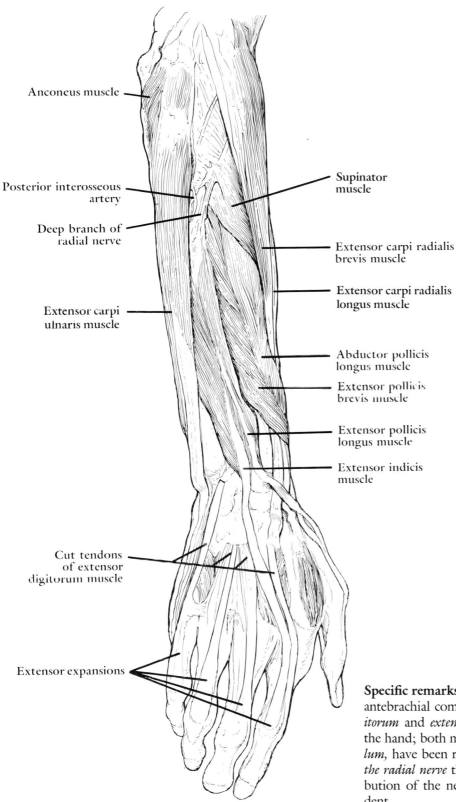

Anconeus muscle

Posterior interosseous artery

Deep branch of radial nerve

Extensor carpi ulnaris muscle

Cut tendons of extensor digitorum muscle

Extensor expansions

Supinator muscle

Extensor carpi radialis brevis muscle

Extensor carpi radialis longus muscle

Abductor pollicis longus muscle

Extensor pollicis brevis muscle

Extensor pollicis longus muscle

Extensor indicis muscle

Specific remarks: To show deeper muscles in the posterior antebrachial compartment, the tendons of the *extensor digitorum* and *extensor digiti minimi muscles* have been cut in the hand; both muscles, together with the *extensor retinaculum*, have been removed. The passage of the *deep branch of the radial nerve* through the *supinator muscle* and the distribution of the nerve to the extensor muscles are well evident.

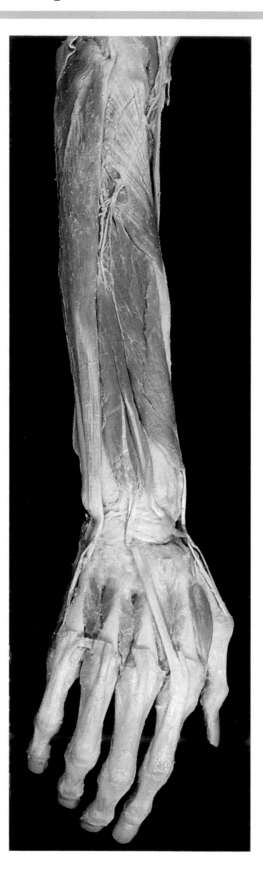

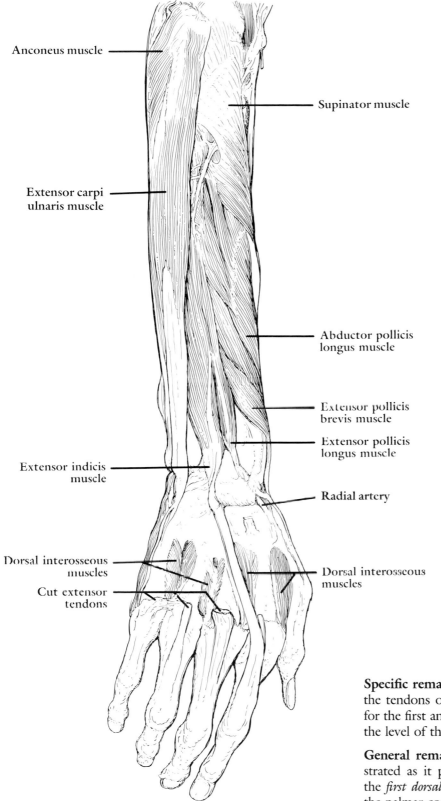

Anconeus muscle

Supinator muscle

Extensor carpi ulnaris muscle

Abductor pollicis longus muscle

Extensor pollicis brevis muscle

Extensor pollicis longus muscle

Extensor indicis muscle

Radial artery

Dorsal interosseous muscles

Dorsal interosseous muscles

Cut extensor tendons

Specific remarks: To expose the *dorsal interosseous muscles,* the tendons of the extensors, with the exception of those for the first and second digits, have been removed to about the level of the *metacarpophalangeal joints.*

General remarks: Now the *radial artery* can be demonstrated as it passes through the anatomical snuffbox and the *first dorsal interosseous muscle* to become continuous in the palmar compartment with the *deep palmar arch.*

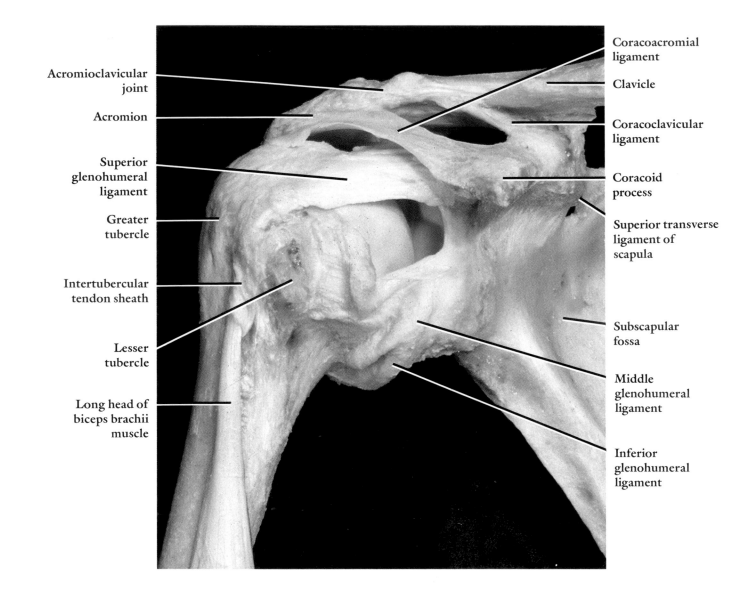

Coracoacromial ligament

Clavicle

Coracoclavicular ligament

Coracoid process

Superior transverse ligament of scapula

Subscapular fossa

Middle glenohumeral ligament

Inferior glenohumeral ligament

Acromioclavicular joint

Acromion

Superior glenohumeral ligament

Greater tubercle

Intertubercular tendon sheath

Lesser tubercle

Long head of biceps brachii muscle

General remarks: The large gap of the *articular capsule* between the *superior* and *middle glenohumeral ligaments* is the opening through which the *subscapular bursa* usually communicates with the articular space. The tendon of the *long head of the biceps brachii muscle* perforates the articular capsule to become attached to the *supraglenoid tubercle*.

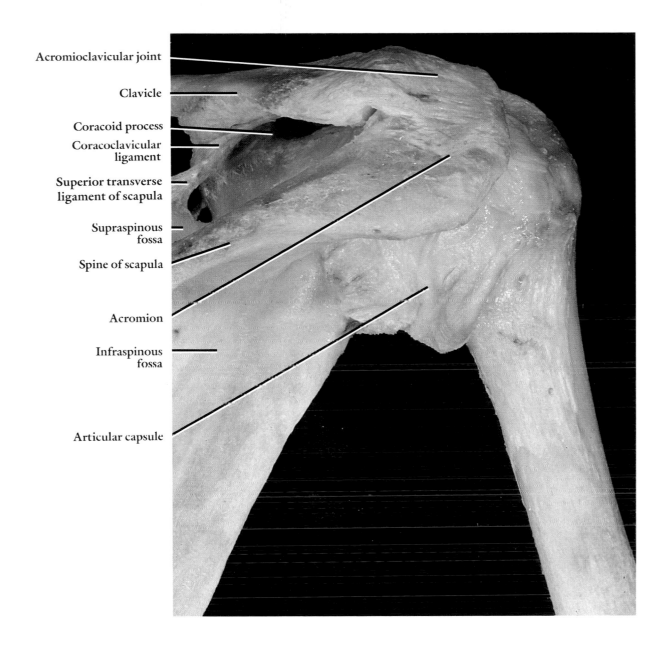

Acromioclavicular joint

Clavicle

Coracoid process

Coracoclavicular ligament

Superior transverse ligament of scapula

Supraspinous fossa

Spine of scapula

Acromion

Infraspinous fossa

Articular capsule

General remarks: The *articular capsule of the glenohumeral joint* has no distinct ligaments and is thinner on this side.

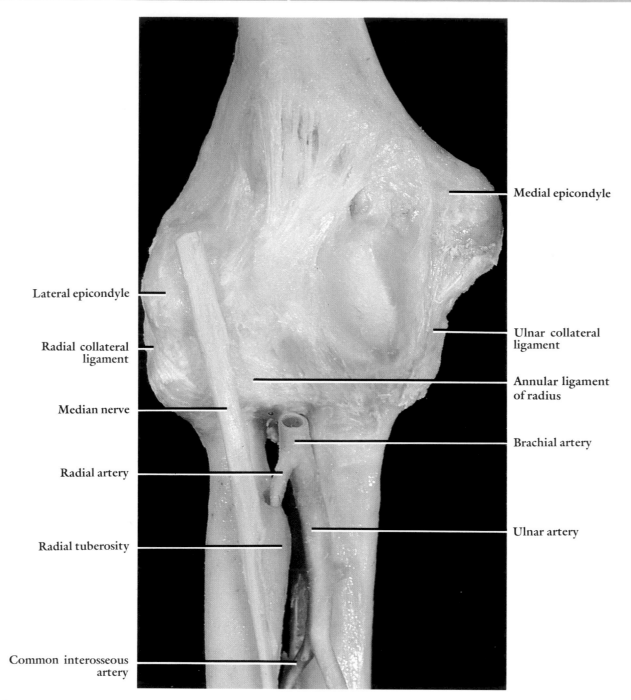

Medial epicondyle

Lateral epicondyle

Radial collateral
ligament

Ulnar collateral
ligament

Median nerve

Annular ligament
of radius

Radial artery

Brachial artery

Radial tuberosity

Ulnar artery

Common interosseous
artery

Specific remarks: In removing the musculature from all around the elbow region, two structures have been kept on the anterior aspect as points of reference: the *median nerve* and the *brachial artery*. The initial part of the *radial artery*, the *ulnar artery*, and the *common interosseous artery* are also shown.

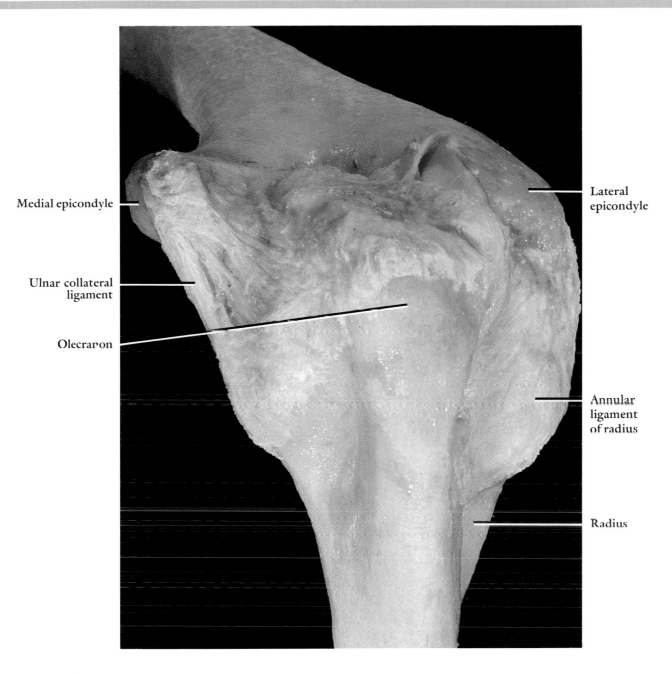

Medial epicondyle

Ulnar collateral ligament

Olecranon

Lateral epicondyle

Annular ligament of radius

Radius

Anterior aspect of the right wrist joint

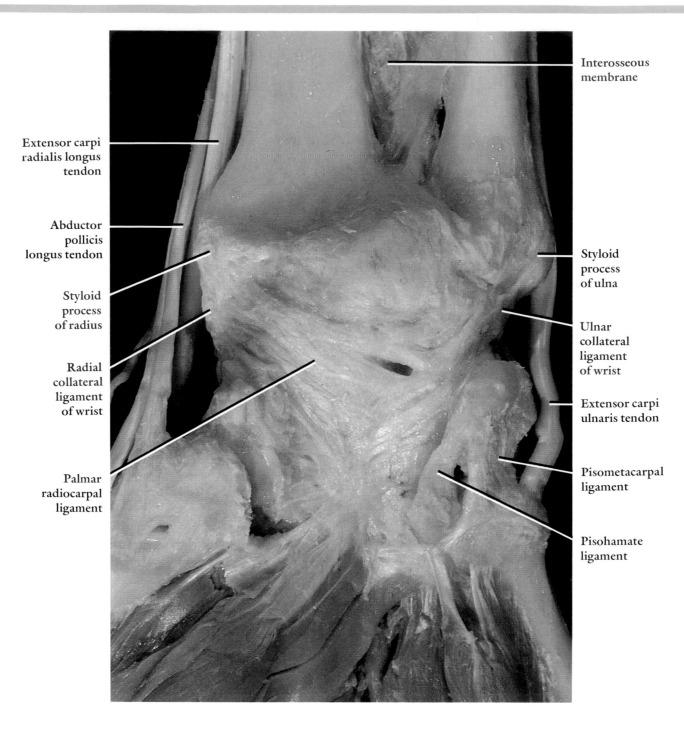

Extensor carpi radialis longus tendon

Abductor pollicis longus tendon

Styloid process of radius

Radial collateral ligament of wrist

Palmar radiocarpal ligament

Interosseous membrane

Styloid process of ulna

Ulnar collateral ligament of wrist

Extensor carpi ulnaris tendon

Pisometacarpal ligament

Pisohamate ligament

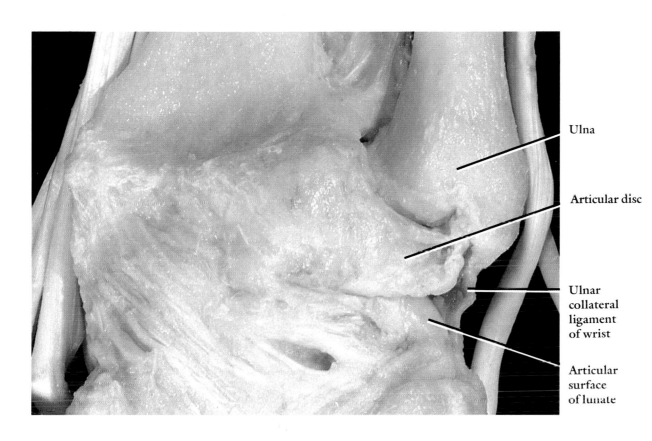

Ulna

Articular disc

Ulnar
collateral
ligament
of wrist

Articular
surface
of lunate

Specific remarks: The *articular capsule* has been opened anteriorly to show the *articular disc* between the *ulna* and *carpal bones*.

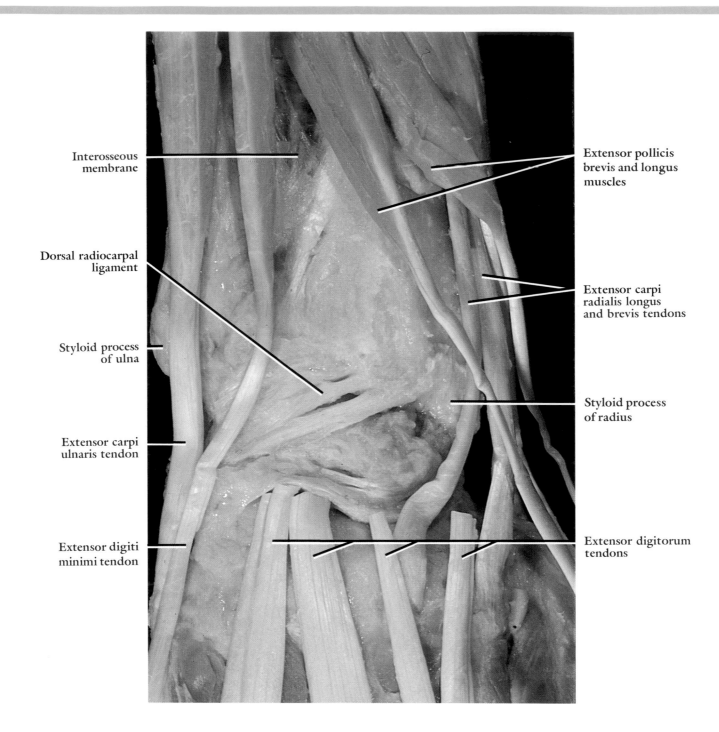

Interosseous
membrane

Dorsal radiocarpal
ligament

Styloid process
of ulna

Extensor carpi
ulnaris tendon

Extensor digiti
minimi tendon

Extensor pollicis
brevis and longus
muscles

Extensor carpi
radialis longus
and brevis tendons

Styloid process
of radius

Extensor digitorum
tendons

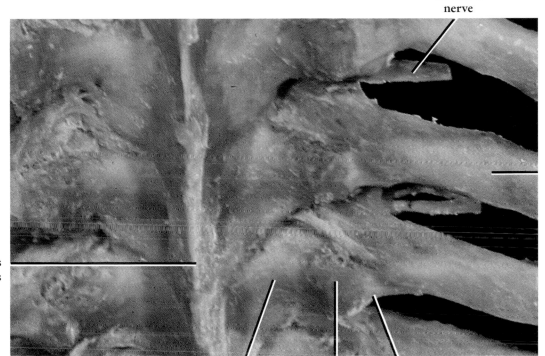

Intercostal
nerve

Rib

Spinous
process

Lamina

Transverse
process

Lateral
costotransverse
ligament

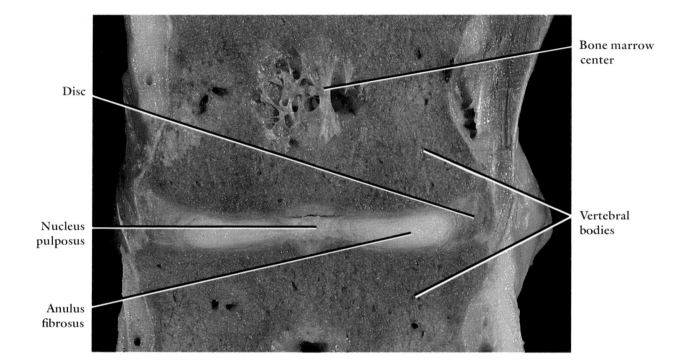

Bone marrow
center

Disc

Vertebral
bodies

Nucleus
pulposus

Anulus
fibrosus

General remarks: Vertebral bodies are viable centers for the production of blood cells. If deformities of the vertebral structure occur during adolescence, the *intervertebral discs,* which independently undergo degenerative changes, may be dislocated, usually in a posterolateral direction, to compress the neighboring nerves and consequently to cause local muscular spasm.

References

99

Ashley, G.T.: Morphological and pathological significance of synostoses at the manubrio-sternal joint, Thorax **9**:159, 1954.

Ashley, G.T.: The relationship between the pattern of ossification and the definitive shape of the mesosternum in man, J. Anat. **90**:87, 1956.

100

Davis, T.R.: Human lower lumbar vertebrae: some mechanical and osteological considerations, J. Anat. **95**:337, 1961.

108

Profeus, C.J.: The olecranon epiphyses, J. Anat. **94**:286P, 1960.

109

An, K.N., et al.: Normative model of human hand for biomechanical analysis, J. Biomech. **12**:775, 1979.

O'Rahilly, R.: Developmental deviations in the carpus and tarsus, Clin. Orthop. **10**:9, 1956.

Singh, I.: Variations in the metacarpal bones, J. Anat. **93**:262, 1959.

110

Garn, S.M., and Rohmann, C.G.: Variability in the order of ossification of the bony centers of the hand and wrist, Am. J. Phys. Anthropol. **18**:219, 1960.

Krogman, W.M.: The human skeleton in forensic medicine, Springfield, Ill., 1962, Charles C Thomas, Publisher.

112

Wolstenholme, G.E.W., and Knight, J., editors: Lactogenic hormones, Ciba Foundation Symposium, Edinburgh and London, 1972, Churchill-Livingstone.

114

Turner-Warwick, R.T.: The lymphatics of the breast, Br. J. Surg. **46**:574, 1959.

115

Ashley, G.T.: The manner of insertion of the pectoralis major muscle in man, Anat. Rec. **113**:301, 1952.

Greig, H.W., Anson, B.G., and Budinger, J.M.: Variations in the form and attachments of the biceps brachii muscle, J. Bull. Northwestern U. Med. School **26**:241, 1952.

116

Catton, W.T., and Gray, J.E.: Electromyographic study of the action of the serratus anterior muscle in respiration, J. Anat. **85**:412P, 1951.

Guijarro de Pablos, J.E., et al.: Variacion anatomica bilateral del nervio musculocutaneo suinteres en la practica quirurgica, Ann. Anat. **31**:225, 1982.

Harris, W.: The morphology of the brachial plexus, London, 1939, Oxford University Press.

117

De Troyer, A., Kelly, S., and Zin, W.A.: Mechanical action of the intercostal muscles on the ribs, Science **220**:87, 1983.

Hoshiko, M.: Electromyographic investigation of the intercostal muscles during speech, Arch. Phys. Med. **43**:115, 1962.

Taylor, A.: The contribution of the intercostal muscles to the effort of respiration in man, J. Physiol. **151**:390, 1960.

118

Bronk, D.W., and Ferguson, L.K.: The nervous control of intercostal respiration, Am. J. Physiol. **110**:700, 1935.

120

Miller, M.R., Rolston, H.J., and Kasahara, M.: The pattern of cutaneous innervation of the human hand, Am. J. Anat. **102**:183, 1958.

Sayfi, Y.: Note sur l'innervation des dos de la main, Arch. Anat. Pathol. **15**:139, 1967.

122

Bromes, M.F., and Wilgis, E.F.S.: Anatomical variations of the palmaris longus causing carpal tunnel syndrome, Plast. Reconstr. Surg. Nov. 1978, p. 798.

Reimann, A.F., et al.: The palmaris longus muscle and tendon: a study of 1600 extremities, Anat. Rec. **89**:495, 1944.

123

Jamieson, R.W., and Anson, B.J.: The relation of the median nerve to the heads of origin of the pronator teres muscle: a study of 300 specimens, Quart. Bull. Northwest. Univ. Med. Sch. **26**:34, 1952.

124

Person, R.S., and Roshchina, N.A.: Electromiograficheskoe issledovanie koordinatsii deiatelnosti myshtsantagonistov pri dvzhenii paltsev ruki cheloveka, Fiziol. Zh. SSSR **44**:455, 1958.

125

Basmajian, J.V., and Travill, A.A.: Electromyography of the pronator muscles in the forearm, Anat. Rec. **139**:45, 1961.

126

Coleman, S.S., and Anson, B.J.: Arterial patterns in the hand based upon a study of 650 specimens, Surg. Gynecol. Obstet. **113**:409, 1961.

Harness, D., and Sekeles, E.: The double anastomotic innervation of thenar muscles, J. Anat. **109**:461, 1971.

Papathanassion, B.T.: A variant of the motor branch of the median nerve in the hand, J. Bone Joint Surg. **50B**:156, 1968.

127

Day, M.H., and Napier, J.R.: The two heads of flexor pollicis brevis, J. Anat. **95**:123, 1961.

Mehta, H.J., and Gardner, W.U.: A study of lumbrical muscles in the human hand, Am. J. Anat. **109**:227, 1961.

128

Braithwaite, F., et al.: The applied anatomy of the lumbricals and interosseous muscles of the hand, Guy's Hosp. Rep. **97**:185, 1948.

Harness, D., and Sekeles, E.: The double anastomotic innervation of thenar muscles, J. Anat. **109**:461, 1971.

129

Bearn, J.G.: An electromyographic study of the trapezius, deltoid, pectoralis major, biceps, and triceps muscles during static loading of the upper limb, Anat. Rec. **140**:103, 1961.

131

Huelke, D.F.: The dorsal scapular artery—a proposed term for the artery to the rhomboid muscles, Anat. Rec. **142**:57, 1962.

133

Coleman, S.S., McAffee, D.K., and Anson, B.J.: The insertion of the abductor pollicis longus muscle: an anatomical study of 175 specimens, Quart. Bull. Northwestern U. Med. School **27:**117, 1953.

134

McFarland, G.B., Jr., Krusen, U.L., and Weathersby, H.T.: Kinesiology of selected muscles acting on the wrist: electromyographic study, Arch. Phys. Med. **43:**165, 1962.

135

Apfelberg, D.B., and Larson, S.J.: Dynamic anatomy of the ulnar nerve at the elbow, Plast. Reconstr. Surg. **51:**76, 1973.

136

Inman, V.T., et al.: Observations on the function of the shoulder joint, J. Bone Joint Surg. **26:**1, 1944.

137

Engín, A.E.: On the biomechanics of the shoulder complex, J. Biomech. **13:**575, 1980.

Saha, K.: Theory of shoulder mechanism, Springfield, Ill., 1961, Charles C Thomas, Publisher.

139

Martin, B.F.: The annular ligament of the superior radioulnar joint, J. Anat. **92:**473, 1958.

Tillmann, B.: Entwicklung und functionelle Anatomie des Ellenbogengelenkes, Z. Orthoped. **116:**392, 1978.

141

Lewis, O.J., Hamshere, R.J., and Bucknill, T.M.: The anatomy of the wrist joint, J. Anat. **106:**539, 1970.

Toft, R., and Berme, N.: A biomechanical analysis of the joints of the thumb, J. Biomech. **13:**353, 1980.

144

Hendry, N.G.C.: The hydration of the nucleus pulposus and its relation to intervertebral disc derangement, J. Bone Joint Surg. **40B:**132, 1958.

Peacock, A.: Observation on the postnatal structure of the intervertebral disc in man, J. Anat. **86:**162, 1952.

Tandury, G.: Entwicklungsgeschichte und Fehlbildungen der Wirbelsaule, Stuttgart, 1958.

Part Three
THORAX

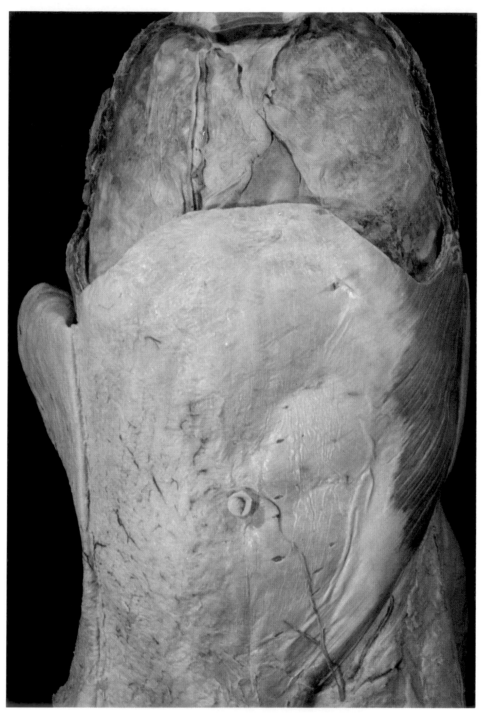

146

External inguinal ring and its contents in a female

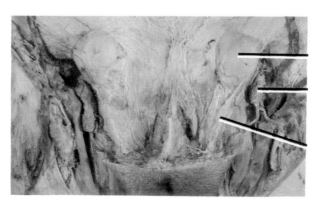

Superficial inguinal ring

Superficial inguinal lymph nodes

Round ligament

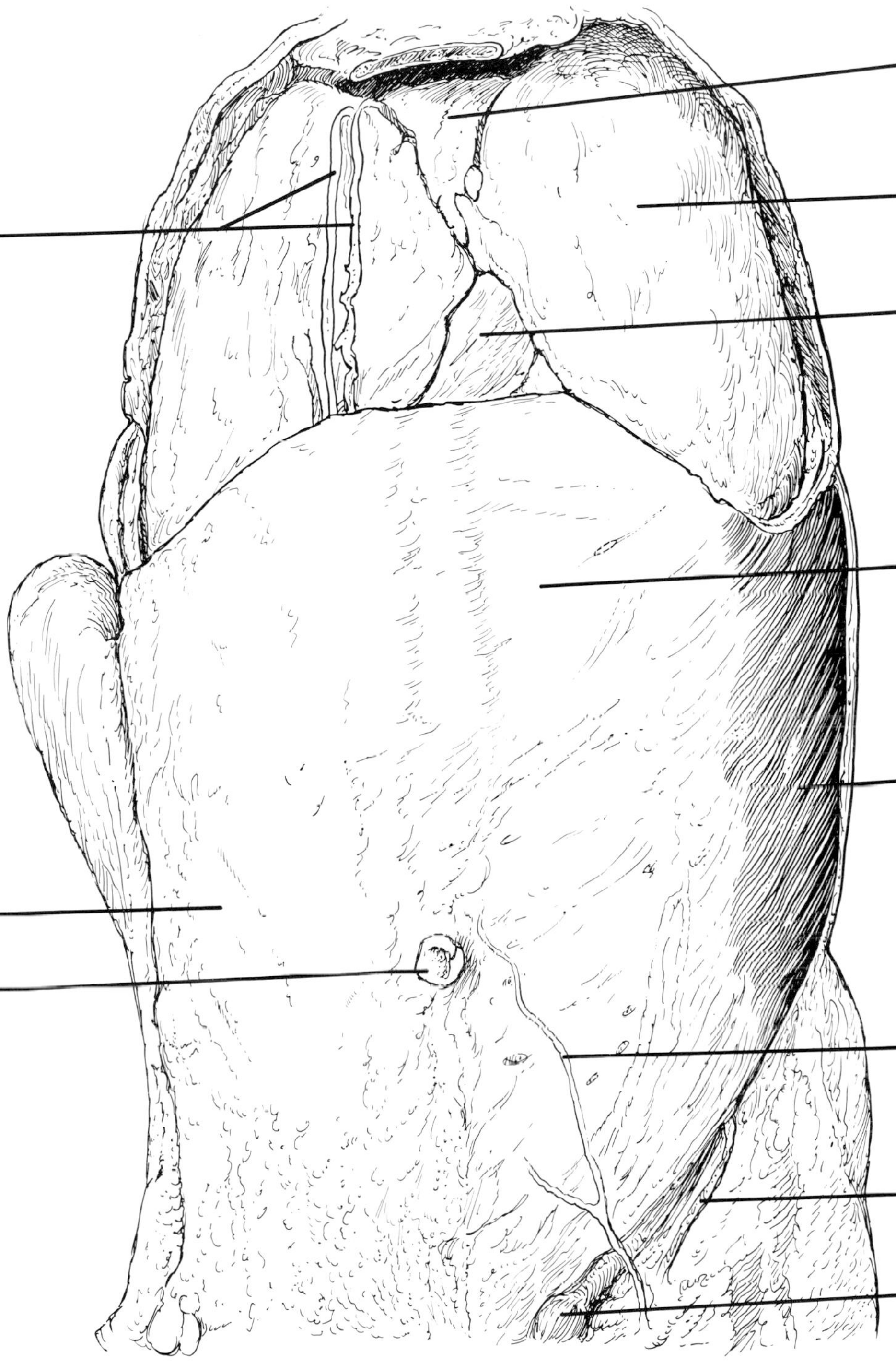

Remnants of thymus

Pleura

Internal thoracic
vessels

Pericardium

Rectus sheath

External oblique
muscle of
abdomen

Superficial
fascia

Umbilicus

Superficial
epigastric
vessels

Superficial iliac
circumflex vessels

Spermatic cord

Specific remarks: The ribs and intercostal contents have been cut vertically at the midaxillary lines and then horizontally at the *xiphoid process* level; the anterior thoracic wall has been removed. In addition to the skin having been reflected from the entire anterolateral abdominal wall, the subcutaneous tissue and the *abdominal fascia* have been removed from the left half of the region to demonstrate the *external oblique muscle of the abdomen*.

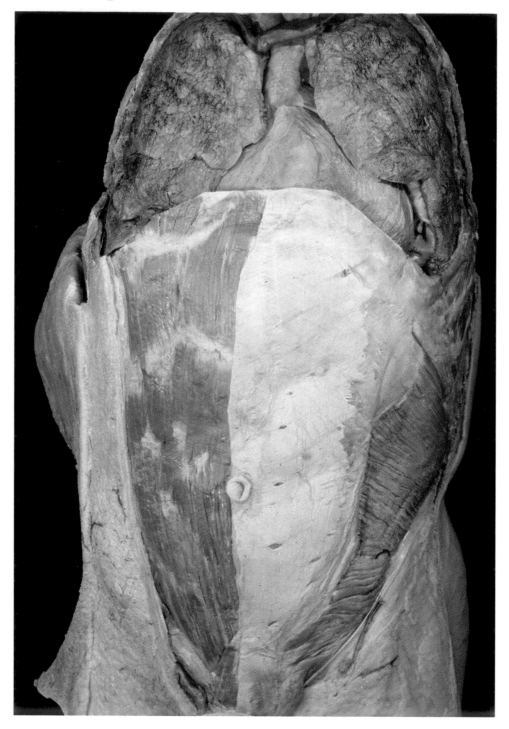

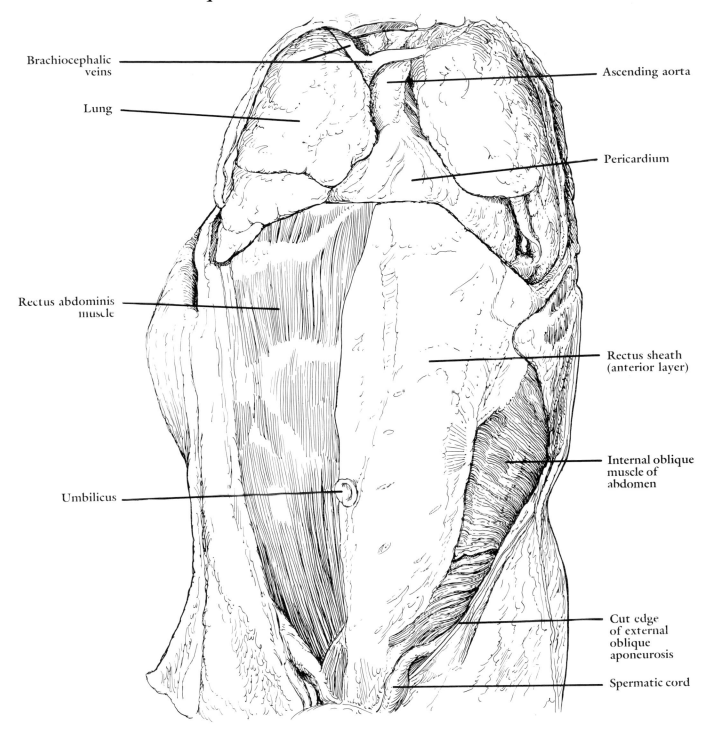

Brachiocephalic veins

Lung

Rectus abdominis muscle

Umbilicus

Ascending aorta

Pericardium

Rectus sheath (anterior layer)

Internal oblique muscle of abdomen

Cut edge of external oblique aponeurosis

Spermatic cord

Specific remarks: The pleural sheaths *(parietal pleura)* have been removed from both lungs and the connective tissue from the *pericardial sac*. On the right side of the abdominal wall the *rectus sheath* has been incised longitudi-nally and reflected laterally to expose the *rectus muscle*. On the left side the *external oblique muscle* has been dissected away; the rectus sheath has been preserved. The *internal oblique muscle of the abdomen* is exposed.

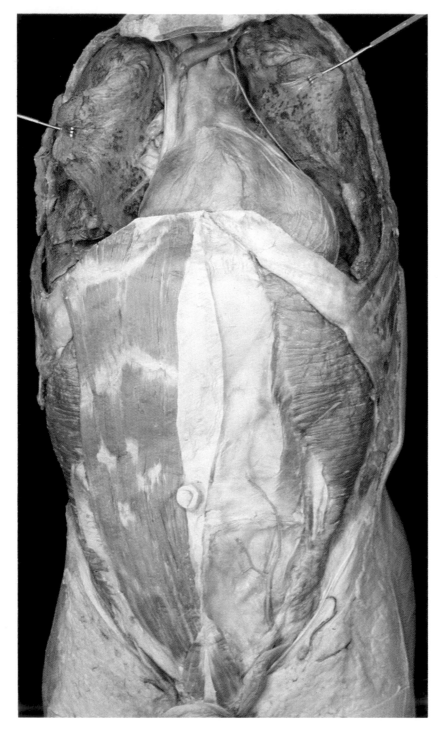

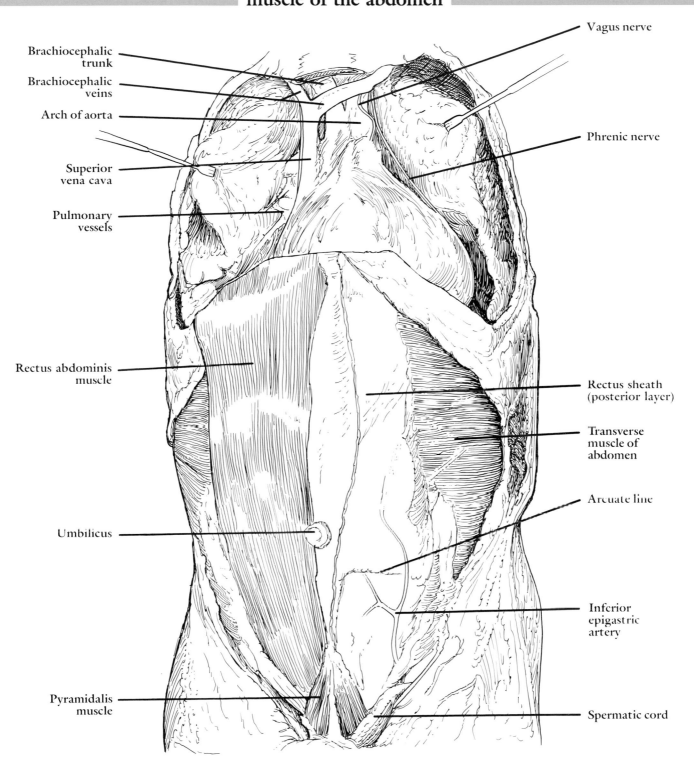

Vagus nerve

Brachiocephalic trunk

Brachiocephalic veins

Arch of aorta

Phrenic nerve

Superior vena cava

Pulmonary vessels

Rectus abdominis muscle

Rectus sheath (posterior layer)

Transverse muscle of abdomen

Arcuate line

Umbilicus

Inferior epigastric artery

Pyramidalis muscle

Spermatic cord

Specific remarks: To demonstrate the large blood vessels in the *mediastinum* and the *left vagus* and *phrenic nerves*, both lungs have been retracted laterally. The right *transverse muscle* of the abdomen is shown in relation to the *rectus abdominis muscle*. On the left, after the rectus muscle has been removed, the transverse muscle is demonstrated in relation to the posterior layer of the *rectus sheath, arcuate line,* and *transversalis fascia.*

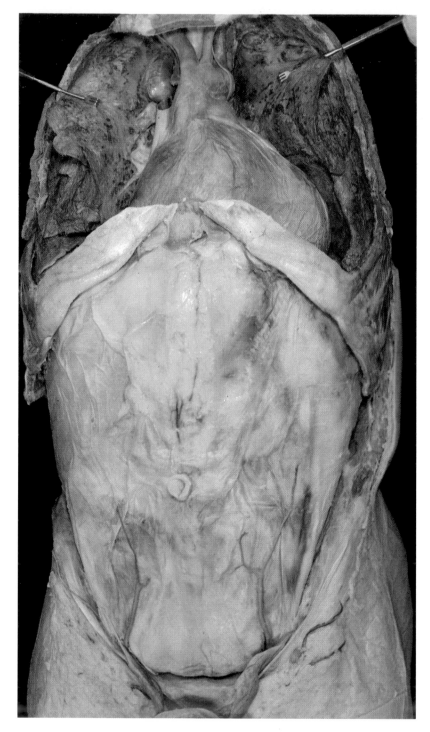

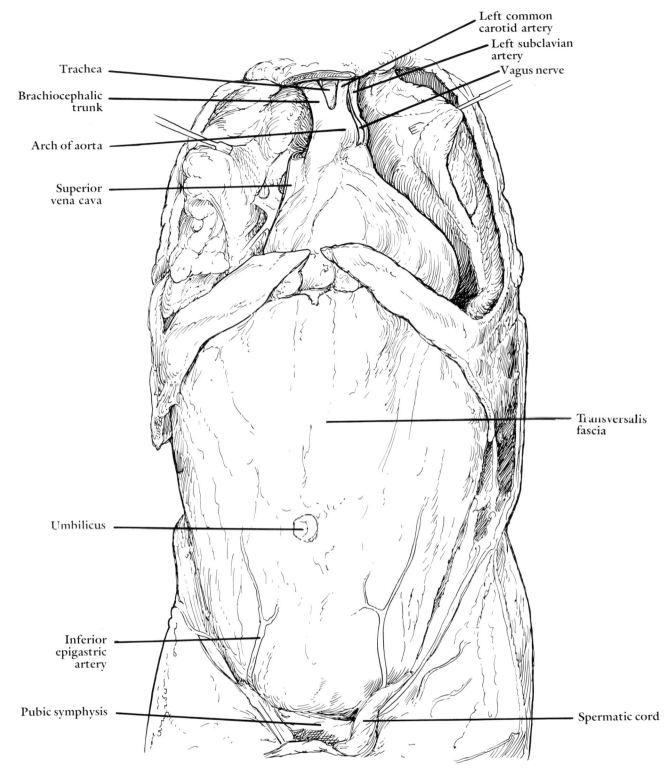

Left common
carotid artery

Left subclavian
artery

Vagus nerve

Trachea

Brachiocephalic
trunk

Arch of aorta

Superior
vena cava

Transversalis
fascia

Umbilicus

Inferior
epigastric
artery

Pubic symphysis

Spermatic cord

Specific remarks: Both *phrenic nerves,* the *brachiocephalic veins,* and a segment of the *superior vena cava* have been removed from the *mediastinum* to demonstrate the *arch of the aorta* and the three branches. From right to left they are the *brachiocephalic trunk,* the *left common carotid,* and the *left subclavian*. All muscles, together with their aponeuroses, have been removed from the anterolateral aspect of the abdomen to expose the *transversalis fascia*.

General remarks: The transversalis fascia adheres to the underlying portion of the *parietal peritoneum*.

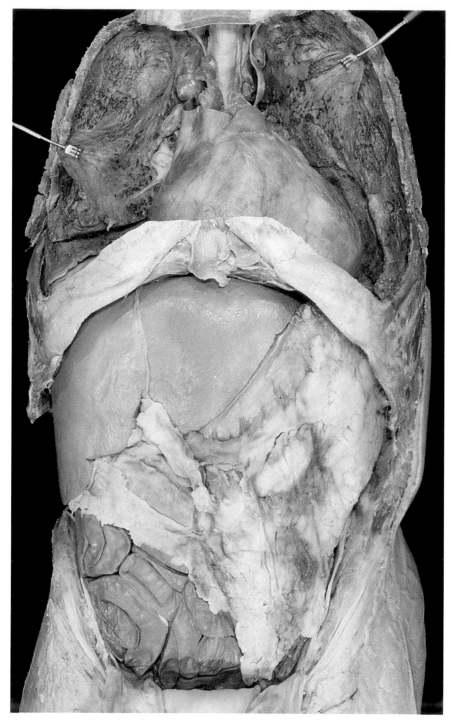

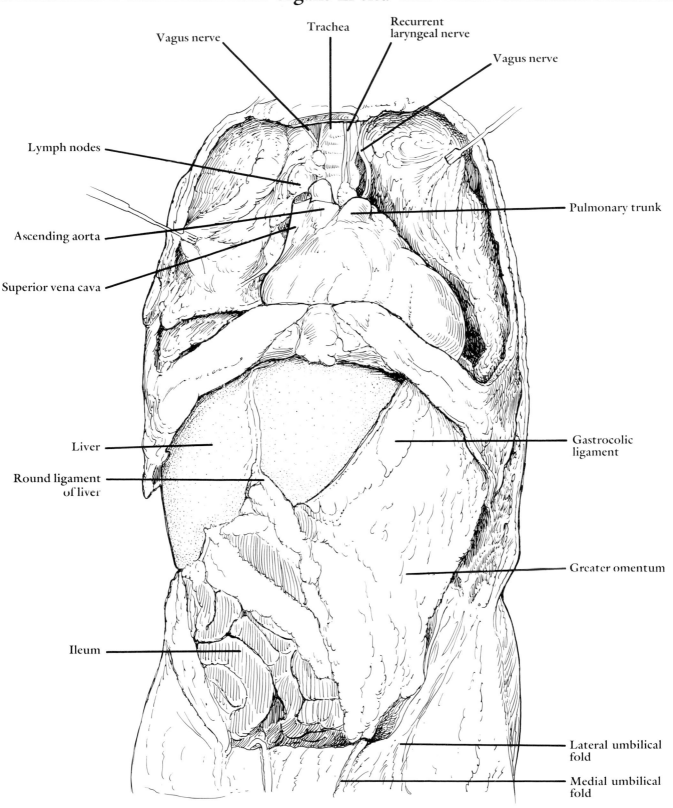

Vagus nerve

Trachea

Recurrent
laryngeal nerve

Vagus nerve

Lymph nodes

Pulmonary trunk

Ascending aorta

Superior vena cava

Liver

Gastrocolic
ligament

Round ligament
of liver

Greater omentum

Ileum

Lateral umbilical
fold

Medial umbilical
fold

Specific remarks: In this view the *aortic arch* and the *pulmonary trunk* have been cut close to their origins and removed to show the *trachea* with associated *lymph nodes, vagi*, and the *left recurrent (inferior) laryngeal nerve*. The abdominal organs are exposed after the *transversalis fascia* and the *parietal peritoneum* have been reflected from the anterolateral wall inferiorly.

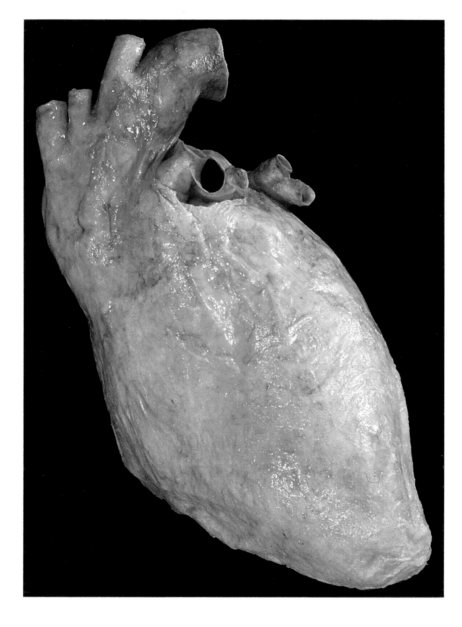

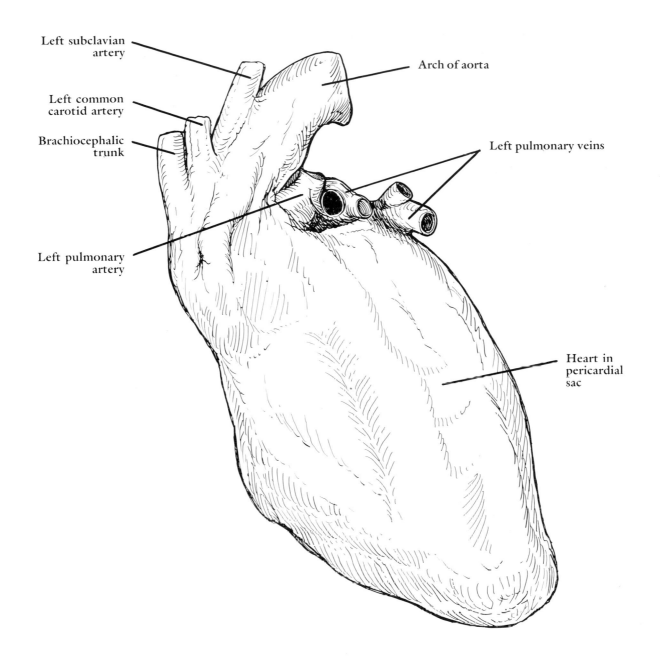

Left subclavian artery

Left common carotid artery

Brachiocephalic trunk

Left pulmonary artery

Arch of aorta

Left pulmonary veins

Heart in pericardial sac

Specific remarks: For this and for subsequent views of the heart the *aortic arch* has been cut just distal to the origin of the *left subclavian artery*, the *pulmonary trunk* close to its origin, and the *superior* and *inferior venae cavae* and *pulmonary veins* close to their entries into the *pericardium*. Subsequently the organ was removed from the *mediastinum*.

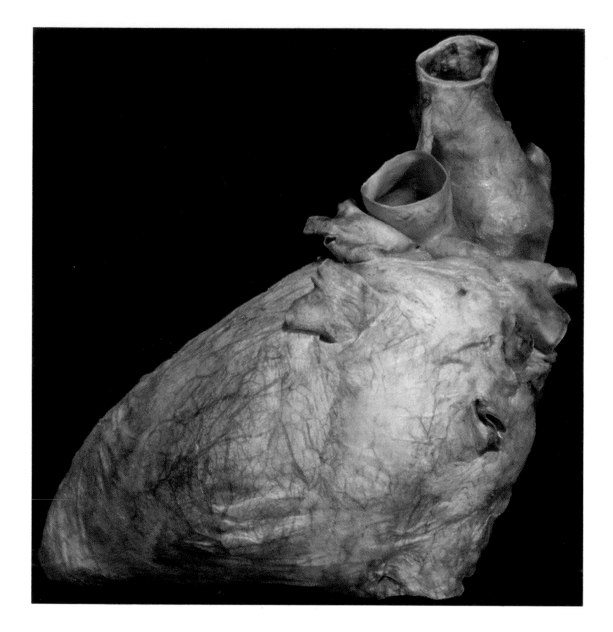

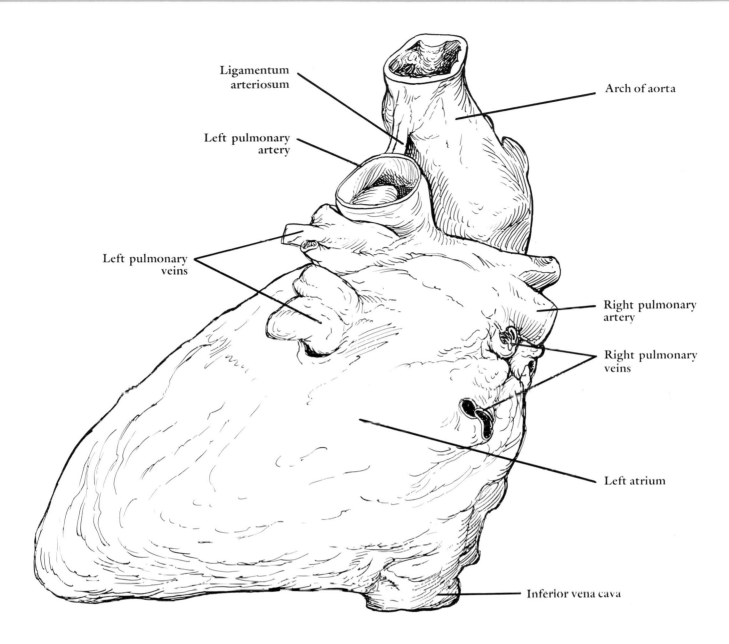

Ligamentum arteriosum

Left pulmonary artery

Arch of aorta

Left pulmonary veins

Right pulmonary artery

Right pulmonary veins

Left atrium

Inferior vena cava

General remarks: In this view both *pericardial sinuses,* the *transverse* and *oblique,* can be appreciated. The former sinus extends between the arterial compartment anteriorly and superiorly and the venous compartment inferiorly and posteriorly. The oblique sinus is confined among the *pulmonary veins* and blindly ends superiorly where the *parietal pericardium* reflects onto the cardiac surface.

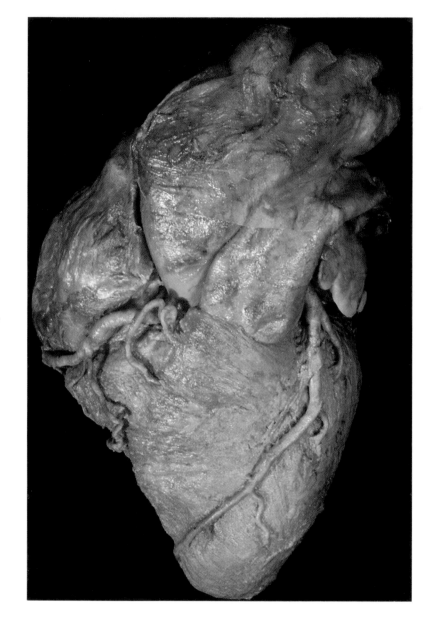

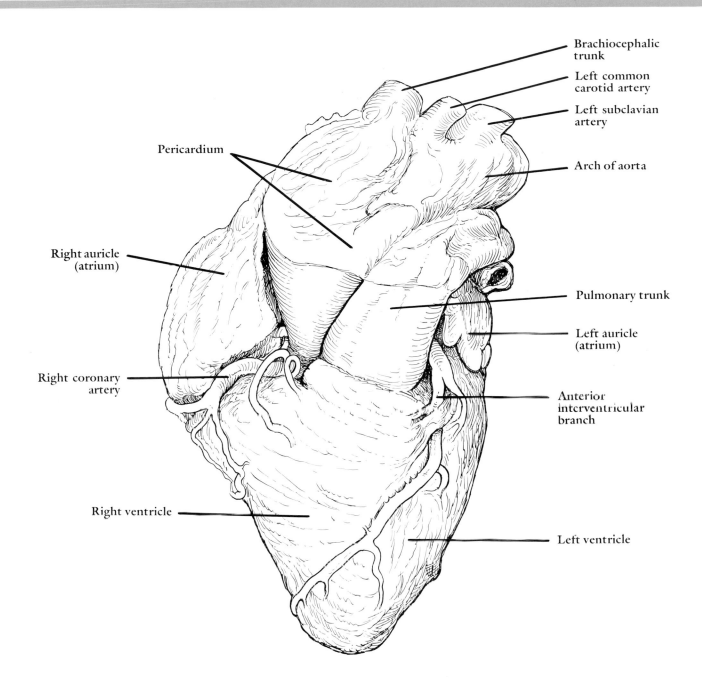

Brachiocephalic trunk

Left common carotid artery

Left subclavian artery

Arch of aorta

Pericardium

Right auricle (atrium)

Pulmonary trunk

Left auricle (atrium)

Right coronary artery

Anterior interventricular branch

Right ventricle

Left ventricle

Specific remarks: Following the removal of the *pericardium* and *epicardium* the muscular layer of the heart and the *coronary blood vessels* are shown.

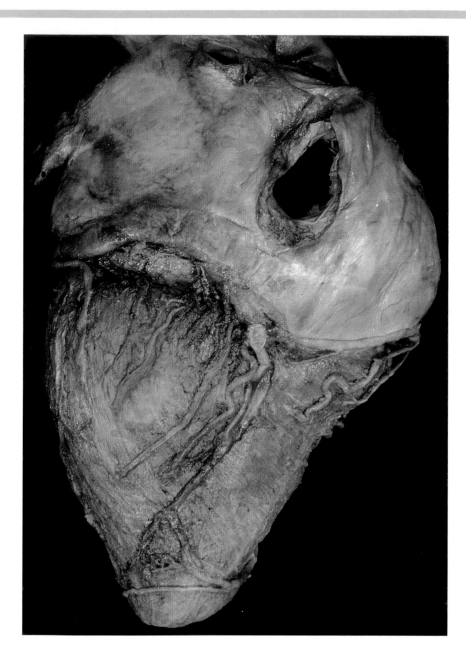

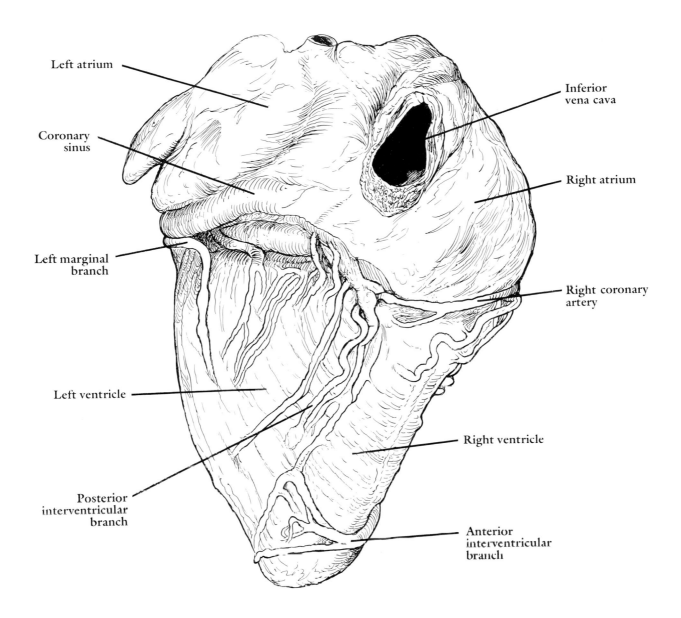

Left atrium

Coronary sinus

Left marginal branch

Left ventricle

Posterior interventricular branch

Inferior vena cava

Right atrium

Right coronary artery

Right ventricle

Anterior interventricular branch

General remarks: Most of the venous drainage from the heart is conveyed to the *right atrium* by way of the *coronary sinus*.

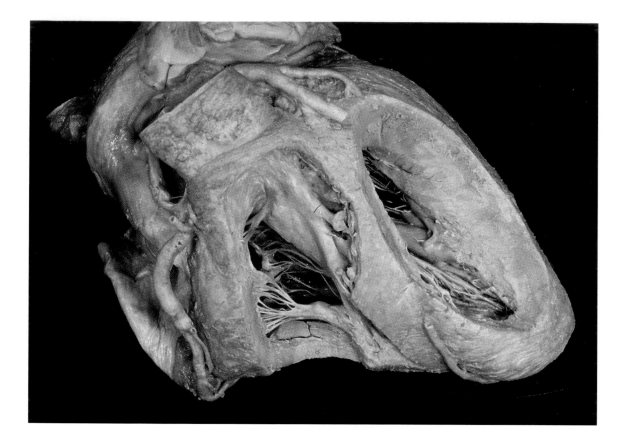

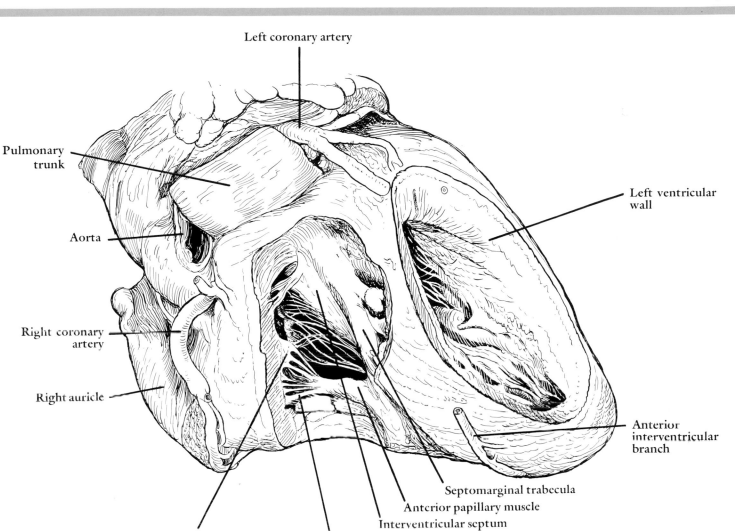

Left coronary artery

Pulmonary trunk

Aorta

Right coronary artery

Right auricle

Left ventricular wall

Anterior interventricular branch

Septomarginal trabecula

Anterior papillary muscle

Interventricular septum

Anterior cusp

Chordae tendineae

Specific remarks: A part of the anterior and left sides of the heart has been removed to show the internal structure of the *ventricles*. The *septomarginal trabecula* is demonstrated in the *right ventricle* from the *interventricular septum* to the base of the *anterior papillary muscle*. This trabecula transmits the right limb of the *atrioventricular bundle* to the right ventricular musculature.

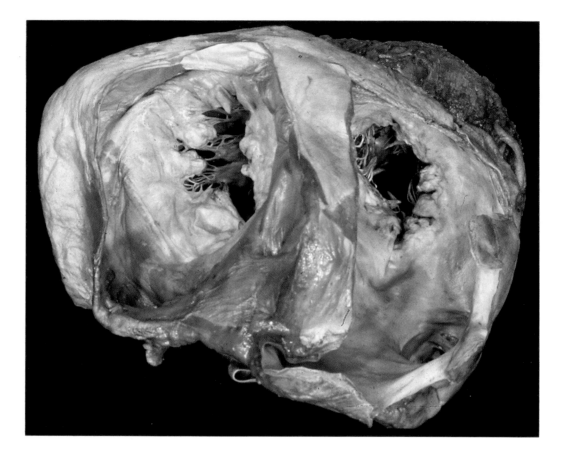

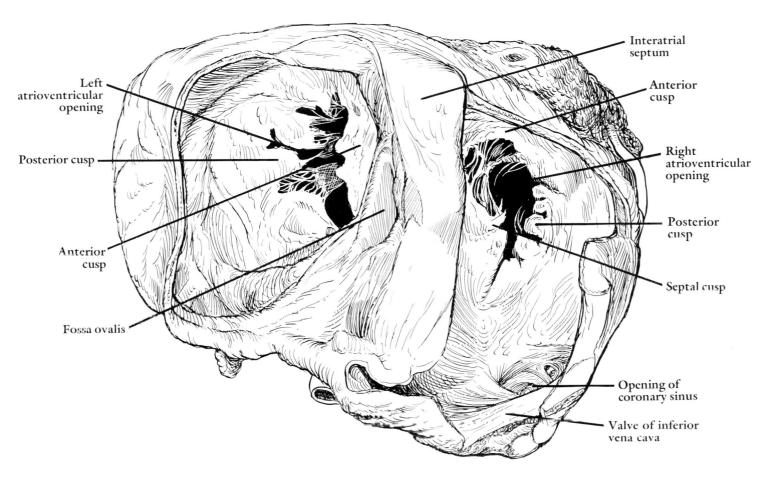

Left atrioventricular opening

Posterior cusp

Anterior cusp

Fossa ovalis

Interatrial septum

Anterior cusp

Right atrioventricular opening

Posterior cusp

Septal cusp

Opening of coronary sinus

Valve of inferior vena cava

Specific remarks: The internal atrial structure and the *interatrial septum* are demonstrated here, after the posterior wall of these chambers has been circularly cut and separated from the rest of heart.

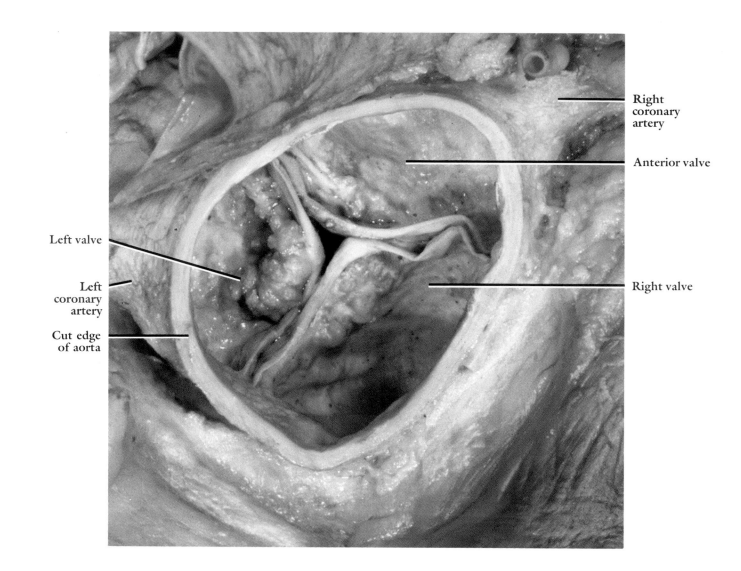

Right coronary artery

Anterior valve

Left valve

Left coronary artery

Cut edge of aorta

Right valve

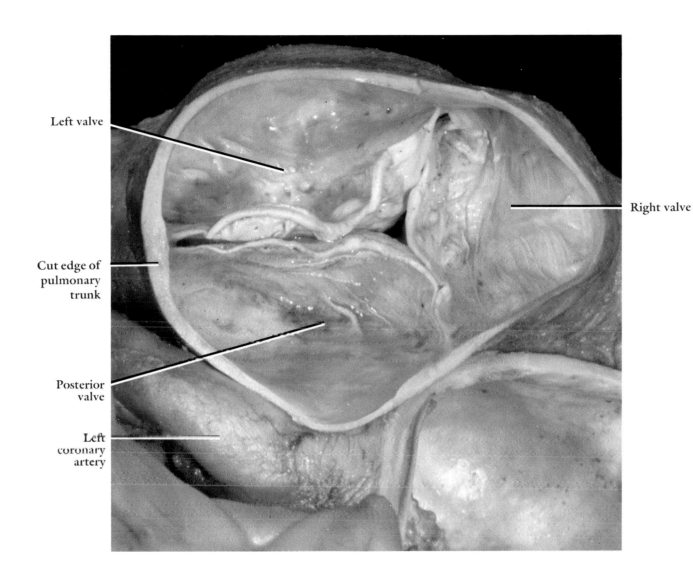

Left valve

Right valve

Cut edge of
pulmonary
trunk

Posterior
valve

Left
coronary
artery

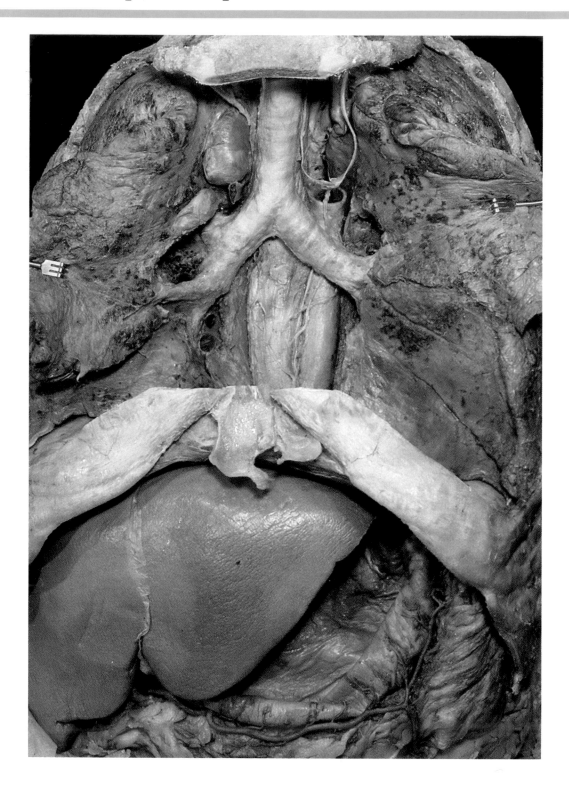

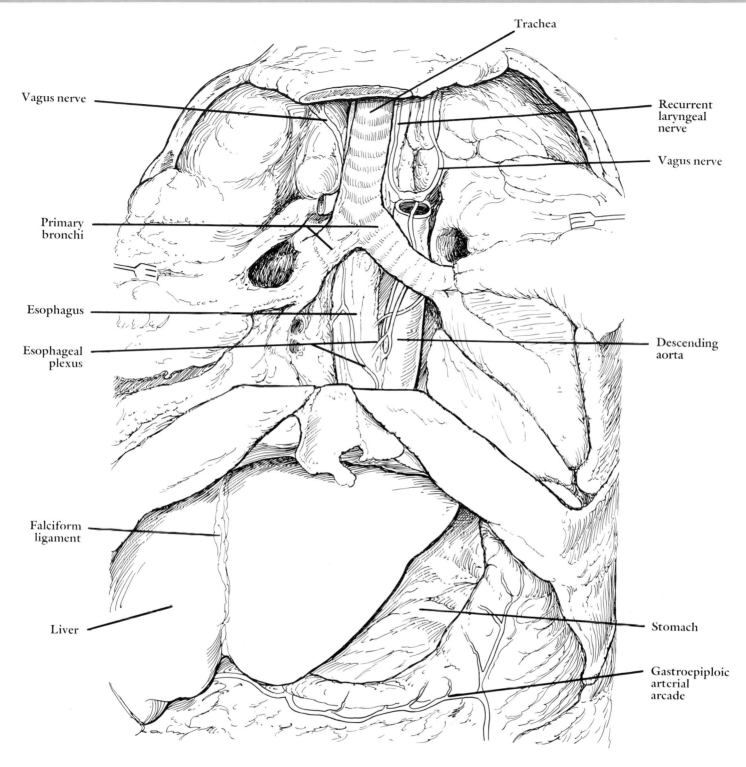

Trachea

Vagus nerve

Recurrent
laryngeal
nerve

Vagus nerve

Primary
bronchi

Esophagus

Descending
aorta

Esophageal
plexus

Falciform
ligament

Liver

Stomach

Gastroepiploic
arterial
arcade

Specific remarks: Immediately posterior to large medias-tinal blood vessels and the *pericardium,* which have been removed from this view, are the *trachea* and *bronchi, esoph-agus,* and the *descending aorta.* The *vagus nerves* are shown as they descend posterior to the primary *bronchi* toward the esophageal wall. The *left recurrent (inferior) laryngeal nerve* branches off the vagus, loops inferior to the *arch of the aorta,* and then ascends in the groove between the trachea and esophagus.

General remarks: Both vagus nerves, while passing through the mediastinal compartment, contribute their components to the thoracic organs, i.e., trachea, bronchi, lungs, esophagus, heart.

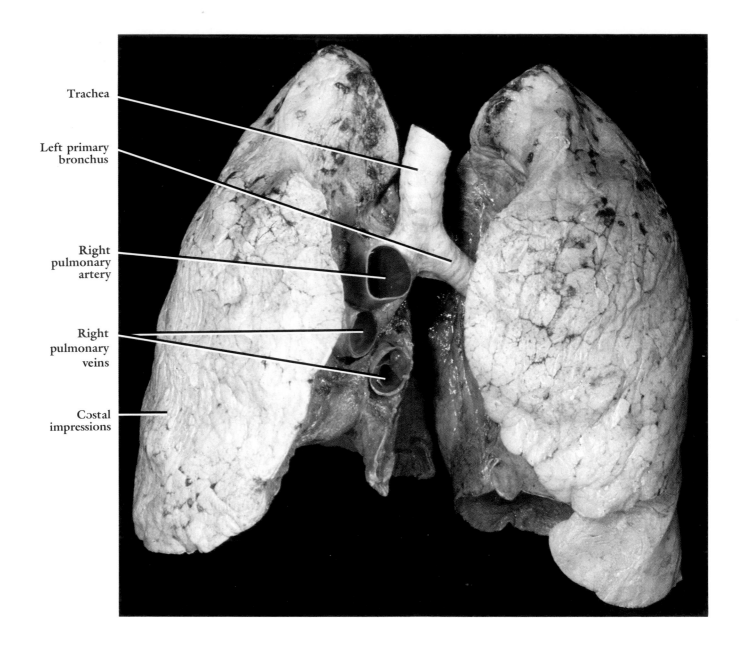

Trachea

Left primary
bronchus

Right
pulmonary
artery

Right
pulmonary
veins

Costal
impressions

Specific remarks: For this and for the next view all pulmonary blood vessels have been separated from the heart, and the *trachea* has been transected and, together with *lungs,* removed from the *thoracic cavity.*

Trachea

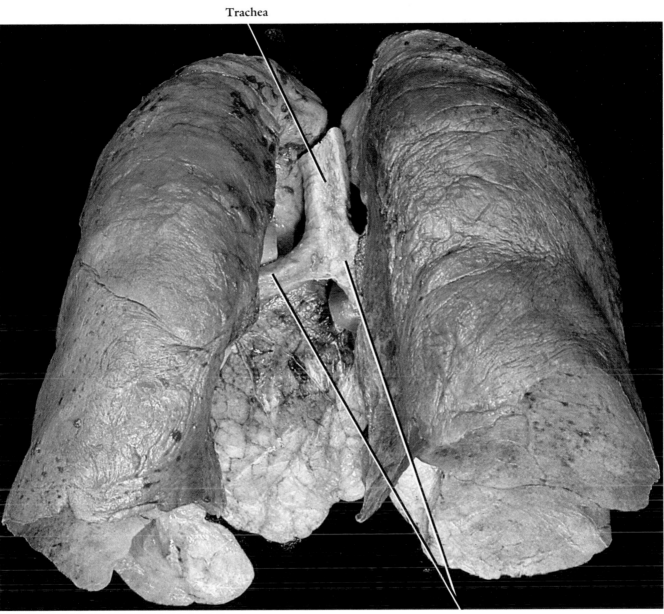

Primary
bronchi

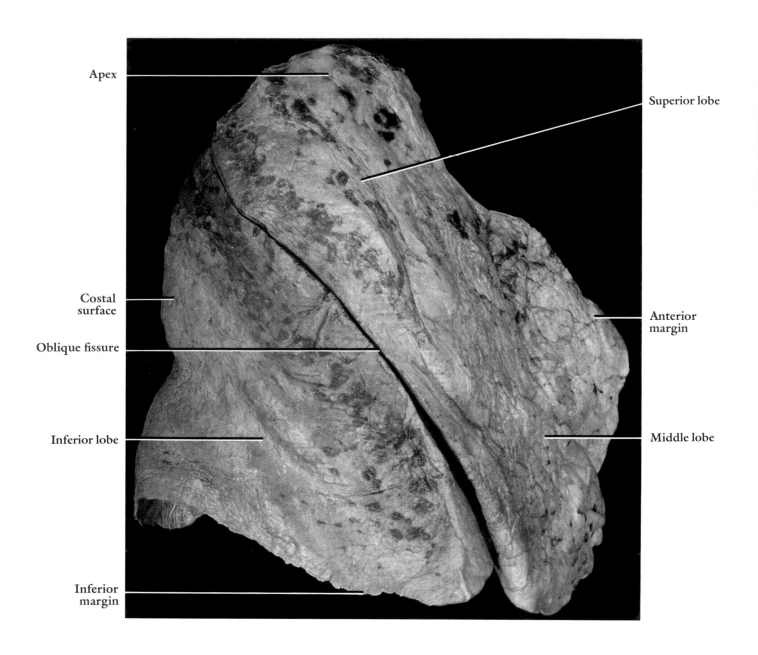

Apex

Superior lobe

Costal
surface

Oblique fissure

Anterior
margin

Inferior lobe

Middle lobe

Inferior
margin

Specific remarks: For this and for the three subsequent views the *pulmonary vessels* and *primary bronchi* have been cut close to the *hilum* and the two lungs separated.

General remarks: The *horizontal fissure* is not apparent in this specimen. When present it represents the borderline between the *superior* and *middle lobes*.

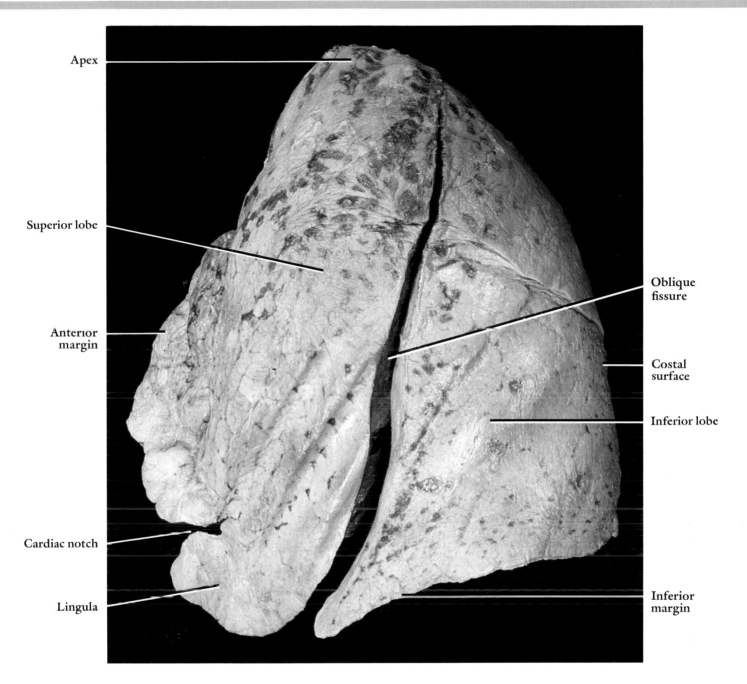

Apex

Superior lobe

Anterior margin

Cardiac notch

Lingula

Oblique fissure

Costal surface

Inferior lobe

Inferior margin

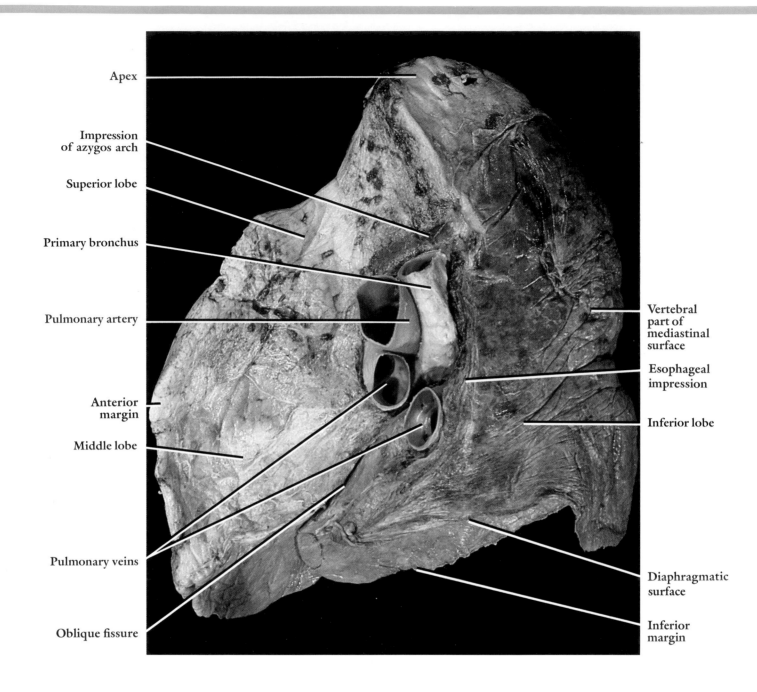

Apex

Impression
of azygos arch

Superior lobe

Primary bronchus

Pulmonary artery

Anterior
margin

Middle lobe

Pulmonary veins

Oblique fissure

Vertebral
part of
mediastinal
surface

Esophageal
impression

Inferior lobe

Diaphragmatic
surface

Inferior
margin

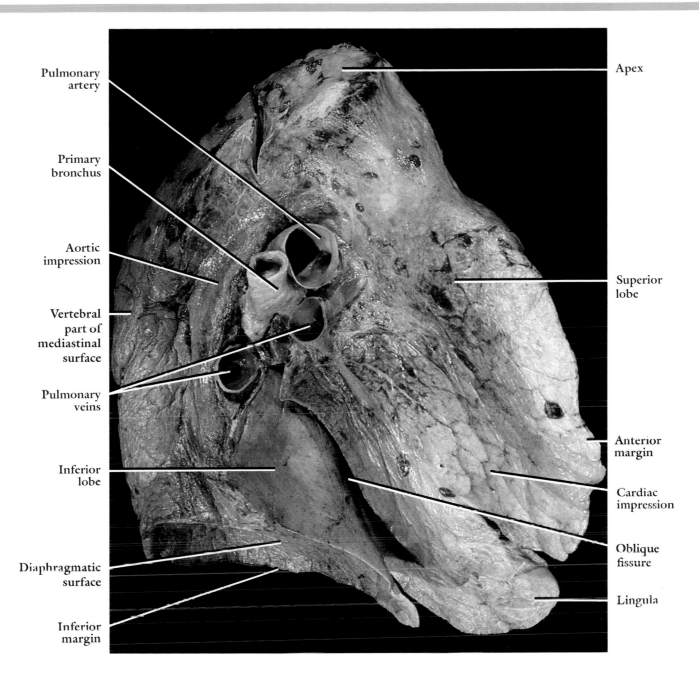

Pulmonary
artery

Primary
bronchus

Aortic
impression

Vertebral
part of
mediastinal
surface

Pulmonary
veins

Inferior
lobe

Diaphragmatic
surface

Inferior
margin

Apex

Superior
lobe

Anterior
margin

Cardiac
impression

Oblique
fissure

Lingula

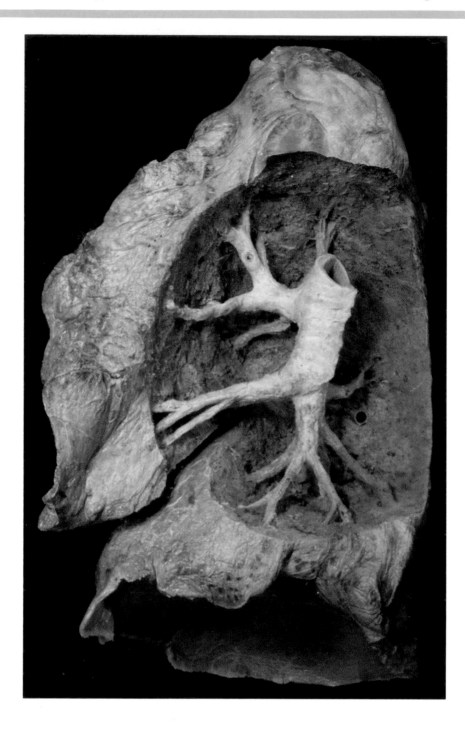

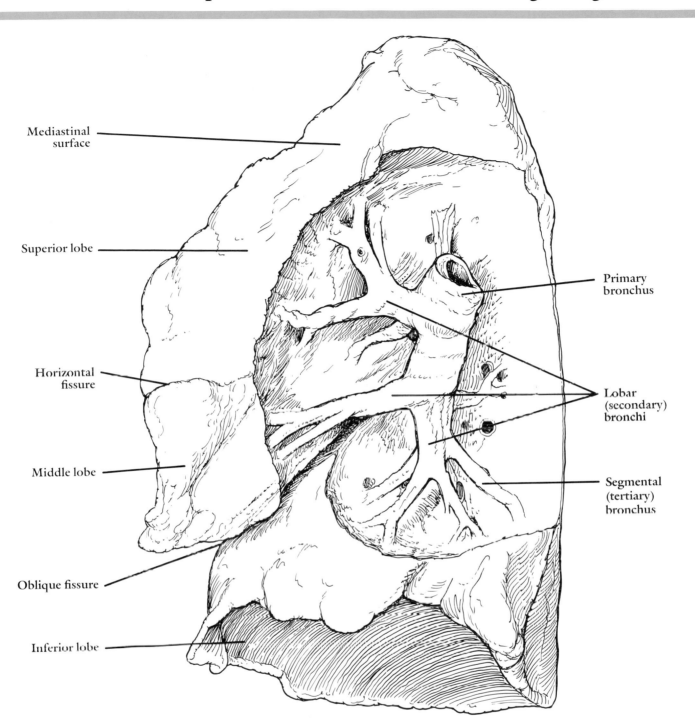

Mediastinal surface

Superior lobe

Horizontal fissure

Middle lobe

Oblique fissure

Inferior lobe

Primary bronchus

Lobar (secondary) bronchi

Segmental (tertiary) bronchus

Specific remarks: *Primary, secondary (lobar),* and *tertiary (segmental) bronchi* are demonstrated after the surrounding *parenchyma* and *pulmonary blood vessels* have been removed from the mediastinal aspect of the lung. It is apparent that each lobe relates to one secondary bronchus, and from there each secondary bronchus supplies a tertiary bronchus to the corresponding *bronchopulmonary segment.*

General remarks: There are ten bronchopulmonary segments in the right lung. Three of them are confined to the *superior lobe,* two to the *middle lobe,* and five to the *inferior lobe.*

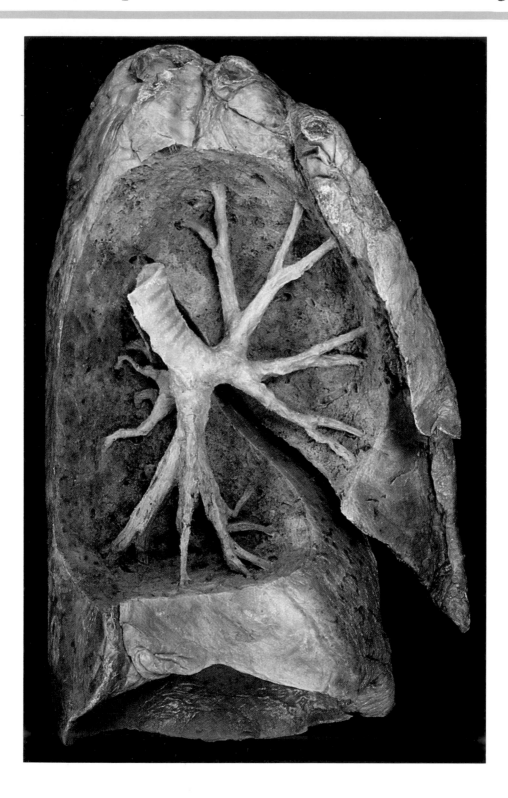

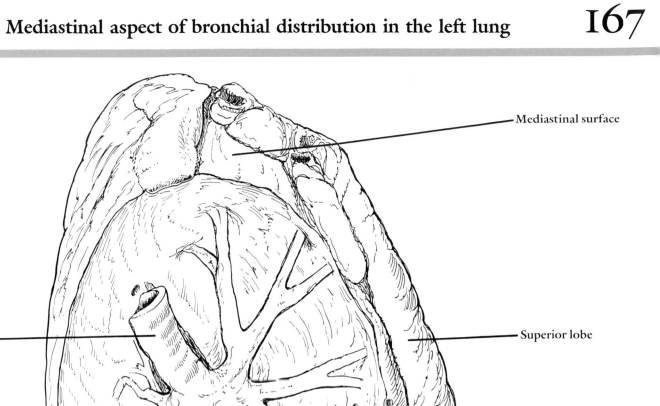

Mediastinal surface

Primary
bronchus

Superior lobe

Lobar
(secondary)
bronchus

Segmental
(tertiary)
bronchus

Oblique fissure

Lingula of
left lung

Inferior lobe

Specific remarks: *Primary, secondary (lobar), and tertiary (segmental) bronchi* are demonstrated after the surrounding *parenchyma* and *pulmonary blood vessels* have been removed from the mediastinal aspect of the lung. There are two secondary bronchi, one for each lobe, in the left lung. The upper secondary bronchus, however, is distributed similarly to the upper and middle bronchi together in the right lung.

General remarks: There are ten *bronchopulmonary segments* in the left lung. Five of them are confined to the *superior lobe* and five to the *inferior lobe*.

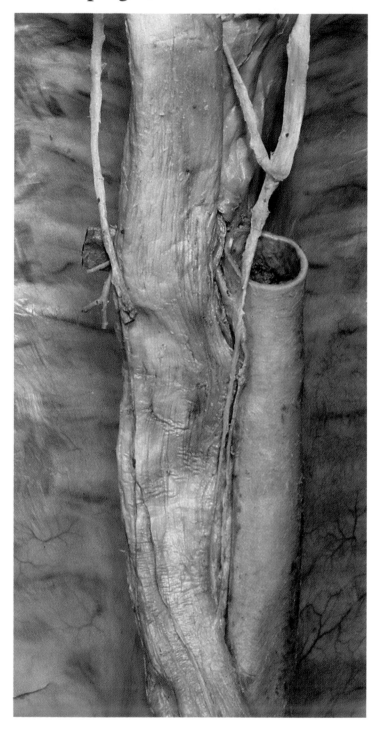

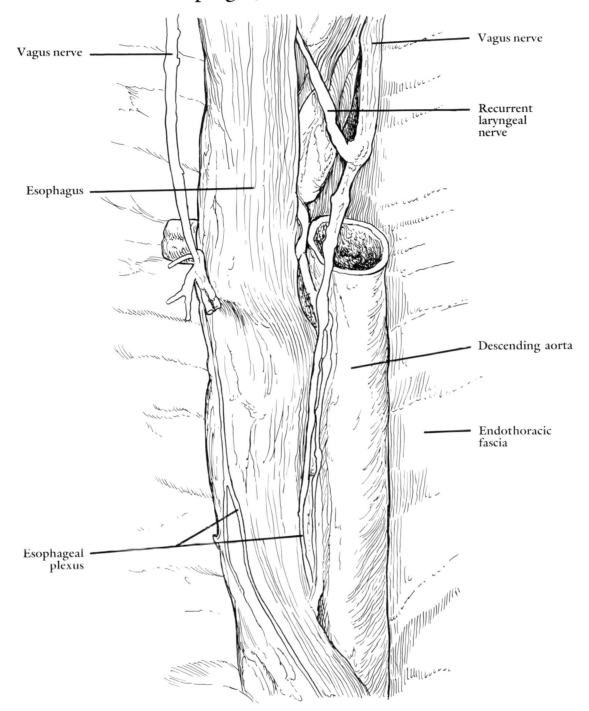

Vagus nerve

Vagus nerve

Recurrent laryngeal nerve

Esophagus

Descending aorta

Endothoracic fascia

Esophageal plexus

Specific remarks: Following the removal of the *heart, arch of the aorta,* large blood vessels, *trachea, bronchi,* and the *lungs* from the *thoracic cavity,* the *esophagus, vagi,* and *descending aorta* become exposed. The internal aspect of the posterior thoracic wall is covered by the *endothoracic fascia.*

General remarks: The right and left vagus nerves branch as they approach the esophageal wall. The former nerve predominates in the *posterior esophageal plexus,* and the latter nerve predominates in the *anterior esophageal plexus.* These plexuses, together with the esophagus, pass through the *esophageal hiatus of the diaphragm* to supply visceromotor components to the abdominal viscera.

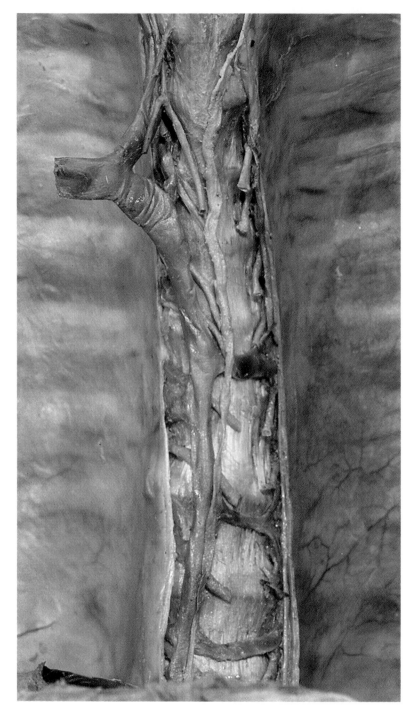

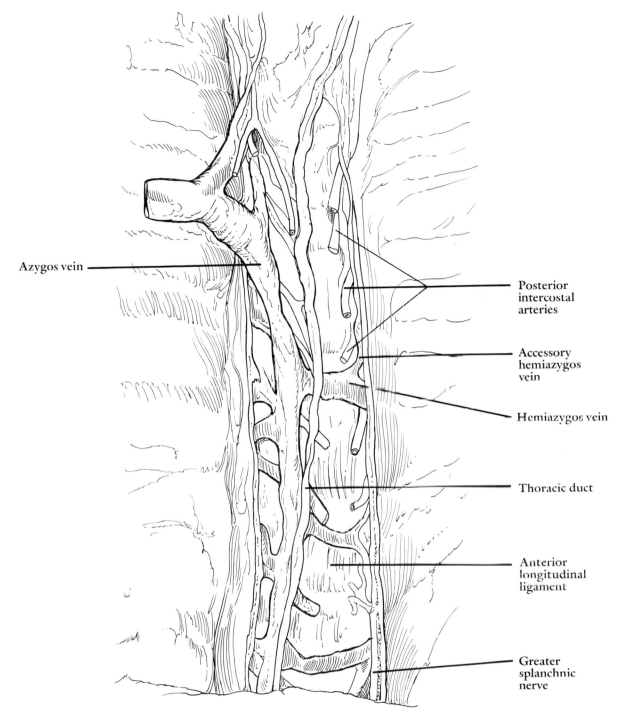

Azygos vein

Posterior intercostal arteries

Accessory hemiazygos vein

Hemiazygos vein

Thoracic duct

Anterior longitudinal ligament

Greater splanchnic nerve

Specific remarks: Immediately posterior to the *esophagus* and *descending aorta,* which together with the *vagus nerves* have been removed from this view, are the *azygos vein, hemiazygos vein, accessory hemiazygos vein,* and the *thoracic duct.*

General remarks: The thoracic duct is the largest lymphatic vessel to transport lymph from the *cisterna chyli* to the major veins on the left side of the root of the neck. One group of *gastric veins* drains into the *portal system* and the other into the hemiazygos vein. Numerous anastomoses between these two groups of veins establish an important collateral pathway from the portal to the systemic circulation. This, or the other similar pathways, becomes functionally viable during obstruction of the portal vein or hepatic parenchymal degenerative or neoplastic changes.

170

Anterior aspect of the azygos veins, thoracic duct, left sympathetic trunk, and the contents of the left intercostal spaces

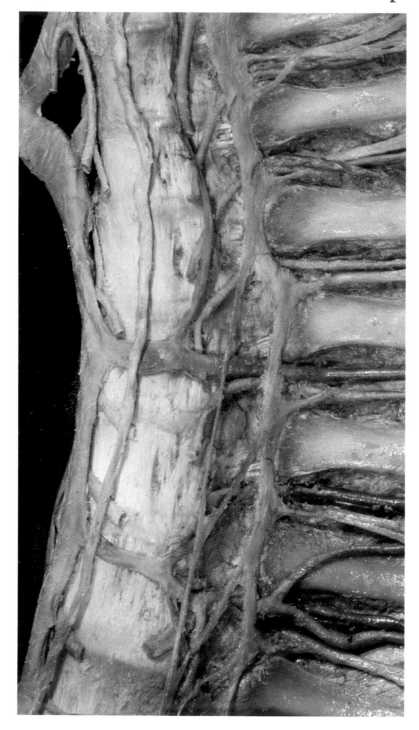

Anterior aspect of the azygos veins, thoracic duct, left sympathetic trunk, and the contents of the left intercostal spaces

I70

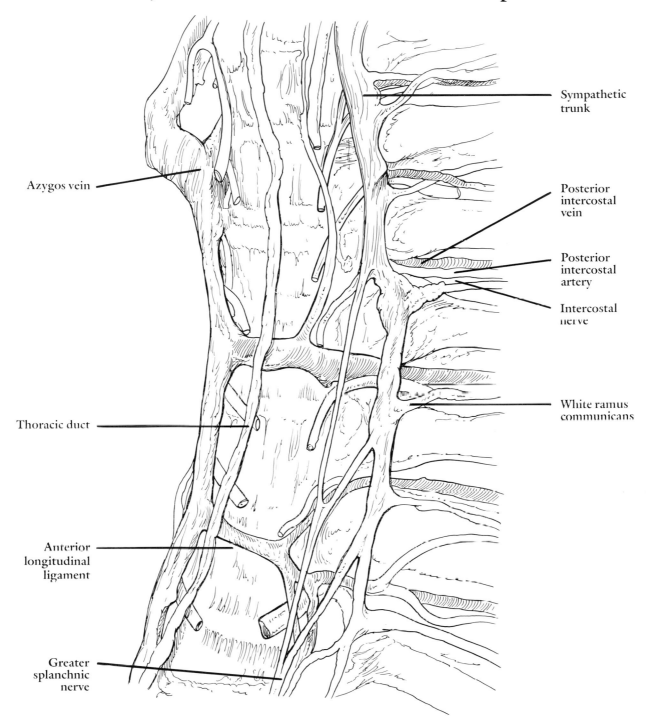

Sympathetic trunk

Azygos vein

Posterior intercostal vein

Posterior intercostal artery

Intercostal nerve

Thoracic duct

White ramus communicans

Anterior longitudinal ligament

Greater splanchnic nerve

Specific remarks: The *endothoracic fascia* and *internal intercostal membranes* have been removed from several intercostal levels on the left side, while the *sympathetic ganglia, interganglionic connections,* and the *greater splanchnic nerve* have been preserved in situ. Lateral connections of the *intercostal nerves* with corresponding sympathetic ganglia, the *white rami,* are demonstrated; the medial connections, the *gray rami,* are overlapped by sympathetic ganglia. Within an intercostal space the *posterior intercostal vein* is superior, the artery is in between, and the nerve is inferior.

General remarks: The white rami carry preganglionic sympathetic axons to the ganglia where most of them synapse. The postganglionic axons are transported back to intercostal nerves by way of the gray rami.

References

146

Anson, B.J., Morgan, E.H., and McVay, C.B.: Surgical anatomy of the inguinal region based upon a study of 500 body-halves, Surg. Gynecol. Obstet. **111:**707, 1960.

Lytle, W.J.: Inguinal anatomy, J. Anat. **128:**581, 1979.

147

Floyd, W.F., and Silver, P.H.S.: Electromyographic study of patterns of activity of the anterior abdominal wall muscles in man, J. Anat. **84:**132, 1950.

Loudon, R.G.: Auscultation of the lung, Clin. Notes Res. Dis. **21:**3, 1982.

McVay, C.B., and Anson, B.J.: Aponeurotic and fascial continuities in the abdomen, pelvis, and thigh, Anat. Rec. **76:**213, 1940.

148

McVay, C.B., and Anson, B.J.: Composition of the rectus sheath, Anat. Rec. 77:213, 1940.

150

Elliot, F.M., and Reid, L.: Some new facts about the pulmonary artery and its branching pattern, Clin. Radiol. **16:**193, 1965.

153

Gross, L.: The blood supply of the heart, London, 1921, Oxford University Press.

155

Truex, R.C., and Smythe, M.Q.: Reconstruction of the human atrioventricular node, Anat. Rec. **158:**11, 1967.

Truex, R.C., Smythe, M.Q., and Taylor, M.J.: Reconstruction of the human sinoatrial node, Anat. Rec. **159:**371, 1967.

156

Walmsley, R.: The orientation of the heart and the appearance of its chambers in adult cadavers, Br. Heart J. **20:**441, 1958.

Wright, R.R., Anson, B.J., and Cleveland, H.C.: The vestigial valves and the interatrial foramen of the adult human heart, Anat. Rec. **100:**331, 1948.

159

Campbell, A.H., and Liddelow, A.G.: Significant variations in the shape of the trachea and large bronchi, Med. J. Aust. **54:**1017, 1967.

163

Bloomer, W.E., Liebow, A.E., and Holes, M.R.: Surgical anatomy of the bronchovascular segments, Oxford, 1960, ??.

Boyden, E.A.: Segmental anatomy of the lung, New York, 1955, McGraw-Hill Book Co., Inc.

165

Fishman, A.P., and Hecht, H.H., editors: The pulmonary circulation and interstitial space, Chicago, 1969, University of Chicago Press.

166

Brock, R.C.: The anatomy of the bronchial tree, London, 1954, Oxford University Press.

168

Doubilet, H., Shafiroff, B.G.P., and Mulholland, J.H.: Anatomy of periesophageal vagi, Ann. Surg. **127:**128, 1948.

169

Kampmeier, O.F.: Evaluation and comparative morphology of the lymphatic system, Springfield, Ill., 1969, Charles C Thomas, Publisher.

170

Davis, F., Gladstone, R.J., and Stibbe, E.P.: The anatomy of the intercostal nerves, J. Anat. **66:**323, 1932.

Pick, J.: The autonomic nervous system, Philadelphia, 1970, J.B. Lippincott Co.

Part Four
ABDOMEN

Anterolateral abdominal wall and inguinal region

Abdominal organs in situ

Isolated segments and internal structure
of gastrointestinal tract

Liver

Spleen

Retroperitoneal region

Horizontal sectional view of abdomen

Kidney

Posterior abdominal wall

Diaphragm

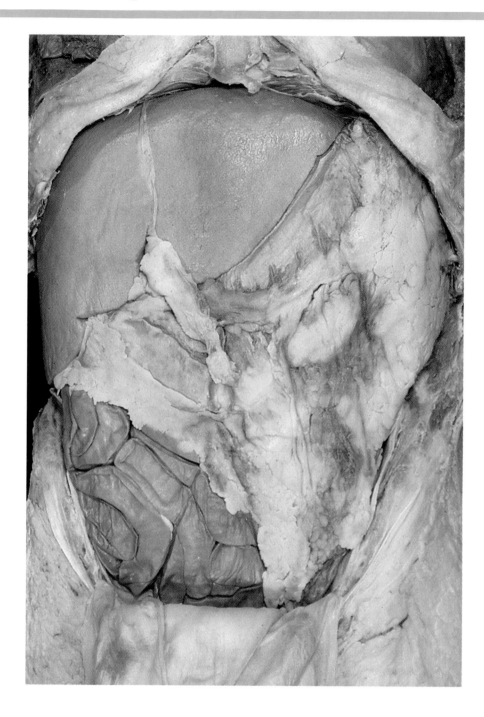

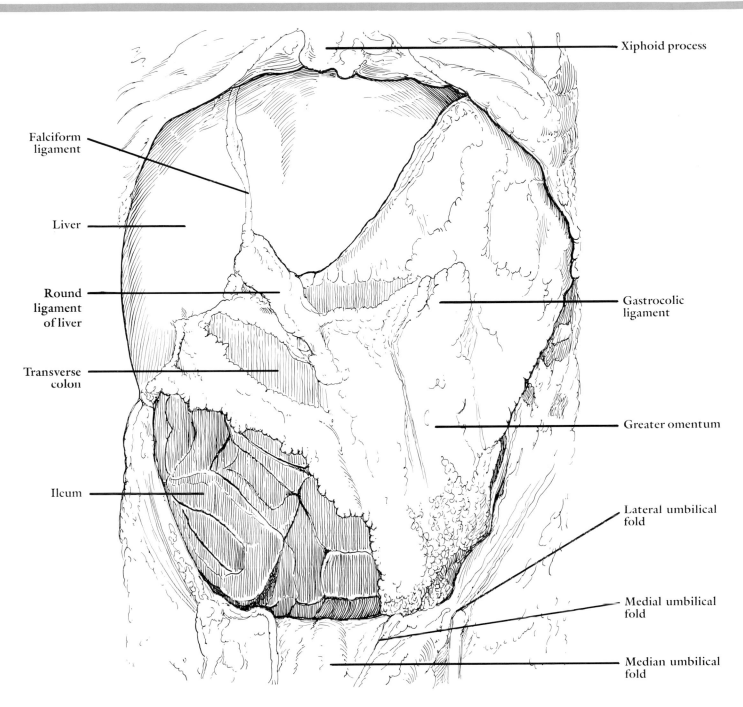

Xiphoid process

Falciform ligament

Liver

Round ligament of liver

Transverse colon

Ileum

Gastrocolic ligament

Greater omentum

Lateral umbilical fold

Medial umbilical fold

Median umbilical fold

General remarks: This is a close-up view of the *abdominal viscera* in Fig. 150. The *falciform ligament*, which represents a reflection of the *visceral peritoneum*, extends from the *umbilicus* superiorly and somewhat to the right to attach the *liver* to the anterior abdominal wall and the *diaphragm*. Although most of the abdominal contents are covered by the *greater omentum*, coils of the *ileum* are exposed in the lower right quadrant. On the deep surface of the inferiorly reflected *parietal peritoneum* the *inguinal folds* and *fossae* are also shown.

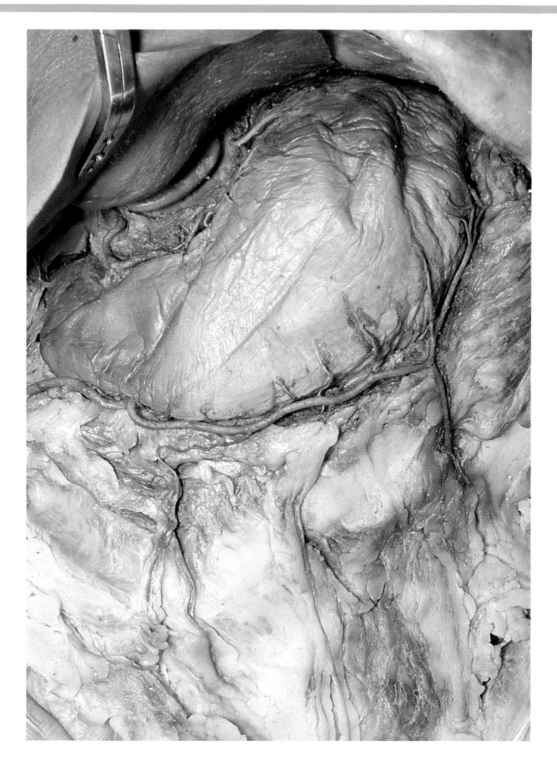

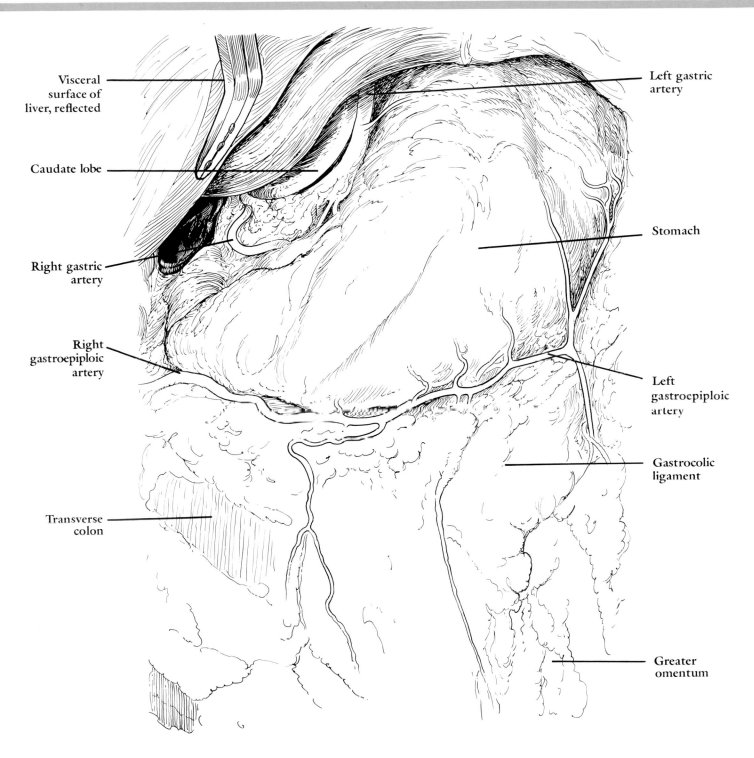

Visceral surface of liver, reflected

Caudate lobe

Right gastric artery

Right gastroepiploic artery

Transverse colon

Left gastric artery

Stomach

Left gastroepiploic artery

Gastrocolic ligament

Greater omentum

Specific remarks: In the upper left quadrant of the abdomen, with the *liver* reflected superiorly, the anterior aspect of the *stomach* is demonstrated. Along the *greater curvature* and within the thickness of the *greater omentum* the *right* and *left gastroepiploic arteries* are shown. Similarly, along the *lesser curvature* and within the thickness of the *lesser omentum* the *right* and *left gastric arteries* are shown.

General remarks: The two gastric arteries (and similarly the two gastroepiploic arteries) anastomose with one another along the corresponding curvature of the stomach. These anastomotic arcades provide a steady circulation to the organ from both sides or from either side during peristalsis.

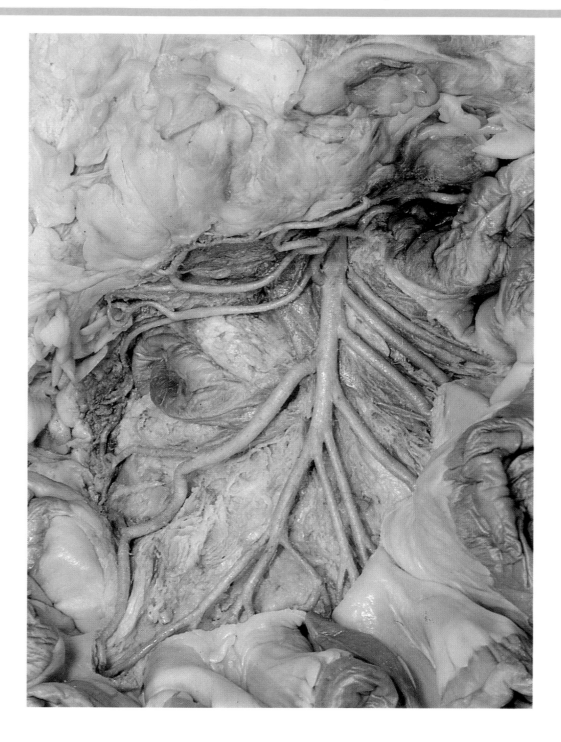

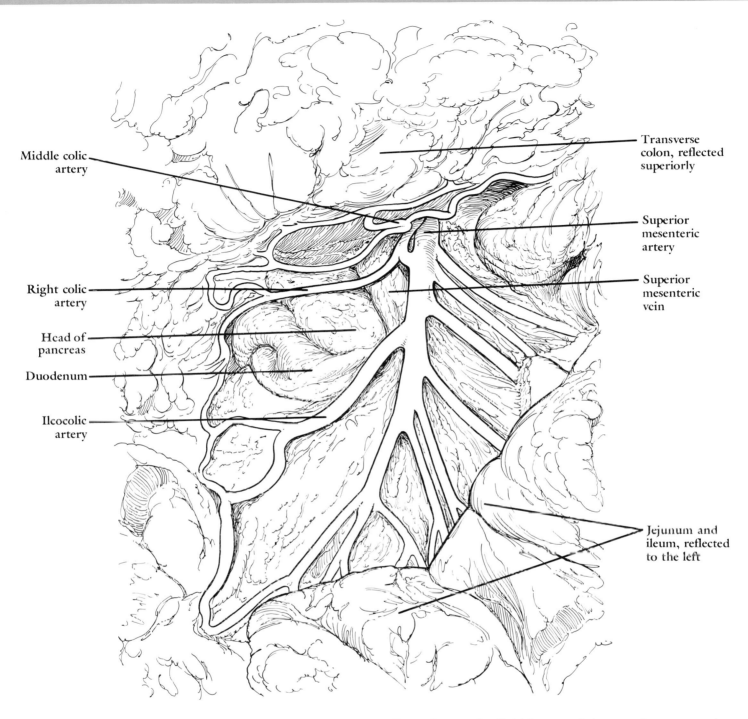

Middle colic artery

Right colic artery

Head of pancreas

Duodenum

Ileocolic artery

Transverse colon, reflected superiorly

Superior mesenteric artery

Superior mesenteric vein

Jejunum and ileum, reflected to the left

Specific remarks: To demonstrate the *superior mesenteric artery* and the branches in the *mesentery* and *mesocolon,* the *greater omentum* with the *transverse colon* has been reflected superiorly, and coils of the small intestine have been displaced to the left and inferiorly.

General remarks: Initial parts of the superior mesenteric artery and vein pass just anterior to the *uncinate process of the pancreas* and *duodenum.* During herniation of the small intestine the artery may be retracted in such a way as to compress the duodenum against the *aorta,* which is immediately posterior to the duodenum. It is demonstrated once again here that the adjacent arteries anastomose to form arcades. The number of arcades—one, two, or many—depends on the segment of the *alimentary tract.*

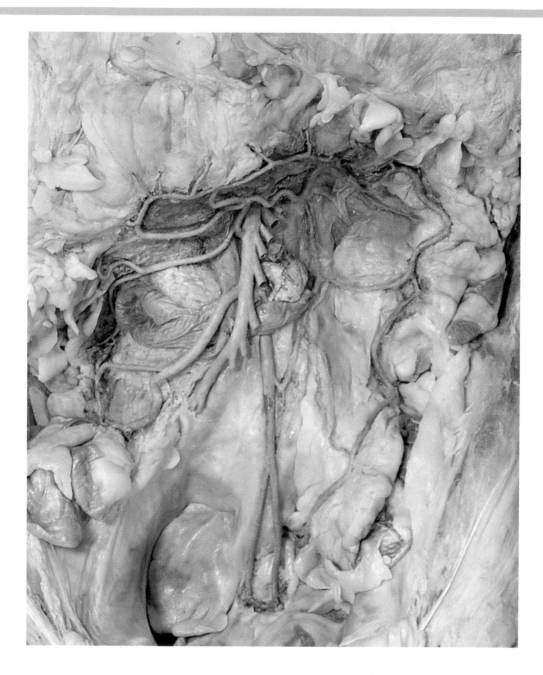

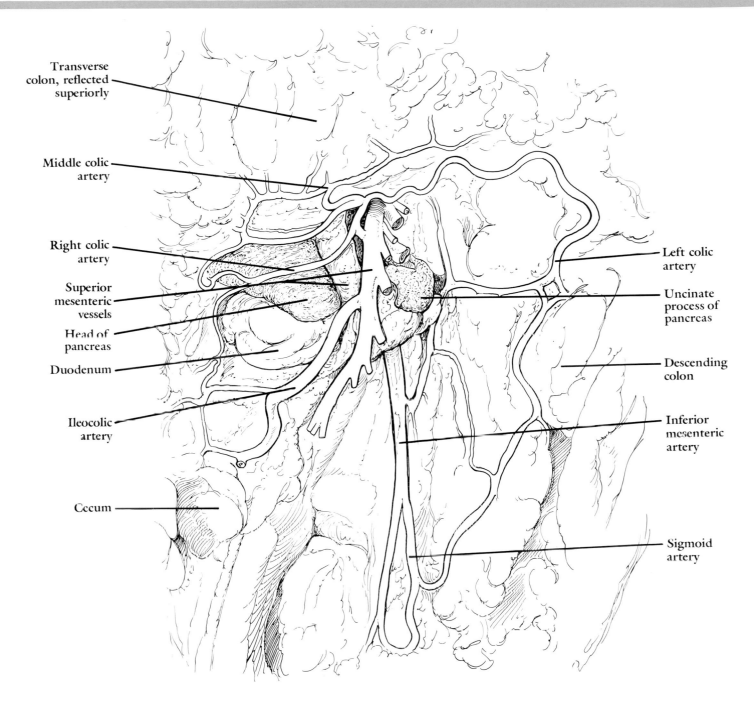

Transverse colon, reflected superiorly

Middle colic artery

Right colic artery

Superior mesenteric vessels

Head of pancreas

Duodenum

Ileocolic artery

Cecum

Left colic artery

Uncinate process of pancreas

Descending colon

Inferior mesenteric artery

Sigmoid artery

Specific remarks: For this view the small intestine has been removed together with corresponding branches of the *superior mesenteric artery* from the *duodenojejunal junction* to close to the *ileocolic junction*. The right branches of the superior mesenteric artery, on the other hand, are kept intact along the *ascending* and *transverse colon*. Distribution of the *inferior mesenteric artery* is shown along the transverse, *descending*, and *sigmoid colons*.

Anterior aspect of the pancreas, spleen, duodenum, and associated structures

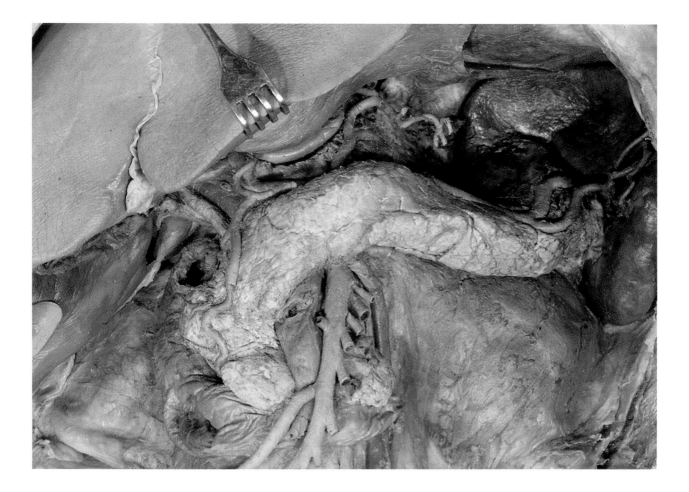

Anterior aspect of the pancreas, spleen, duodenum, and associated structures

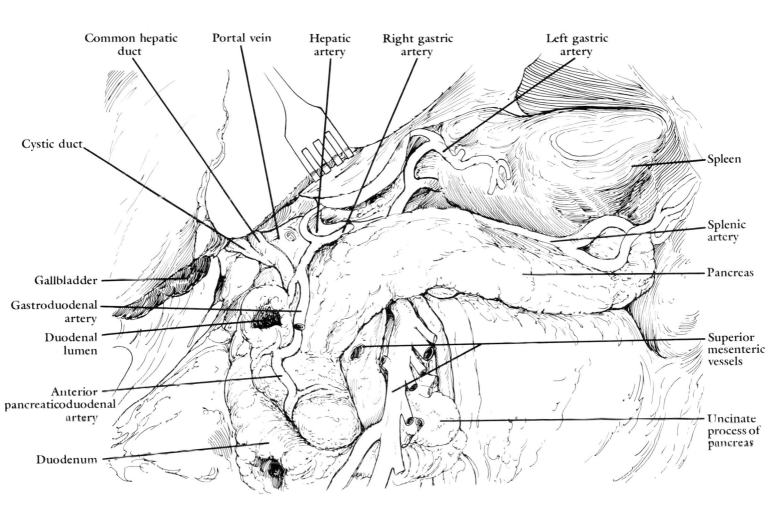

Common hepatic duct

Portal vein

Hepatic artery

Right gastric artery

Left gastric artery

Cystic duct

Spleen

Splenic artery

Gallbladder

Pancreas

Gastroduodenal artery

Duodenal lumen

Superior mesenteric vessels

Anterior pancreaticoduodenal artery

Uncinate process of pancreas

Duodenum

Specific remarks: For this view the *esophagus, stomach,* and a part of the *duodenum* have been removed from the level of the *diaphragm* to the *superior duodenal flexure,* and the *parietal peritoneum* has been removed from the anterior aspect of the *pancreas* and duodenum. The relationships of the *splenic artery* with the pancreas and *splenic hilum* and the *anterior pancreaticoduodenal arcade* are demonstrated.

General remarks: The anterior and *posterior pancreaticoduodenal arcades* are formed by anastomoses of the anterior and posterior branches, respectively, of the *superior* and *inferior pancreaticoduodenal arteries.* The superior artery is a branch of the *gastroduodenal artery,* and the inferior of the *superior mesenteric artery.*

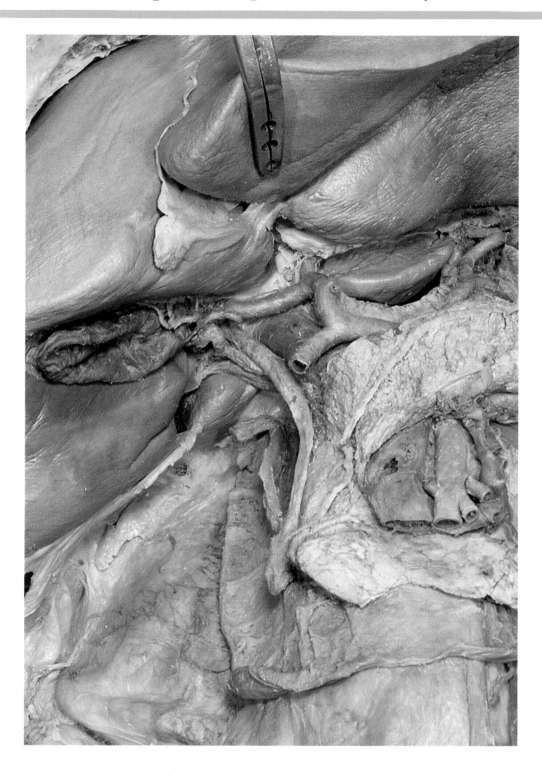

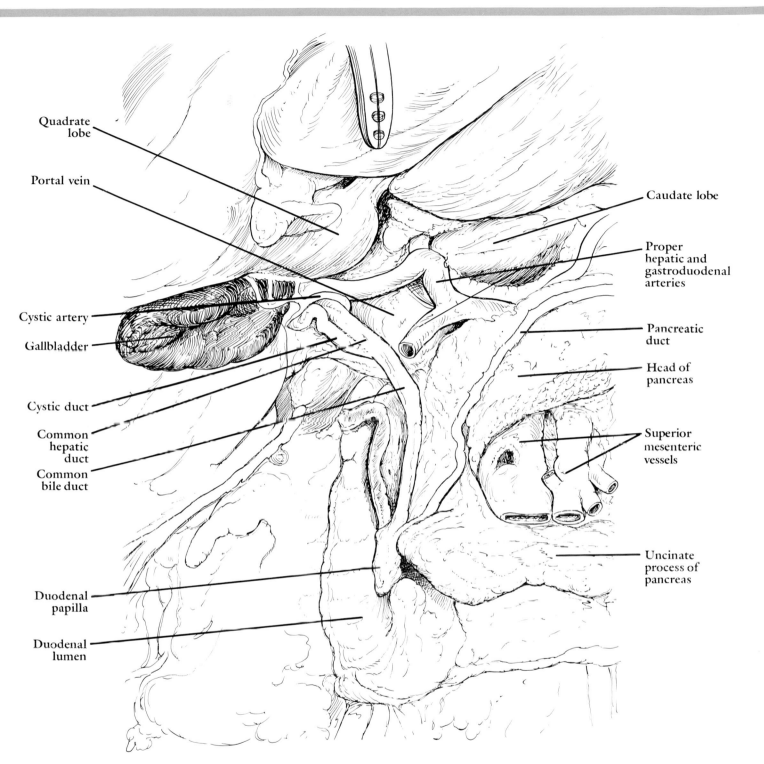

Quadrate lobe

Portal vein

Cystic artery

Gallbladder

Cystic duct

Common hepatic duct

Common bile duct

Duodenal papilla

Duodenal lumen

Caudate lobe

Proper hepatic and gastroduodenal arteries

Pancreatic duct

Head of pancreas

Superior mesenteric vessels

Uncinate process of pancreas

Specific remarks: The *duodenum* has been cut frontally through its middle and the anterior half removed. The entire biliary system, which consists of the *gallbladder, cystic duct, hepatic ducts,* and *common bile duct,* and the *pancreatic duct* inside the *pancreatic parenchyma* have been simultaneously exposed. The relationships between terminal parts of the common bile and pancreatic ducts and their common opening at the *major papilla of the duodenum* are evident.

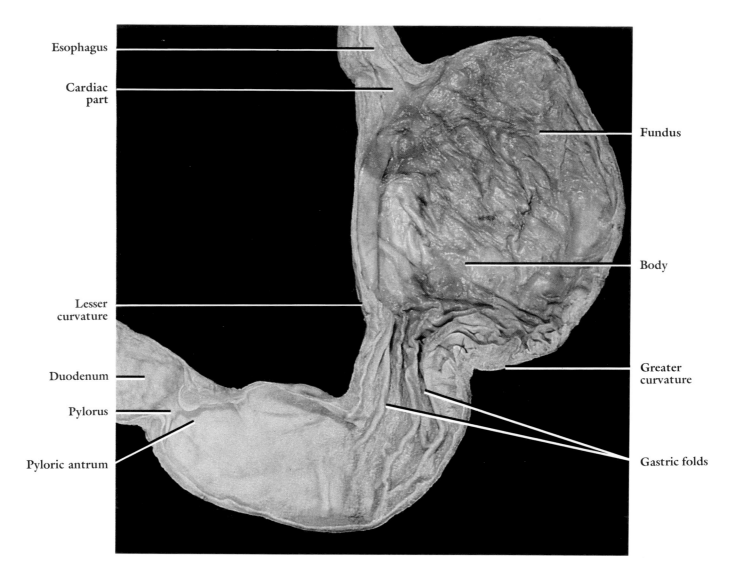

Esophagus

Cardiac part

Fundus

Body

Lesser curvature

Duodenum

Pylorus

Pyloric antrum

Greater curvature

Gastric folds

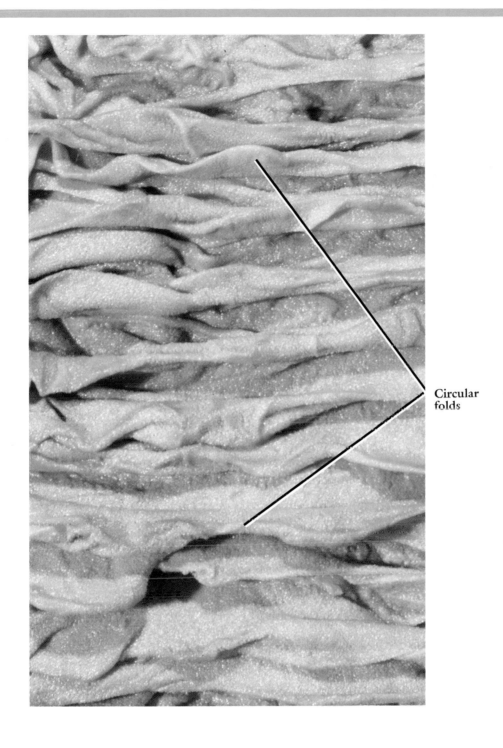

Circular
folds

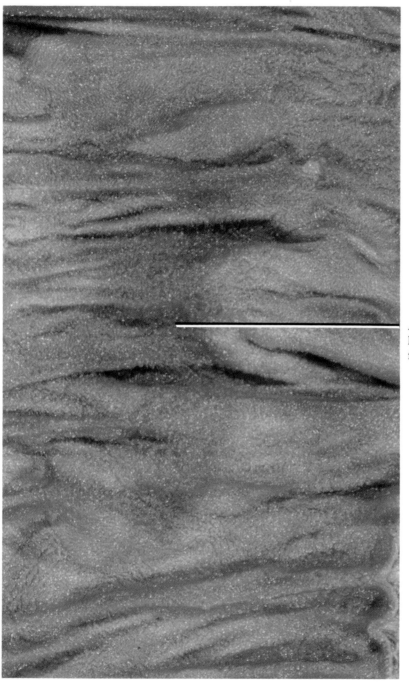

Aggregate
lymphoid
follicles

General remarks: *Peyer's patches* are aggregates of *lymphoid follicles,* which are most numerous in the *ileum*. Their number and size diminish from puberty throughout life.

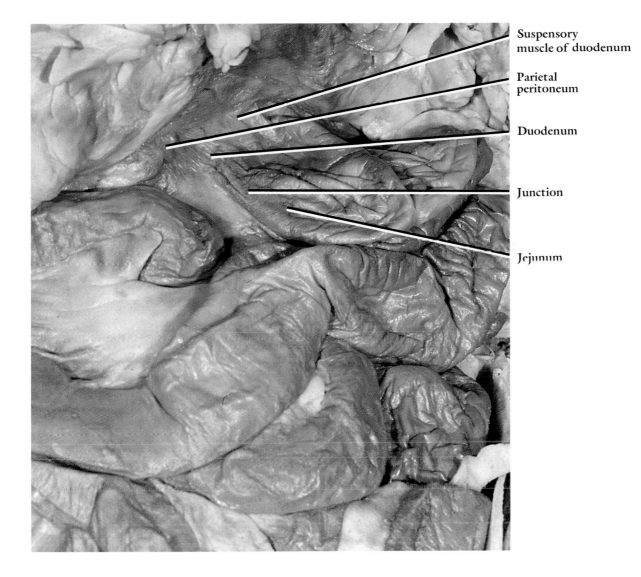

Suspensory muscle of duodenum

Parietal peritoneum

Duodenum

Junction

Jejunum

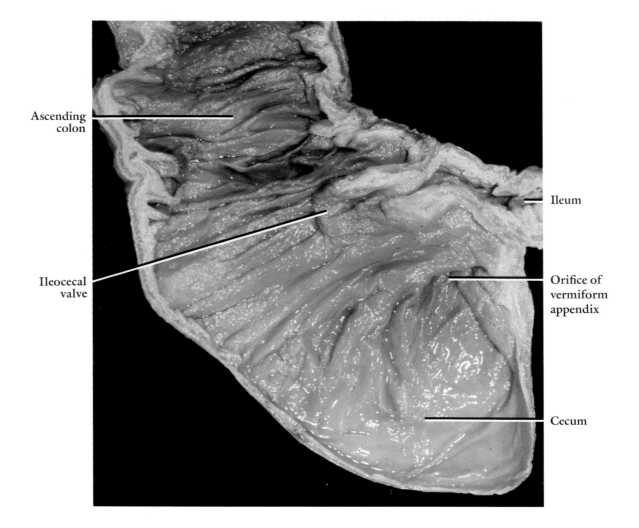

Ascending colon

Ileum

Ileocecal valve

Orifice of vermiform appendix

Cecum

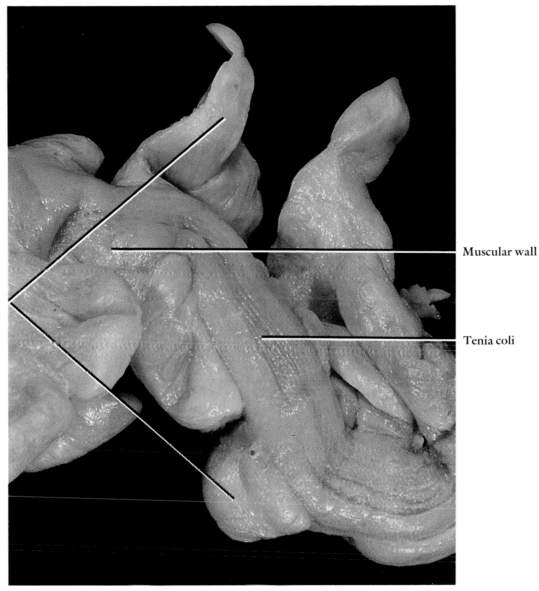

Muscular wall

Tenia coli

Epiploic
appendages

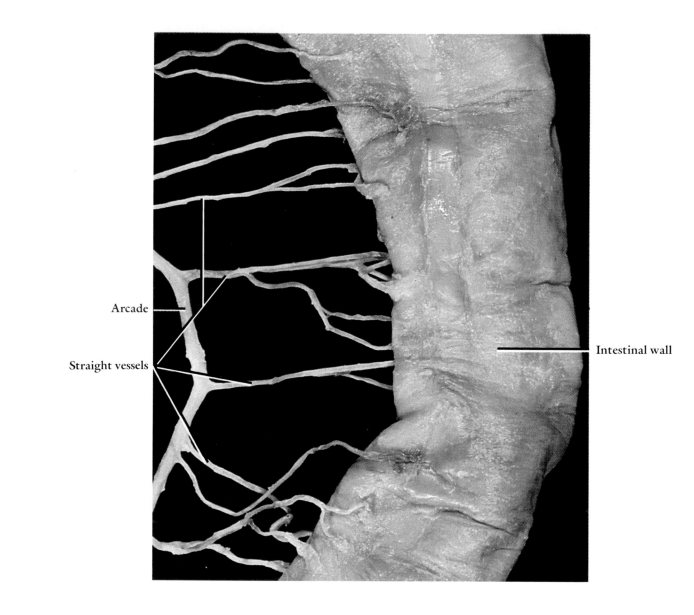

Arcade

Straight vessels

Intestinal wall

General remarks: From the last order of arterial arcades arise the *straight vessels*. Each of these supplies an intestinal ring without anastomosing with the adjacent vessels.

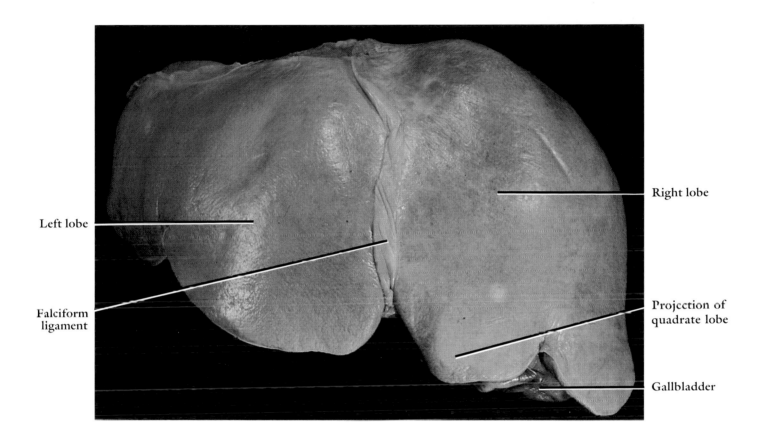

Left lobe

Falciform
ligament

Right lobe

Projection of
quadrate lobe

Gallbladder

Coronary
ligament

Hepatic veins

Right lobe

Left lobe

Left
triangular
ligament

Right
triangular
ligament

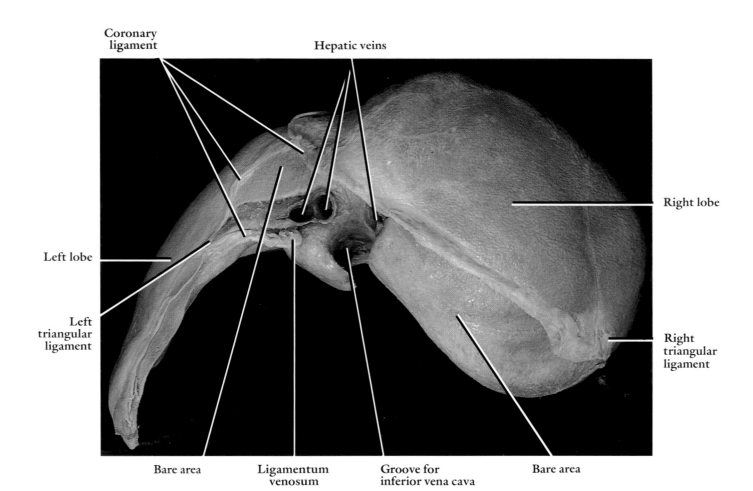

Bare area

Ligamentum
venosum

Groove for
inferior vena cava

Bare area

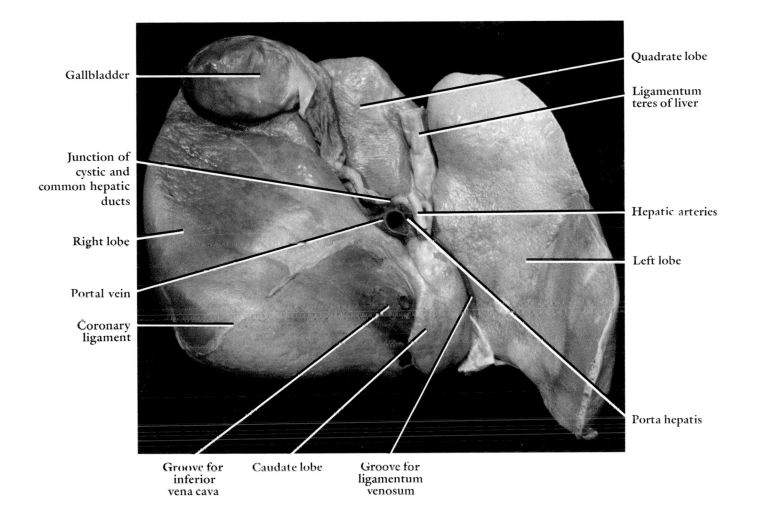

Gallbladder

Junction of
cystic and
common hepatic
ducts

Right lobe

Portal vein

Coronary
ligament

Quadrate lobe

Ligamentum
teres of liver

Hepatic arteries

Left lobe

Porta hepatis

Groove for
inferior
vena cava

Caudate lobe

Groove for
ligamentum
venosum

Superior border

Gastric surface

Splenic vessels

Anterior extremity

Inferior border

Renal surface

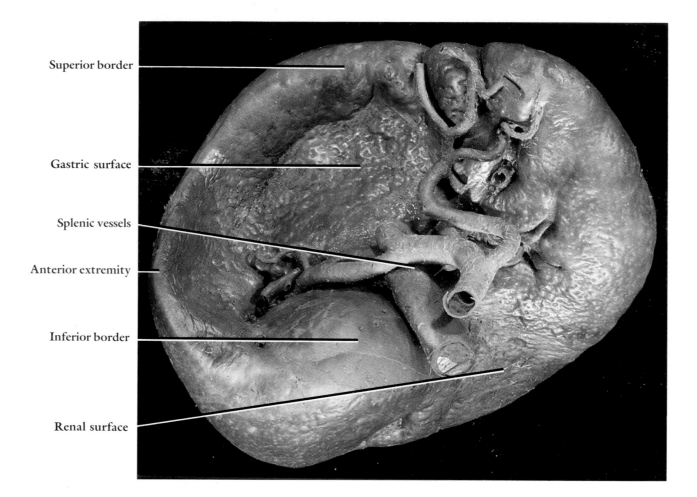

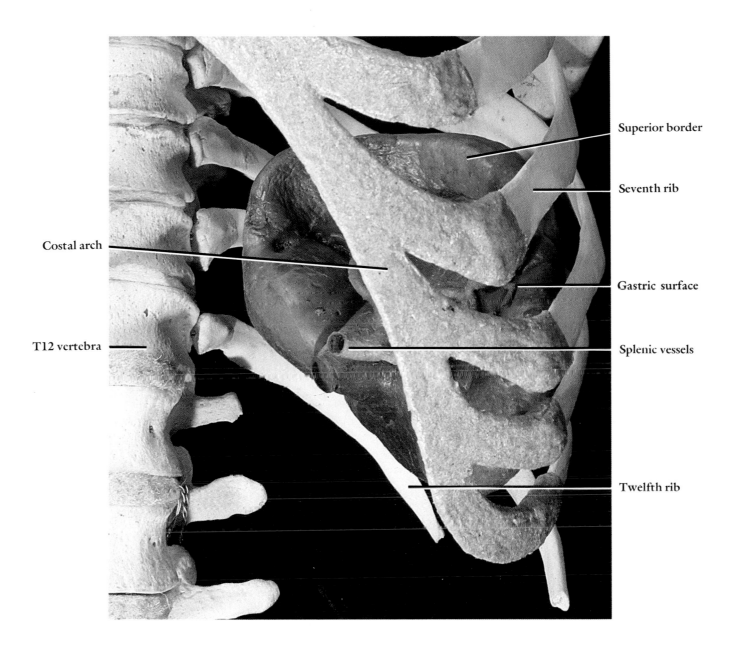

Superior border

Seventh rib

Costal arch

Gastric surface

T12 vertebra

Splenic vessels

Twelfth rib

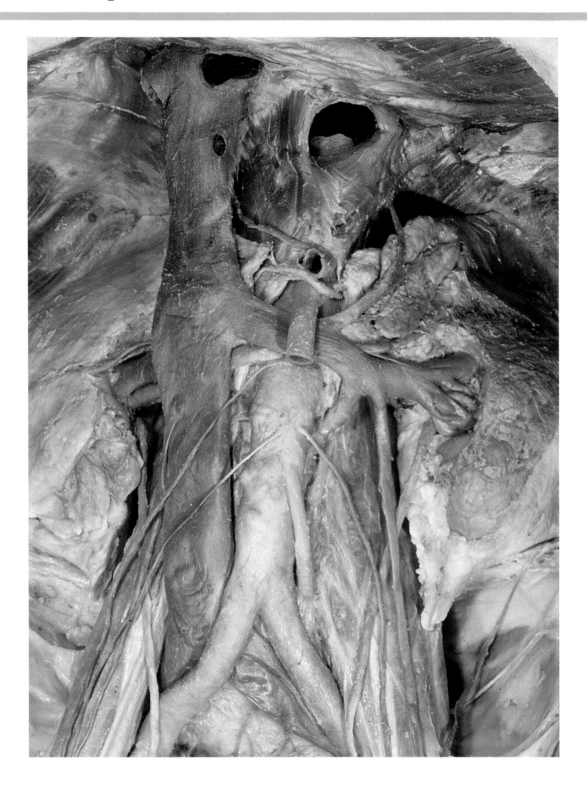

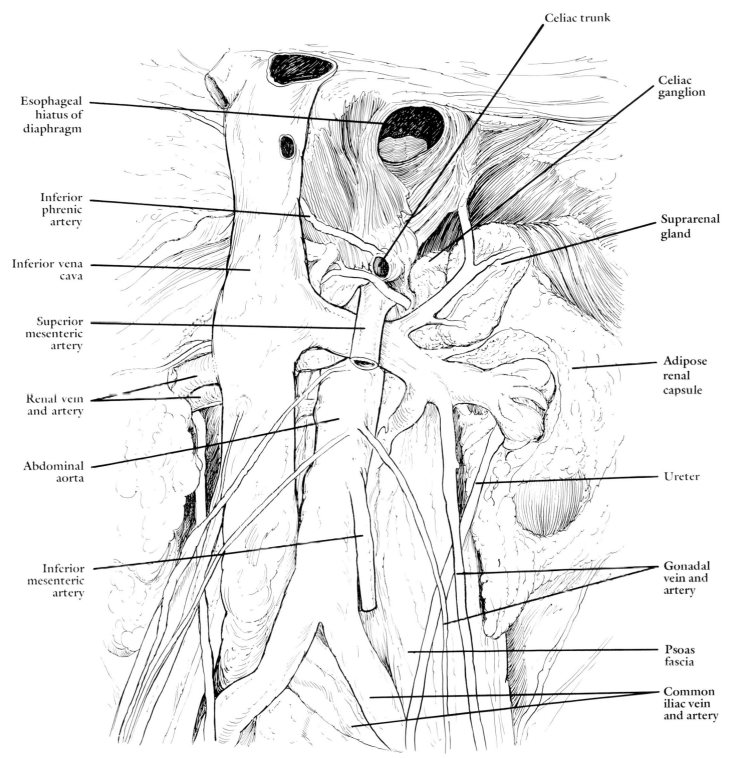

Celiac trunk

Celiac ganglion

Esophageal hiatus of diaphragm

Suprarenal gland

Inferior phrenic artery

Inferior vena cava

Superior mesenteric artery

Adipose renal capsule

Renal vein and artery

Abdominal aorta

Ureter

Inferior mesenteric artery

Gonadal vein and artery

Psoas fascia

Common iliac vein and artery

Specific remarks: The *parietal peritoneum, pancreas,* and retroperitoneal part of the *duodenum* have been removed from the posterior abdominal wall. The *celiac trunk* and the *superior* and *inferior mesenteric arteries* have been cut close to their origins and subsequently removed together with all of their branches. Although the vessels in the middle compartment of retroperitoneal space are fully exposed, the *adipose capsule* is still kept intact around both kidneys. The left *suprarenal gland*, however, is dissected out in relation to corresponding veins and to the *celiac ganglion*.

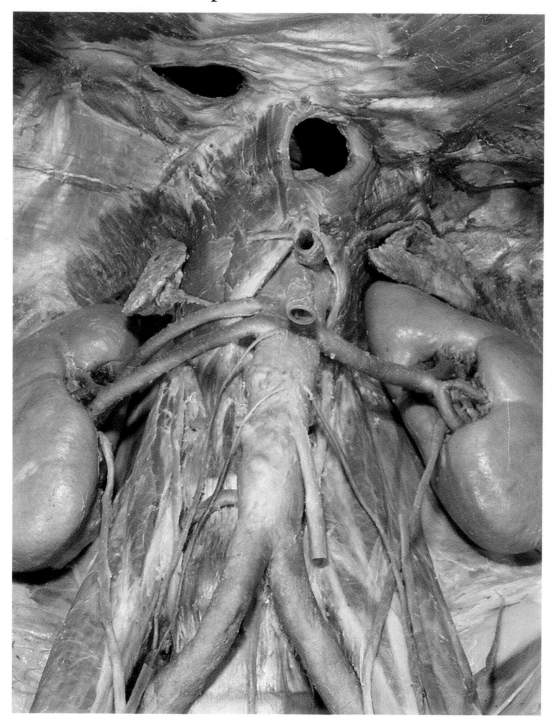

Anterior aspect of the kidneys, suprarenal glands, and retroperitoneal arteries in situ

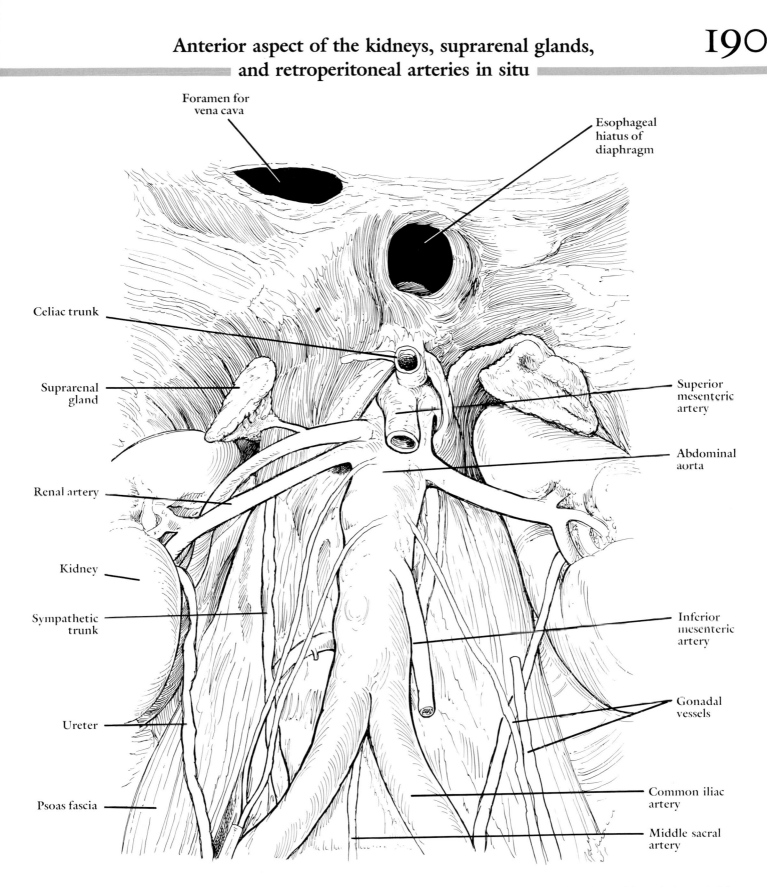

Foramen for vena cava

Esophageal hiatus of diaphragm

Celiac trunk

Suprarenal gland

Renal artery

Kidney

Sympathetic trunk

Ureter

Psoas fascia

Superior mesenteric artery

Abdominal aorta

Inferior mesenteric artery

Gonadal vessels

Common iliac artery

Middle sacral artery

Specific remarks: For this view the *inferior vena cava* with all tributaries and the *renal fascia* together with the *adipose capsule* have been taken away to demonstrate the anterior aspect of the *kidneys* and *suprarenal glands*. The relative positions of the *renal veins* and *arteries* and the *urinary tract* within the *renal hilum* is demonstrated on both sides.

General remarks: The left kidney is positioned about 1.25 cm above the right organ. Left and right renal hili are projected anteriorly just above and below, respectively, the *transpyloric plane*, about 5 cm from the midline.

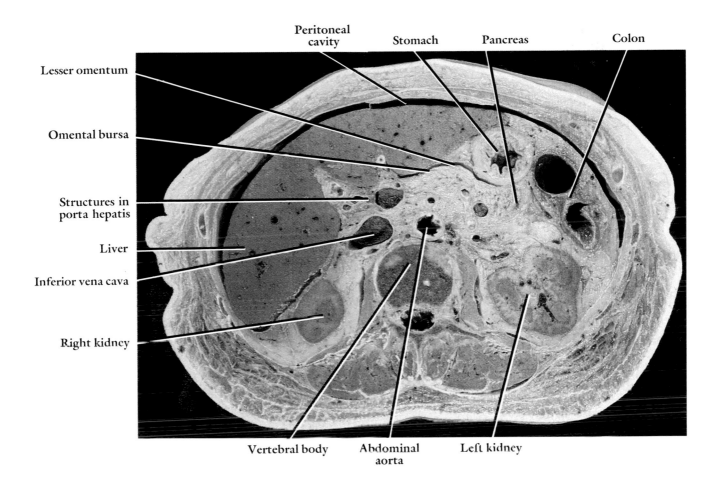

Peritoneal cavity

Stomach

Pancreas

Colon

Lesser omentum

Omental bursa

Structures in porta hepatis

Liver

Inferior vena cava

Right kidney

Vertebral body

Abdominal aorta

Left kidney

Specific remarks: The body has been horizontally cut at the level of the *epiploic foramen*. The upper face of the section is viewed from below.

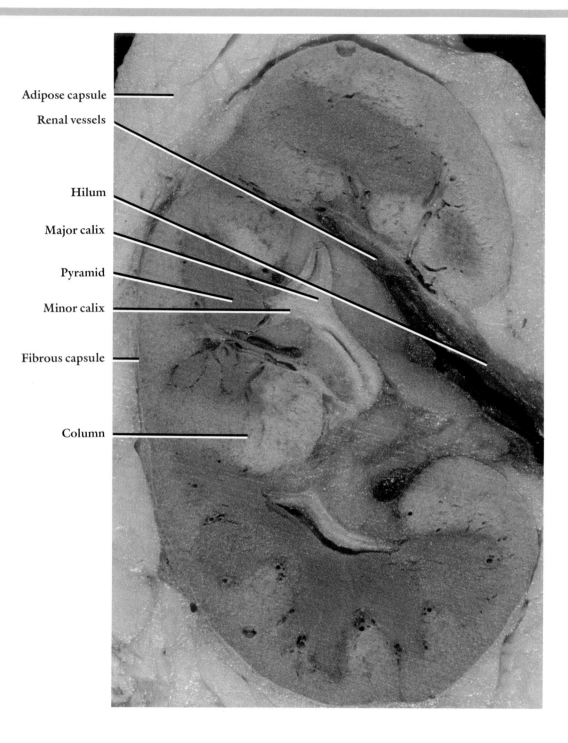

Adipose capsule

Renal vessels

Hilum

Major calix

Pyramid

Minor calix

Fibrous capsule

Column

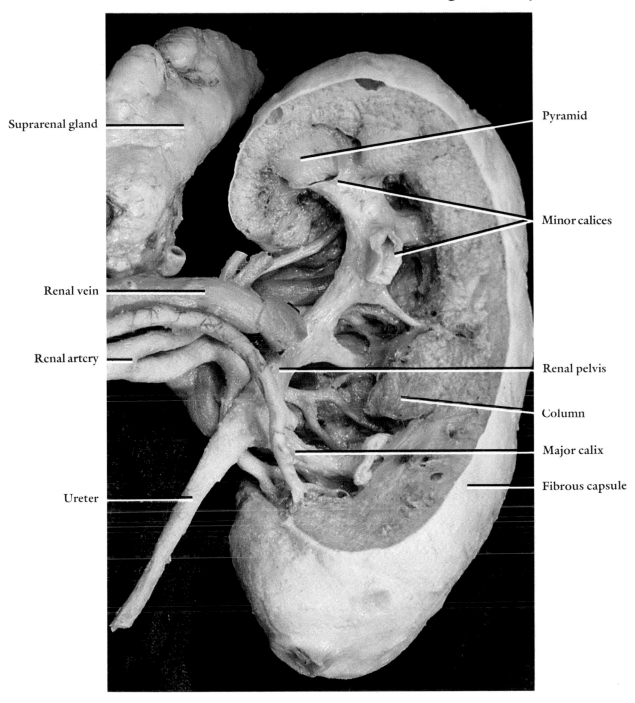

Suprarenal gland

Renal vein

Renal artery

Ureter

Pyramid

Minor calices

Renal pelvis

Column

Major calix

Fibrous capsule

Specific remarks: The *minor* and *major calices,* the *renal pelvis,* and the initial part of the *ureter* have been dissected out through the posterior face of the *renal parenchyma* in relation to the *intrarenal vessels* and *pyramids.*

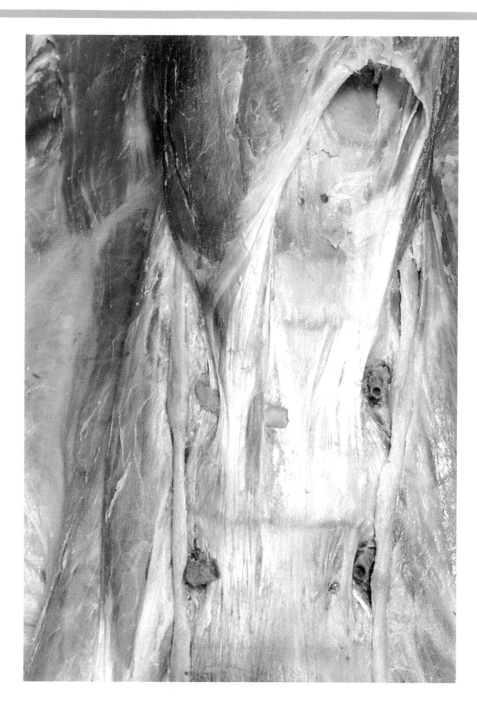

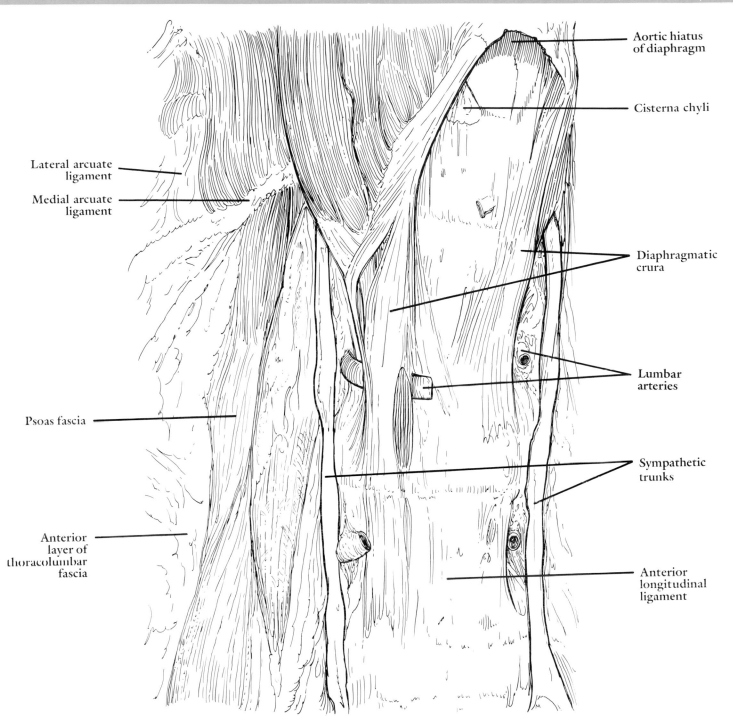

Aortic hiatus
of diaphragm

Cisterna chyli

Lateral arcuate
ligament

Medial arcuate
ligament

Diaphragmatic
crura

Lumbar
arteries

Psoas fascia

Sympathetic
trunks

Anterior
layer of
thoracolumbar
fascia

Anterior
longitudinal
ligament

Specific remarks: All retroperitoneal organs, blood vessels, and nerves have been removed to demonstrate the structure of the posterior abdominal wall on the right side of the body. This wall is formed by the *psoas major, quadratus lumborum,* and *transverse muscle of the abdomen,* together with their fasciae and aponeuroses, from medial to lateral. Attachments of the *diaphragmatic crura* to the *lumbar vertebrae* and the position of the *cisterna chyli* in the *aortic hiatus of the diaphragm* are also shown.

General remarks: Any pus that collects in the thoracolumbar segment of the vertebral column is often channeled into the thigh because of the disposition and structure of the *psoas major fascia.*

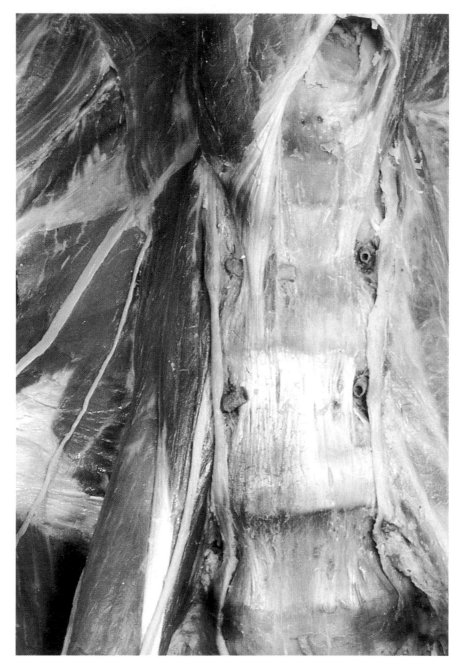

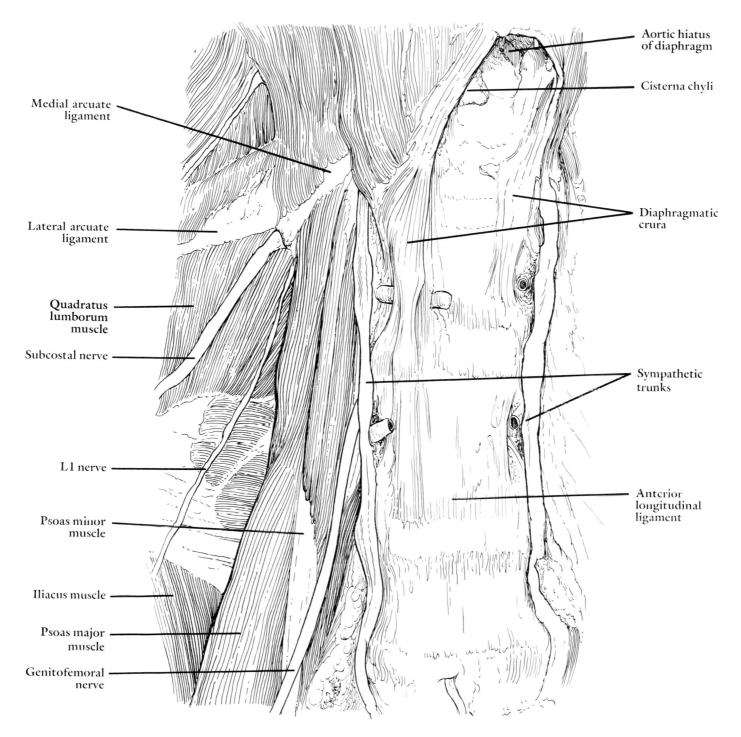

Medial arcuate ligament

Lateral arcuate ligament

Quadratus lumborum muscle

Subcostal nerve

L1 nerve

Psoas minor muscle

Iliacus muscle

Psoas major muscle

Genitofemoral nerve

Aortic hiatus of diaphragm

Cisterna chyli

Diaphragmatic crura

Sympathetic trunks

Anterior longitudinal ligament

Specific remarks: Following the removal of the *psoas major* and *quadratus lumborum fasciae* the two muscles are brought into view. The *medial* and *lateral arcuate ligaments* and branches of the *lumbar plexus* are demonstrated in relation to these muscles.

General remarks: The *psoas minor muscle,* which is shown in this dissection, is developed in about 60% of individuals. Because it reaches inferiorly only to the *pubic pecten* and *iliopectineal eminence,* it acts as a flexor of the trunk.

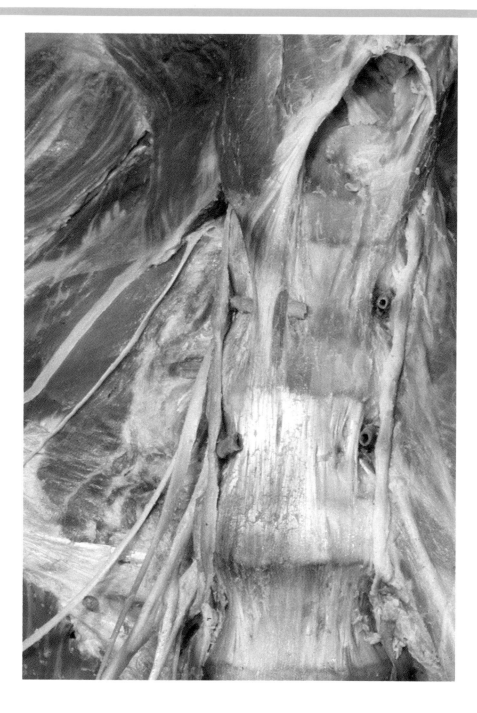

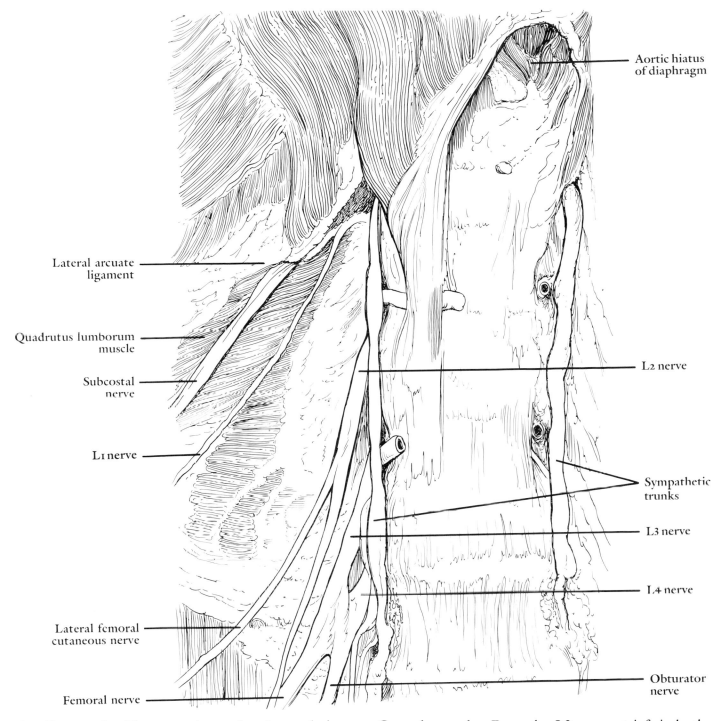

Aortic hiatus
of diaphragm

Lateral arcuate
ligament

Quadrutus lumborum
muscle

Subcostal
nerve

L1 nerve

Lateral femoral
cutaneous nerve

Femoral nerve

L2 nerve

Sympathetic
trunks

L3 nerve

L4 nerve

Obturator
nerve

Specific remarks: The *psoas minor* and *major muscles* have been removed piecemeal during tracing of the peripheral branches of the *lumbar plexus* toward their origins. Distribution of the *lumbar nerves* through the plexus and the course of the terminal branches on the posterior abdominal wall are demonstrated.

General remarks: From the L2 segment inferiorly the *spinal nerves* are connected to the sympathetic ganglia only by way of postganglionic *gray rami*.

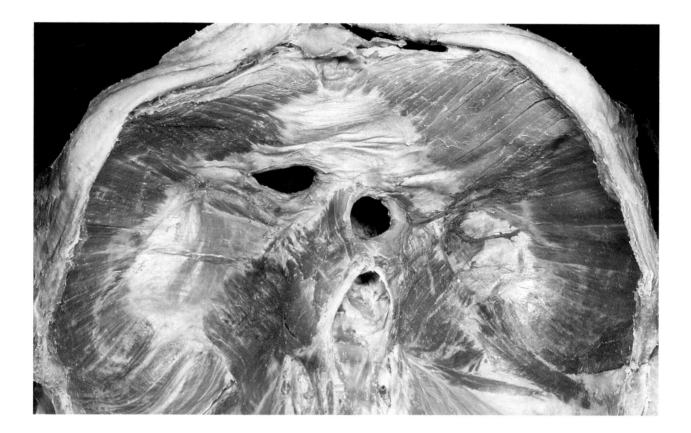

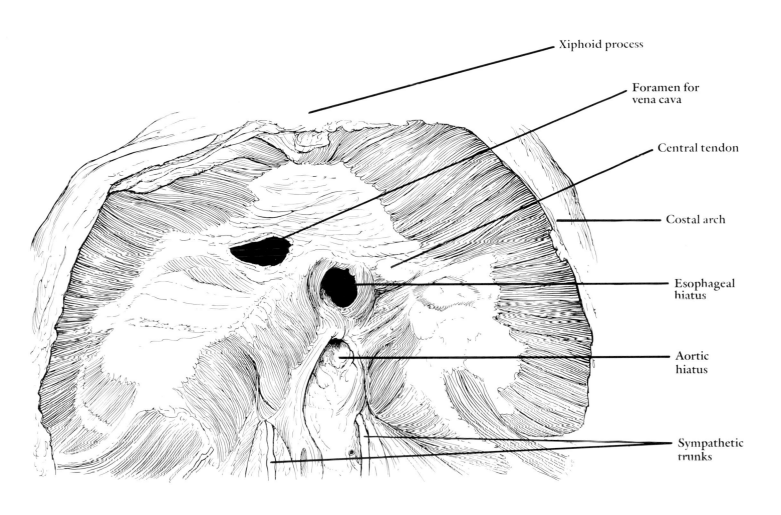

Xiphoid process

Foramen for
vena cava

Central tendon

Costal arch

Esophageal
hiatus

Aortic
hiatus

Sympathetic
trunks

Specific remarks: To show attachments of all parts of the *diaphragm,* the *parietal peritoneum* has been removed from its inferior surface. Those structures passing through the diaphragm have also been removed from their respective openings.

General remarks: Abdominal viscera occasionally herniate through the low resistance points of the diaphragm, such as the *esophageal hiatus,* into the *thorax.*

References

171

Brizon, J., Castaing, J., and Hourtaille, F.C.: Le péritoine, Paris, 1956, Maloine.

172

Barlow, T.E., Bentley, F.H., and Walden, D.N.: Arteries, veins, and arteriovenous anastomoses in the human stomach, Surg. Gynecol. Obstet. **93**:657, 1951.

Horton, R.C.: The gastroepiploic arteries. Guy's Hosp. Rep. **101**:108, 1952.

174

Cokkinis, A.J.: Observations on the mesenteric circulation, J. Anat. **64**:200, 1930.

175

Anson, B.J.: Anatomical considerations in surgery of the gallbladder, Quart. Bull. Northwestern U. Med. School **30**:250, 1956.

Michels, N.A.: The anatomic variations of the arterial pancreaticoduodenal arcades: their import in regional resection involving the gallbladder, bile duct, liver, pancreas, and parts of the small and large intestines, J. Int. Coll. Surg. **37**:13, 1962.

176

Beck, I.T., and Sincler, D.G.: The exocrine pancreas, London, 1971, Churchill Livingstone.

179

Atkinson, M., et al.: Comparison of cardiac and pyloric sphincters: a manometric study, Lancet **2**:918, 1957.

Cornes, J.S.: Number, size, and distribution of Peyer's patches in the human small intestine. II. The development of Peyer's patches, Gut **6**:225, 1965.

180

Argème, M., et al.: Dissection du muscle de Treitz, C.R. Assoc. Anat. **174**:76, 1970.

DiDio, L.J., and Anderson, M.C.: The "sphincters" of the digestive system, Baltimore, 1968, The Williams & Wilkins Co.

186

Elias, H.: Liver morphology, Biol. Rev. **30**:263, 1955.

Koguerman-Lepp, E.P.: Hepatic veins and venous blood outflow from liver segments in man, Arkh. Anat. Gistol. Embriol. **55**:105, 1968.

Outrequin, G., Caix, M., and Casanova, G.: Variations du ligament triangulaire gauche du foie en function du type morphologique, C.R. Assoc. Anat. **136**:756, 1967.

193

Fourman, J., and Moffat, D.B.: The blood vessels of the kidney, Oxford, 1971, Blackwell Scientific Publications.

Schneider, U., Inke, G., and Schneider, J.G.: Zahle, Abstand der Verzweigungsstellen vom Rand des Sinus renalis und Kaliber der extrarenalen Nierengefässe des Menschen, Anat. Anz. **124**:278, 1969.

195

Keagy, R.D., Brumlik, J., and Bergan, J.L.: Direct electromyography of the psoas major muscle in man, J. Bone Joint Surg. **48A**:1377, 1966.

McKiblin, B.: The action of the iliopsoas muscle in the newborn, J. Bone Joint Surg. **50B**:161, 1968.

197

Boyd, W., Blincoe, H., and Heyner, J.C.: Sequence of action of the diaphragm and quadratus lumborum during quiet breathing, Anat. Rec. **151**:579, 1965.

Thornton, M.W., and Schweisthal, M.R.: The phrenic nerve: its terminal divisions and supply to the crura of the diaphragm, Anat. Rec. **164**:283, 1969.

Part Five
PELVIS

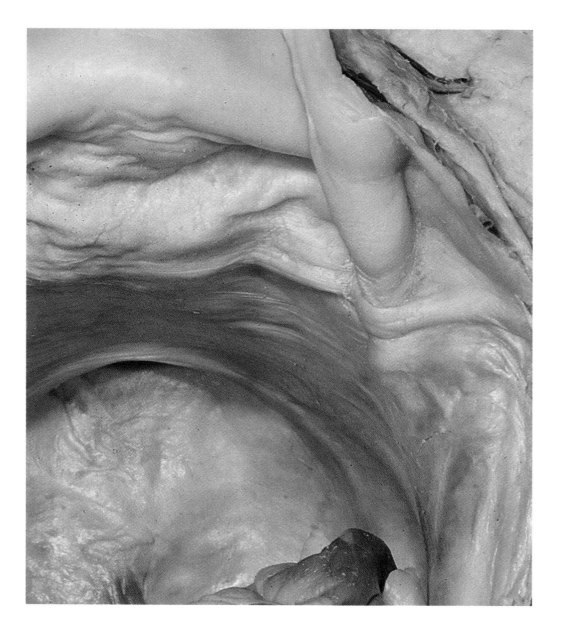

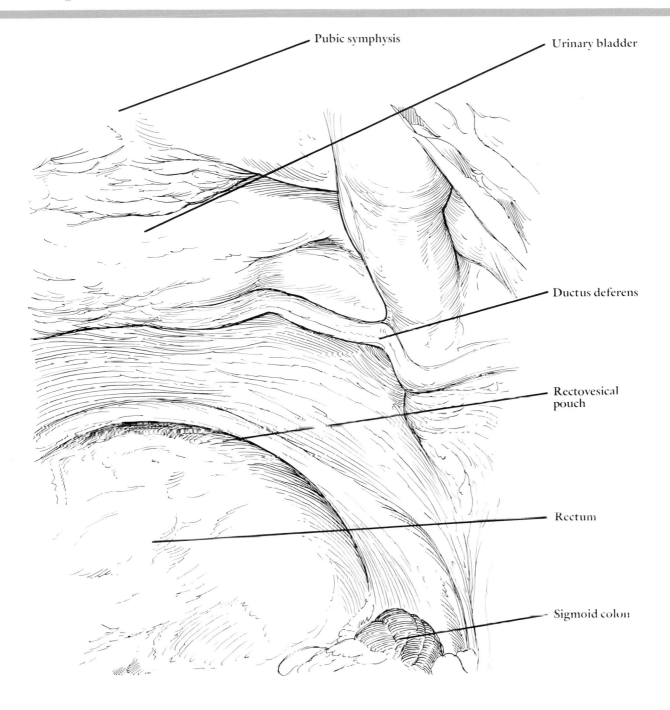

Pubic symphysis

Urinary bladder

Ductus deferens

Rectovesical
pouch

Rectum

Sigmoid colon

Specific remarks: Coils of the small intestine have been removed from the *pelvic inlet* and the *sigmoid colon* reflected superiorly and to the right. The *parietal peritoneum* covering the superior aspect of the *pelvic viscera* is kept intact in this view. Superior and posterior aspects of the *urinary bladder* and the anterior aspect of the *rectum* are demonstrated. The parietal peritoneum, as it reflects from the posterior aspect of the urinary bladder and *seminal vesicles* to the anterior rectal wall, forms the most inferior peritoneal recess—the *rectovesical pouch*.

General remarks: Infectious fluid tends to descend from the general peritoneal cavity into the rectovesical pouch. From there it may be evacuated through the rectum.

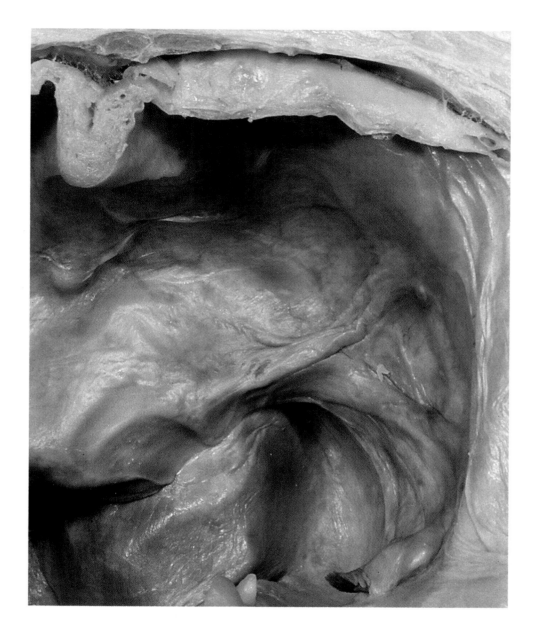

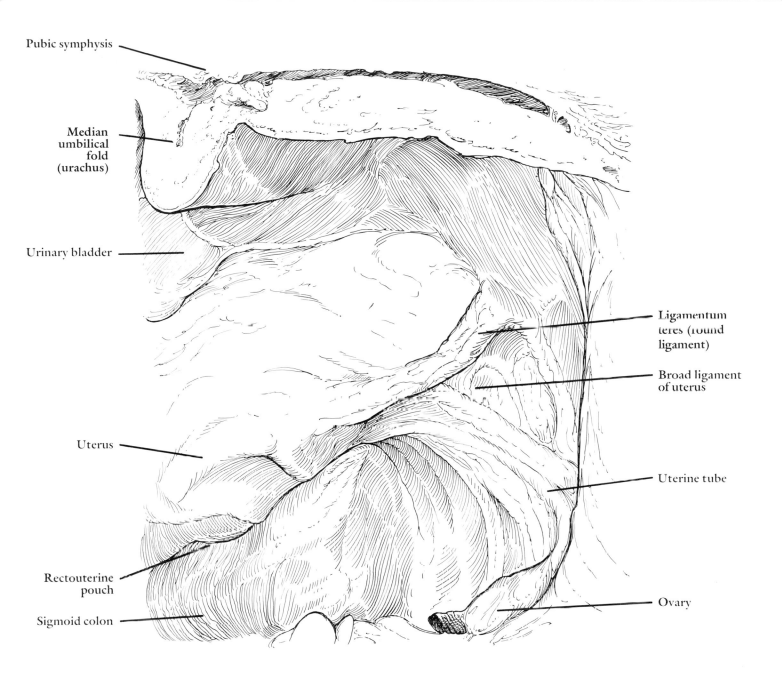

Pubic symphysis

Median umbilical fold (urachus)

Urinary bladder

Uterus

Rectouterine pouch

Sigmoid colon

Ligamentum teres (round ligament)

Broad ligament of uterus

Uterine tube

Ovary

Specific remarks: Coils of the small intestine have been removed from the *pelvic inlet* and the *sigmoid colon* reflected superiorly and to the right. The *parietal peritoneum* and *peritoneal ligaments,* which either cover or relate to the *pelvic viscera,* are kept intact in this view. The superior aspect of the *urinary bladder, uterus, uterine tube,* and the *ovary* and the anterior aspect of the *rectum* are demonstrated. The parietal peritoneum, as it reflects from the posterior aspect of the uterus to the anterior rectal wall, forms the most inferior peritoneal recess—the *rectouterine pouch.*

General remarks: The importance of the rectouterine pouch in the female is comparable to that of the *rectovesical pouch* in the male. Exploration of this space can be achieved through the rectum or through the vagina.

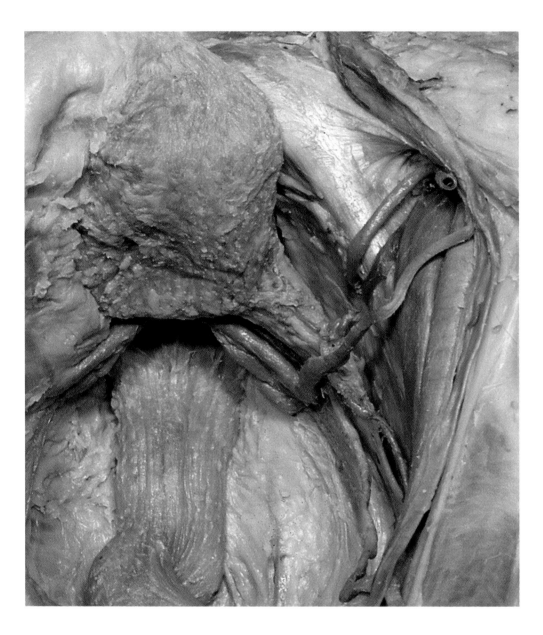

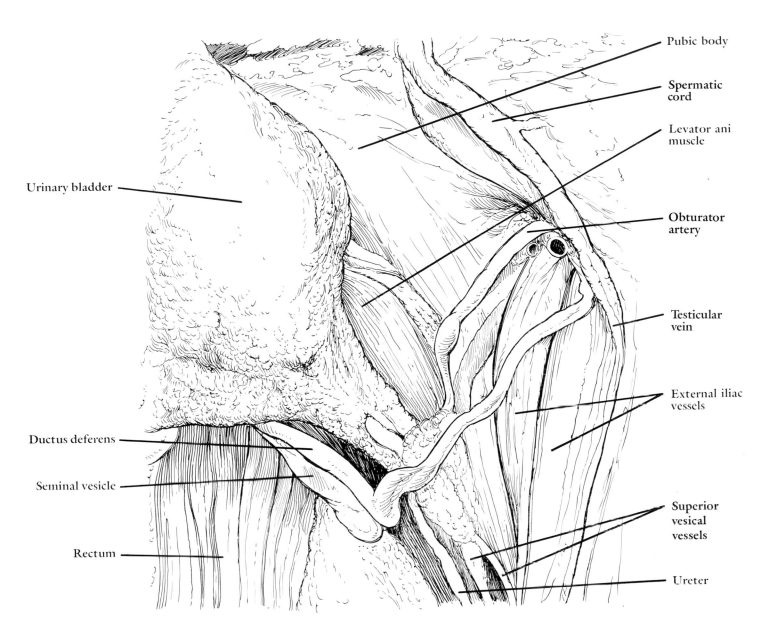

Pubic body

Spermatic cord

Levator ani muscle

Obturator artery

Testicular vein

External iliac vessels

Superior vesical vessels

Ureter

Urinary bladder

Ductus deferens

Seminal vesicle

Rectum

Specific remarks: Following the removal of the *parietal peritoneum* from the pelvic organs it is possible to demonstrate the musculature of the *urinary bladder* and *rectum*. *Ureters, seminal vesicles,* and *ductus deferentes* are demonstrated in relation to the bladder.

General remarks: The ductus deferens extends through the pelvic cavity and then enters the *inguinal canal* along with the *testicular blood vessels*. After exiting the canal at the *superficial inguinal ring*, these elements become incorporated into the *spermatic cord*.

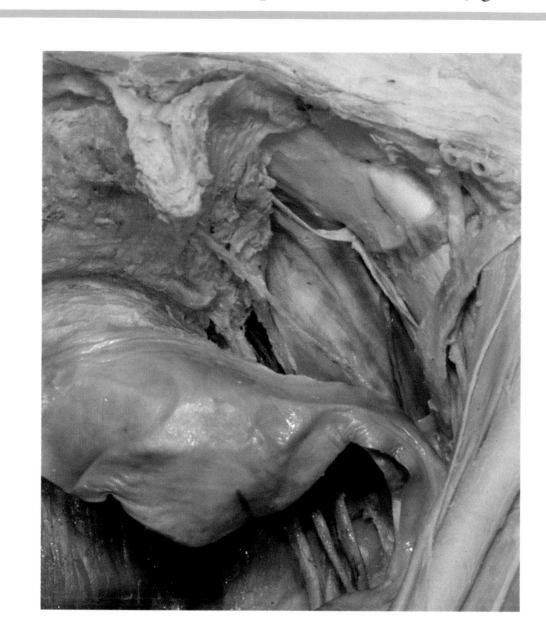

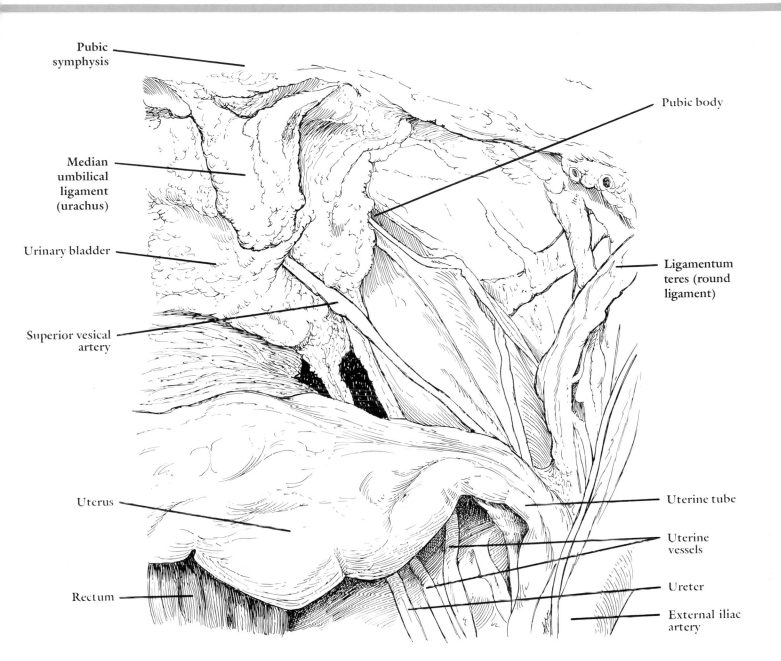

Pubic symphysis

Median umbilical ligament (urachus)

Urinary bladder

Superior vesical artery

Uterus

Rectum

Pubic body

Ligamentum teres (round ligament)

Uterine tube

Uterine vessels

Ureter

External iliac artery

Specific remarks: Following the removal of the *parietal peritoneum* from the *urinary bladder* and the *rectum*, the musculature of these organs is exposed. Peritoneal covering of the *uterus* and *uterine tube* is still in place.

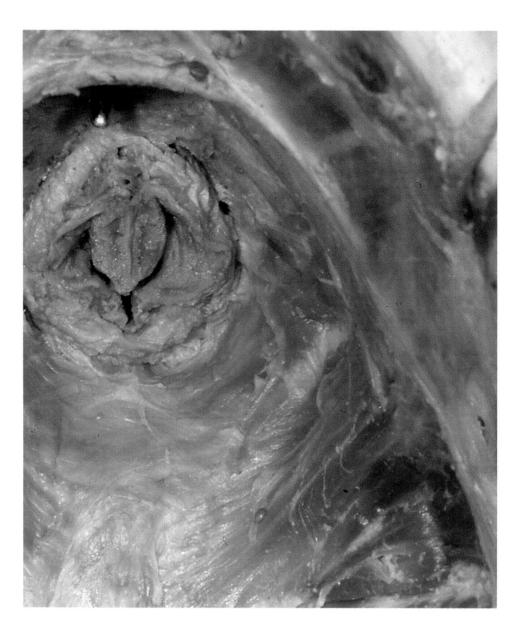

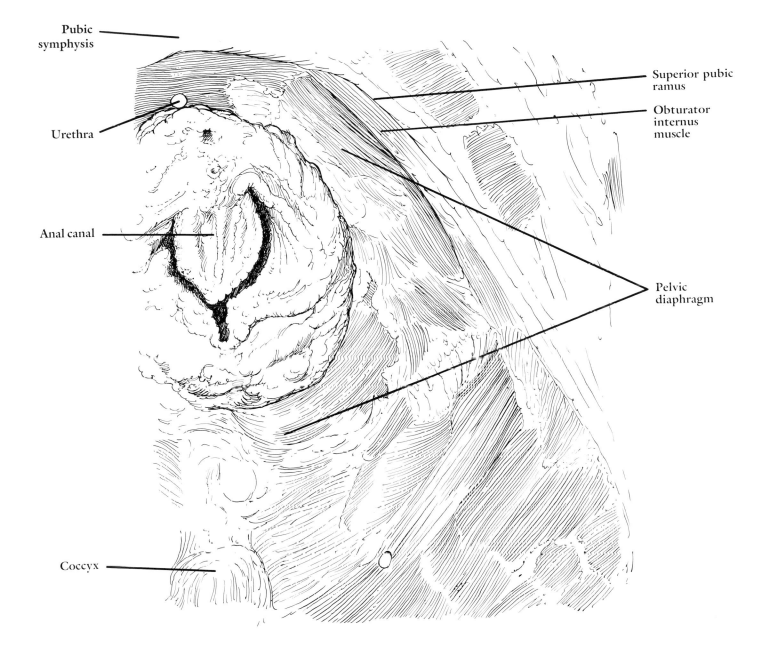

Pubic
symphysis

Superior pubic
ramus

Obturator
internus
muscle

Urethra

Anal canal

Pelvic
diaphragm

Coccyx

Specific remarks: The *anal canal* and *urethra* have been cut just above the level of the *pelvic diaphragm,* and the *pelvic viscera,* blood vessels, nerves, and the *superior fascia of the diaphragm* have been removed from the region. The two openings in the diaphragm are consequently shown: the *urethral,* indicated by a probe, and the *anal.* In addition, the disposition, attachments, and the parts of the *levator ani muscle* are demonstrated.

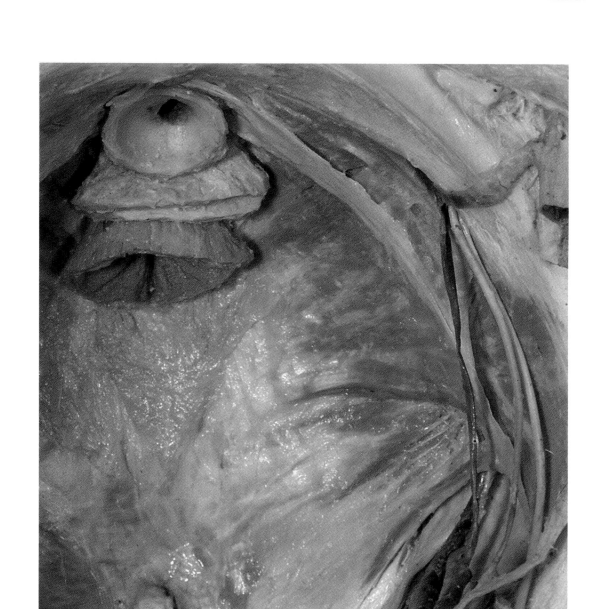

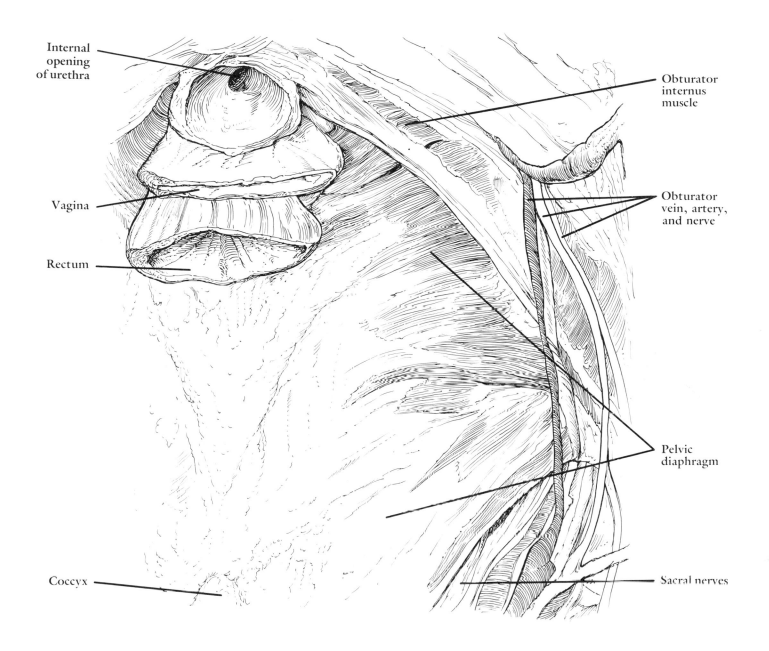

Internal opening of urethra

Obturator internus muscle

Vagina

Obturator vein, artery, and nerve

Rectum

Pelvic diaphragm

Coccyx

Sacral nerves

Specific remarks: The *anal canal, vagina,* and *urethra* have been cut just above the level of the *pelvic diaphragm,* and the *pelvic viscera,* blood vessels, nerves, and the *superior fascia of the diaphragm* have been removed from the region. The three openings in the diaphragm are consequently shown: the *urethral,* the *vaginal,* and the *anal.* In addition, the disposition, attachments, and parts of the *levator ani muscle* are demonstrated.

General remarks: Integrity of the pelvic diaphragm, especially after parturition and damage to the *perineal body,* is important for the maintenance of pelvic viscera in situ. If the resistance of the diaphragm does not meet this requirement, a prolapse of pelvic viscera, in particular those of the *genital tract,* is likely to occur.

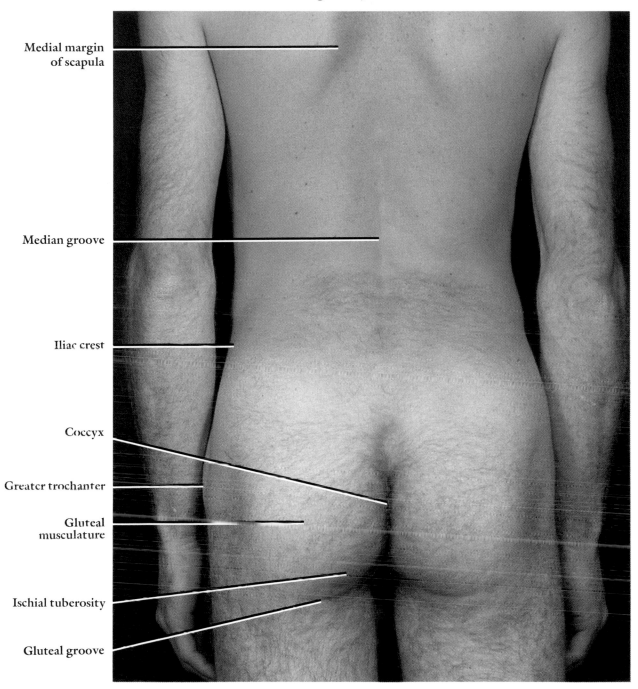

Medial margin
of scapula

Median groove

Iliac crest

Coccyx

Greater trochanter

Gluteal
musculature

Ischial tuberosity

Gluteal groove

General remarks: *Spines* of the *thoracic, lumbar,* and *sacral vertebrae* are readily palpable along the *median sulcus.* The outline of the *scapula,* in particular of the *vertebral border* and the *inferior angle,* is accessible to inspection and palpation, as are the *ribs, iliac crest, greater trochanter of the femur,* and *ischial tuberosity.* In relation to skeletal elements it is possible to ascertain the corresponding muscles.

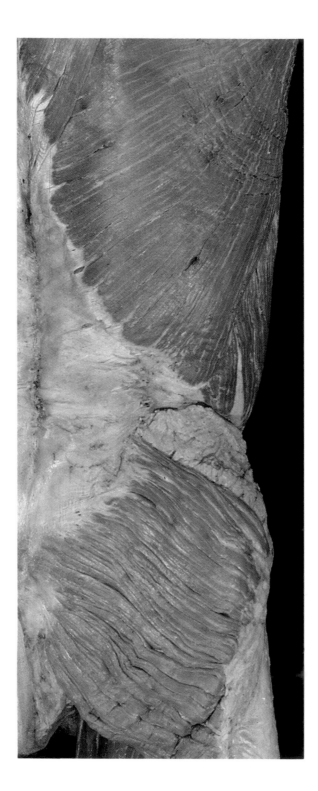

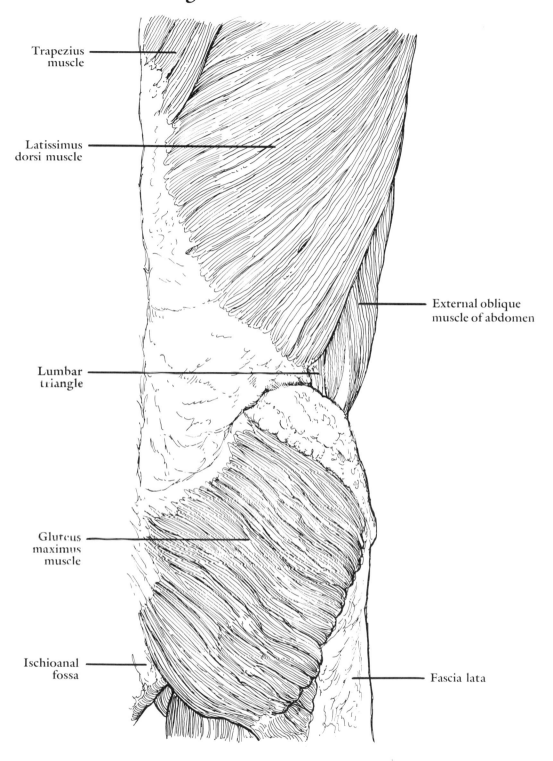

Trapezius muscle

Latissimus dorsi muscle

External oblique muscle of abdomen

Lumbar triangle

Gluteus maximus muscle

Ischioanal fossa

Fascia lata

Specific remarks: Regional skin, subcutaneous tissue, and fascia have been removed to demonstrate the iliolumbar attachment of the *latissimus dorsi muscle,* the posterior part of the *external oblique muscle of the abdomen,* and the *gluteus maximus muscle.* It is apparent in this view how the latter muscle relates laterally to the *greater trochanter* and to the *fascia lata.*

General remarks: The *lumbar triangle* is bounded by the latissimus dorsi muscle superomedially, the external abdominal oblique muscle superolaterally, and by the *iliac crest* inferiorly. The floor of the triangle is made of the *internal abdominal oblique muscle.* Herniation seldom occurs through this triangle.

206

Posterior aspect of the right erector spinae, posterior inferior serratus, and internal abdominal oblique muscles and the middle layer of the gluteal region

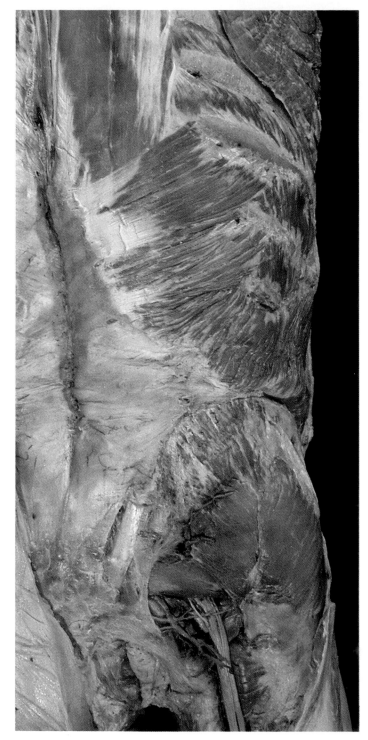

Posterior aspect of the right erector spinae, posterior inferior serratus, 206
and internal abdominal oblique muscles and the middle layer
of the gluteal region

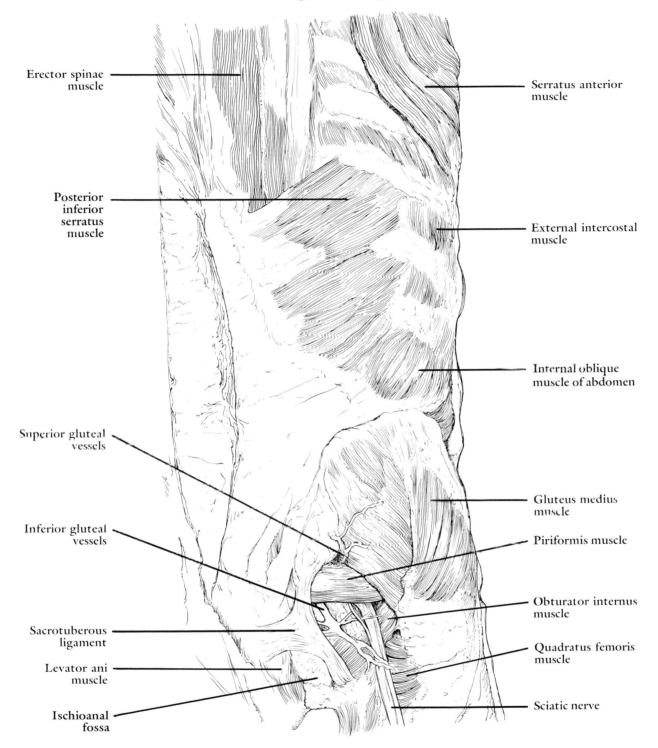

Erector spinae muscle

Posterior inferior serratus muscle

Superior gluteal vessels

Inferior gluteal vessels

Sacrotuberous ligament

Levator ani muscle

Ischioanal fossa

Serratus anterior muscle

External intercostal muscle

Internal oblique muscle of abdomen

Gluteus medius muscle

Piriformis muscle

Obturator internus muscle

Quadratus femoris muscle

Sciatic nerve

Specific remarks: After the *trapezius, latissimus doris, external abdominal oblique,* and *gluteus maximus muscles* have been removed from respective regions, the following muscles are exposed in the lower back region: *posterior inferior serratus, erector spinae,* and *internal abdominal oblique.* Blood vessels and nerves that pass from the pelvic area into the gluteal region are topographically related to the *piriformis muscle.* While the *superior gluteal vessels* and *nerve* enter the gluteal region superior to the muscle, the *inferior gluteal vessels* and *nerve,* the *sciatic nerve,* and the *posterior femoral cutaneous nerve* are related to the inferior border of the muscle.

General remarks: Intramuscular injection is usually done in the superolateral quadrant of the gluteal region to avoid the sciatic nerve and other nerves and blood vessels that are close to it.

Posterior aspect of the right erector spinae, quadratus lumborum, and transversus abdominis muscles and the deep layer of the gluteal region

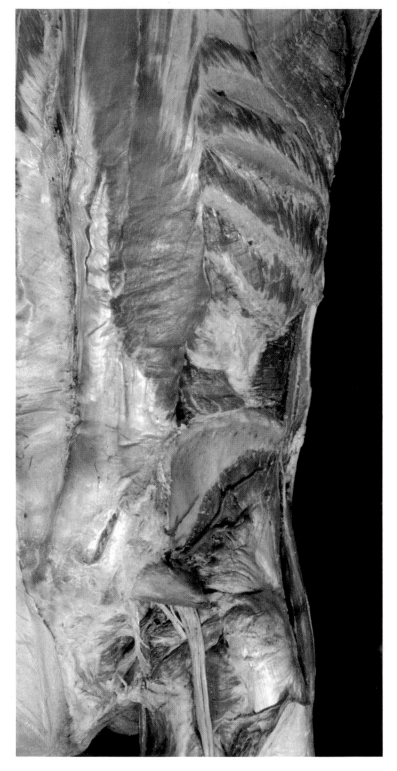

Posterior aspect of the right erector spinae, quadratus lumborum, and transversus abdominis muscles and the deep layer of the gluteal region

207

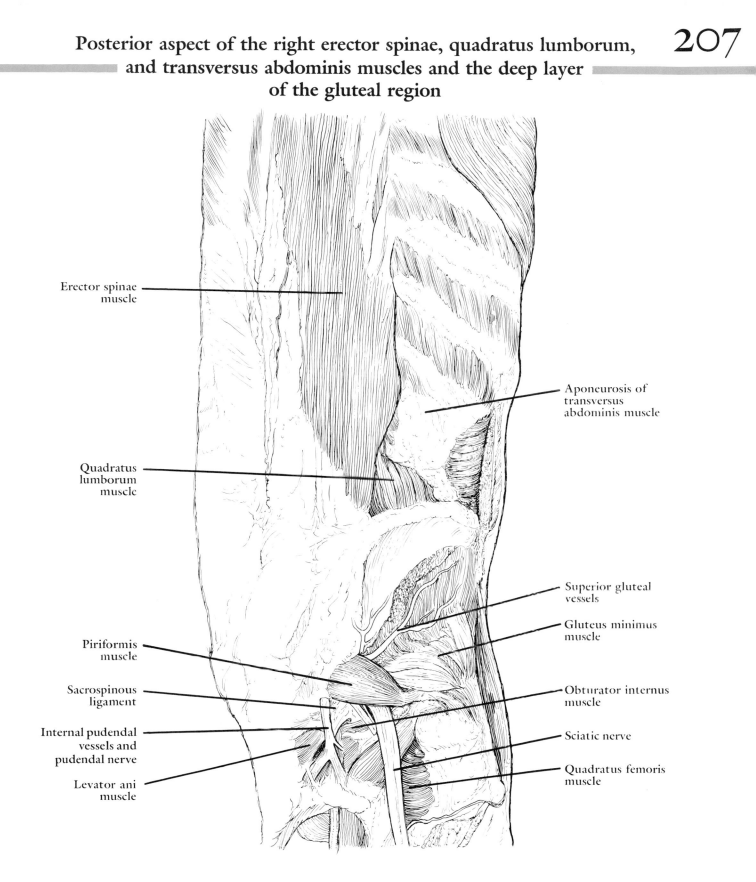

Erector spinae muscle

Quadratus lumborum muscle

Piriformis muscle

Sacrospinous ligament

Internal pudendal vessels and pudendal nerve

Levator ani muscle

Aponeurosis of transversus abdominis muscle

Superior gluteal vessels

Gluteus minimus muscle

Obturator internus muscle

Sciatic nerve

Quadratus femoris muscle

Specific remarks: The following structures have been removed for this view: *posterior inferior serratus muscle, internal abdominal oblique muscle, gluteus medius muscle,* and *sacrotuberous ligament.* Starting from the sacroiliac attachment the *erector spinae muscle* differentiates superiorly into the *iliocostal, longissimus,* and *spinalis* bundles from lateral to medial. With the sacrotuberous ligament removed, both walls of the *ischioanal fossa*—the medial *(levator ani muscle)* and the lateral *(obturator internus muscle)*—are demonstrated.

General remarks: The ischioanal fossa is an infrequent site of herniation.

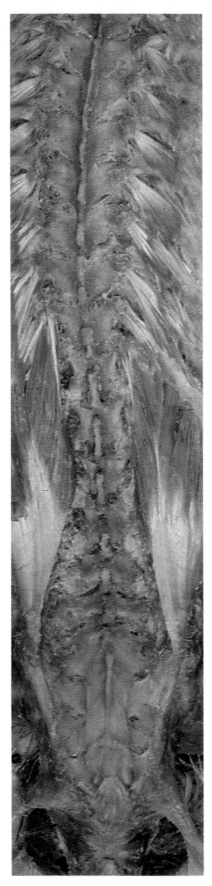

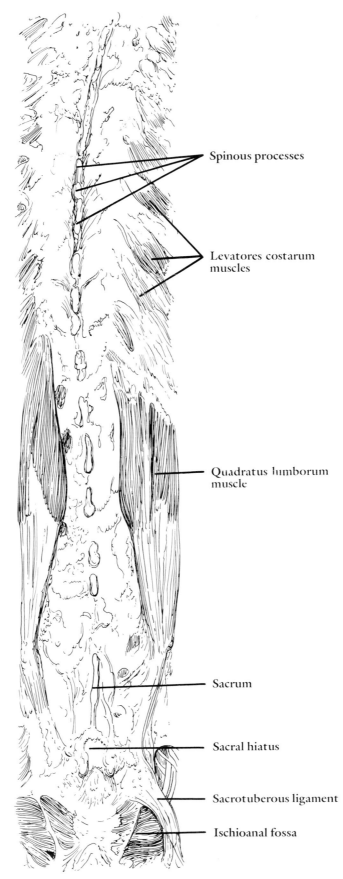

Spinous processes

Levatores costarum muscles

Quadratus lumborum muscle

Sacrum

Sacral hiatus

Sacrotuberous ligament

Ischioanal fossa

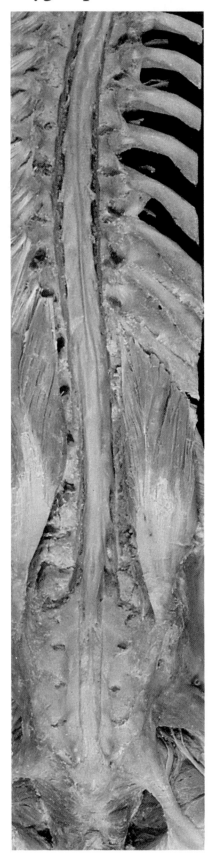

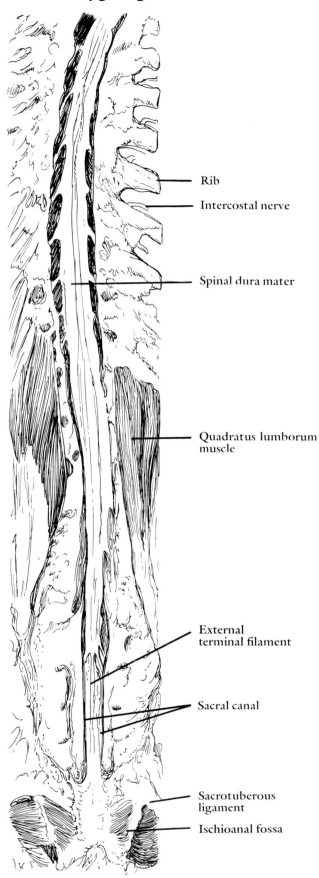

Rib

Intercostal nerve

Spinal dura mater

Quadratus lumborum muscle

External terminal filament

Sacral canal

Sacrotuberous ligament

Ischioanal fossa

210   Posterior aspect of the spinal cord, roots, and ganglia within
the thoracic, lumbar, sacral, and coccygeal parts
of the vertebral canal

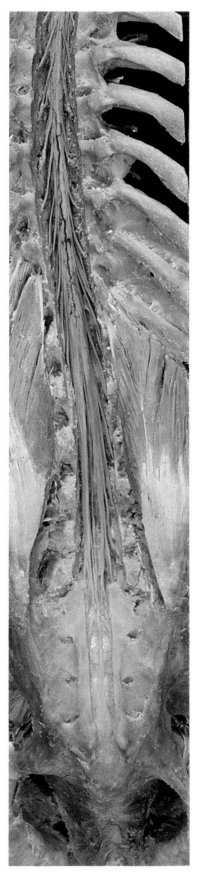

Posterior aspect of the spinal cord, roots, and ganglia within
the thoracic, lumbar, sacral, and coccygeal parts
of the vertebral canal

210

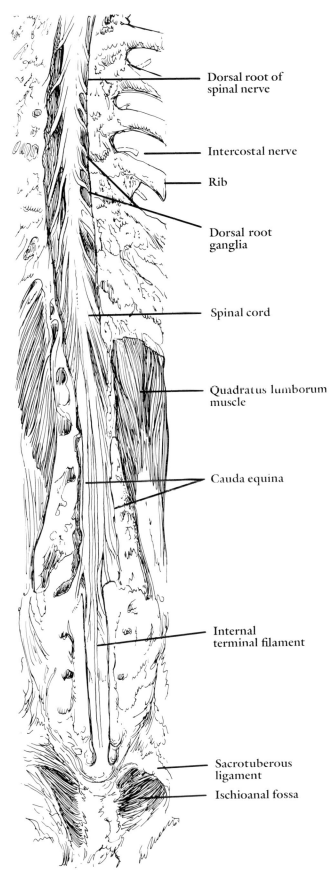

Dorsal root of
spinal nerve

Intercostal nerve

Rib

Dorsal root
ganglia

Spinal cord

Quadratus lumborum
muscle

Cauda equina

Internal
terminal filament

Sacrotuberous
ligament

Ischioanal fossa

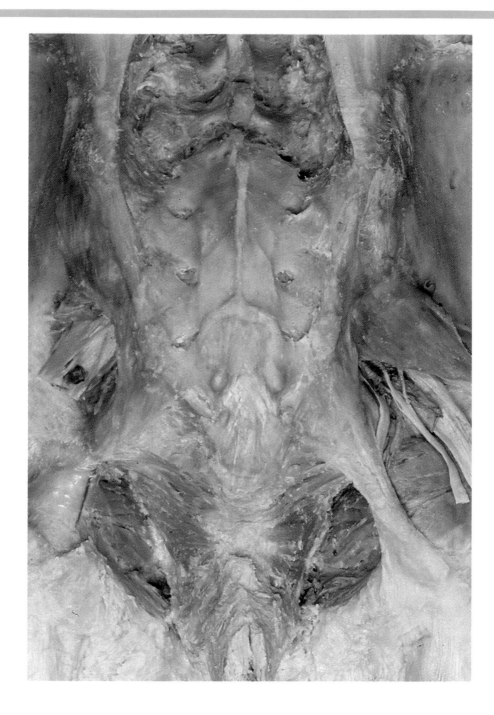

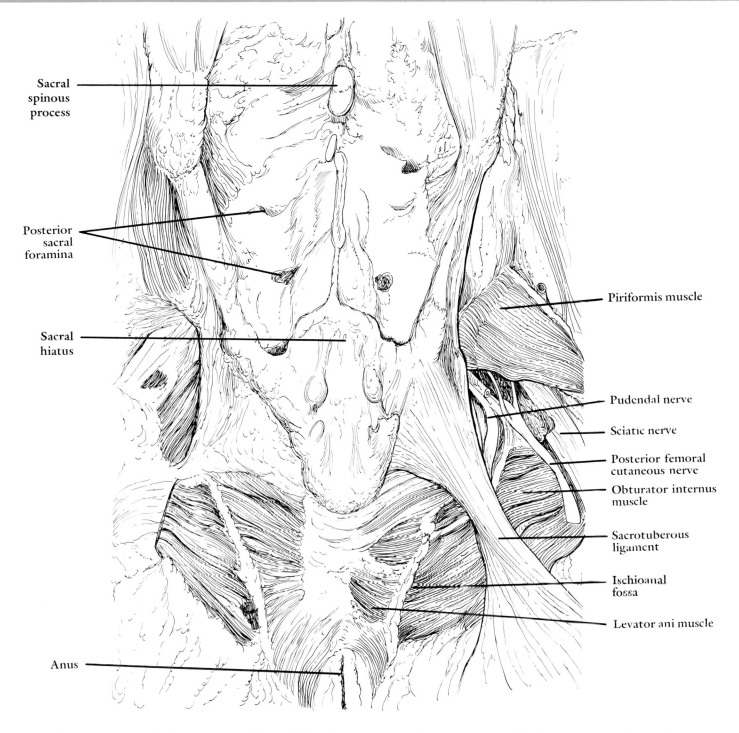

Sacral spinous process

Posterior sacral foramina

Sacral hiatus

Anus

Piriformis muscle

Pudendal nerve

Sciatic nerve

Posterior femoral cutaneous nerve

Obturator internus muscle

Sacrotuberous ligament

Ischioanal fossa

Levator ani muscle

Specific remarks: With the exception of the *piriformis, gemellus superior, obturator internus, gemellus inferior, levator* and *sphincter ani muscles,* the *sacrotuberous ligament,* and the *sciatic, posterior femoral cutaneous,* and *pudendal* nerves, all structures have been removed from the posterior aspect of these regions. The *infrapiriform compartment of the greater sciatic foramen* and its contents are demonstrated. The pudendal nerve, like the *internal pudendal vessels,* passes first through the *greater sciatic foramen,* posterior to the *sacrospinous ligament,* through the *lesser sciatic foramen,* and then continues anteriorly into the *ischioanal fossa.*

General remarks: Because of its deep position the pudendal nerve can be anesthetized by a needle directed from the vaginal wall toward the *ischial spine,* which is palpable through the vaginal wall.

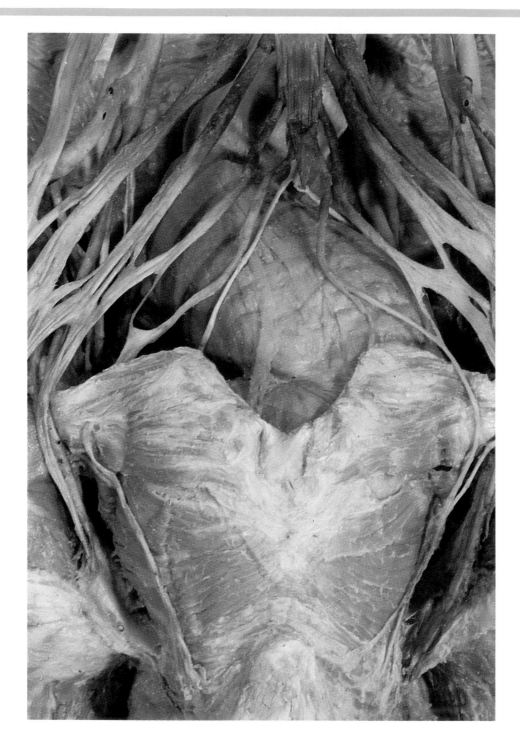

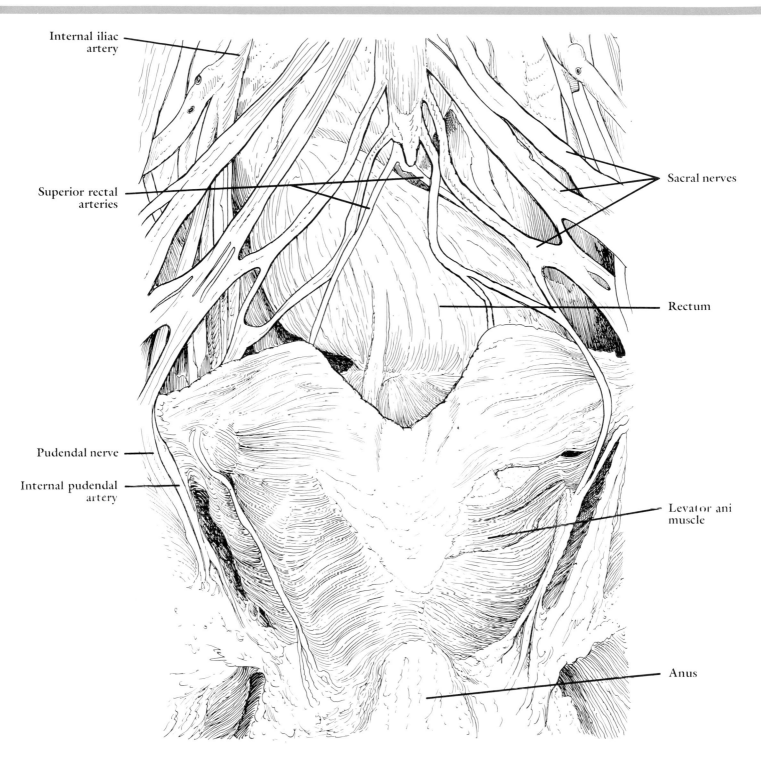

Internal iliac artery

Superior rectal arteries

Pudendal nerve

Internal pudendal artery

Sacral nerves

Rectum

Levator ani muscle

Anus

Specific remarks: The *vertebral column* with adjacent parts of the hip bone and associated ligaments has been removed, whereas the *sacral plexus,* terminal branches of the plexus, and the *levator ani muscle* have been dissected out and preserved in anatomical position. The *rectum* and *rectal blood vessels* are shown in a position anterior to the *sacral nerves*.

General remarks: The superior rectal veins drain into the *portal system;* the middle and inferior rectal veins are tributaries of the systemic circulation. Because of extensive anastomoses among the rectal veins, the portosystemic shunt is readily established when the portal circulation is impaired or occluded. Such conditions cause varicosities in the rectoanal wall.

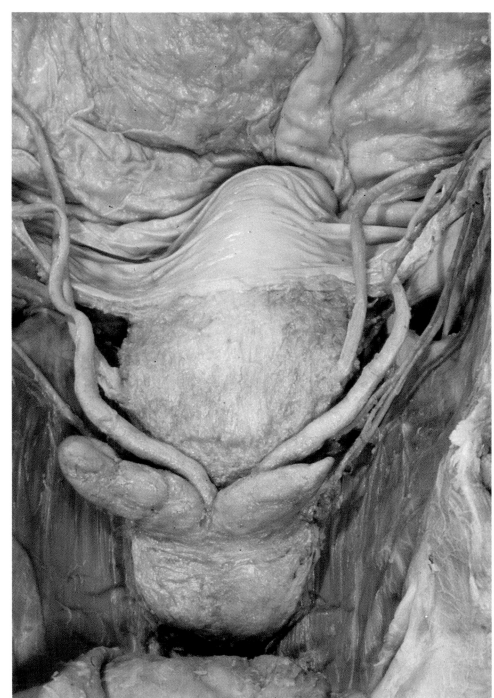

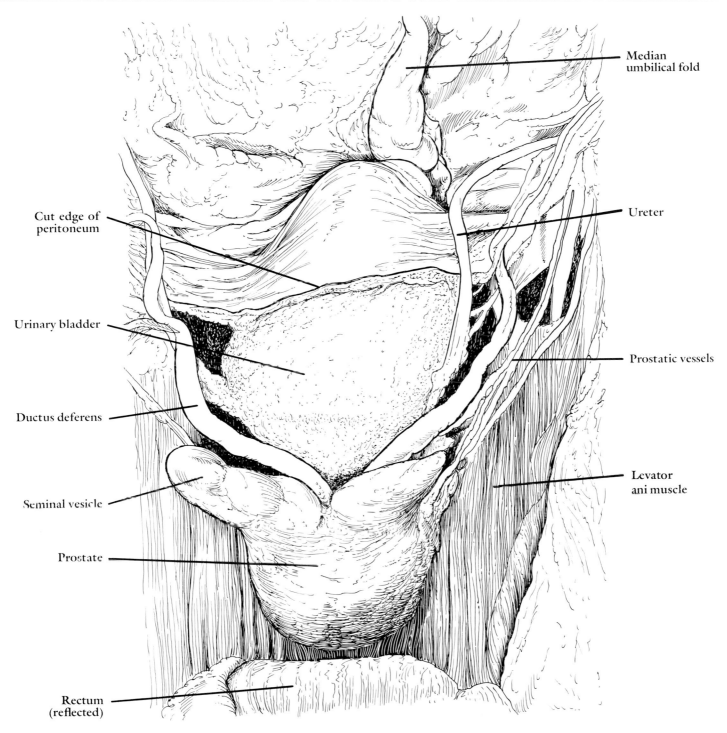

Median umbilical fold

Cut edge of peritoneum

Ureter

Urinary bladder

Ductus deferens

Prostatic vessels

Seminal vesicle

Levator ani muscle

Prostate

Rectum (reflected)

Specific remarks: When the *sacral plexus* is removed and the *rectum* reflected inferiorly, the posterior aspect of the *urinary bladder, seminal vesicles,* and *prostate* become apparent. Although the *parietal peritoneum* is kept intact on the superior aspect of the bladder, the relationship of the latter organ with the *ureters, ductus deferentes,* and *seminal vesicles* is well demonstrated. Pelvic viscera are supported in situ mostly by the *levator ani muscle* together with the *superior* and *inferior fasciae.*

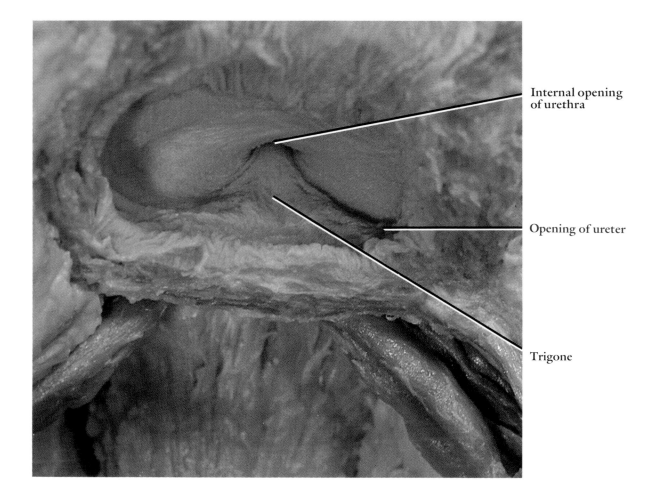

Internal opening
of urethra

Opening of ureter

Trigone

Specific remarks: The *urinary bladder* has been sectioned
horizontally through the middle and the superior segment
of the organ removed.

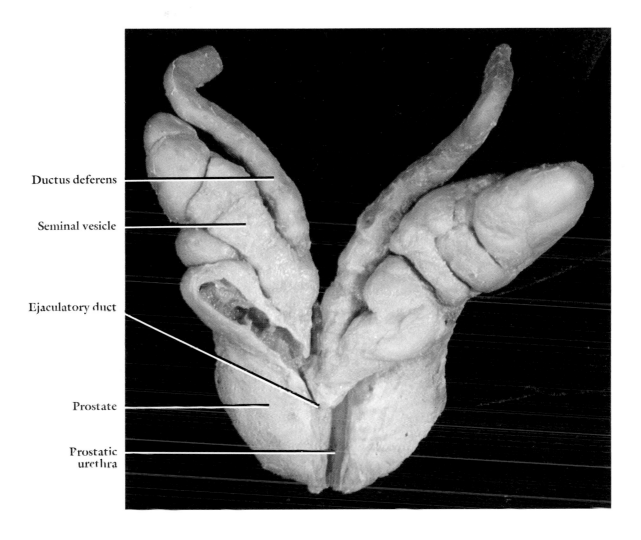

Ductus deferens

Seminal vesicle

Ejaculatory duct

Prostate

Prostatic urethra

Specific remarks: Terminal parts of left *ductus deferens* and *seminal vesicle* have been opened posteriorly to demonstrate their union and formation of the *ejaculatory duct*. The passage of the latter duct in the *prostate* to the point of junction with the *prostatic part of the urethra* is shown.

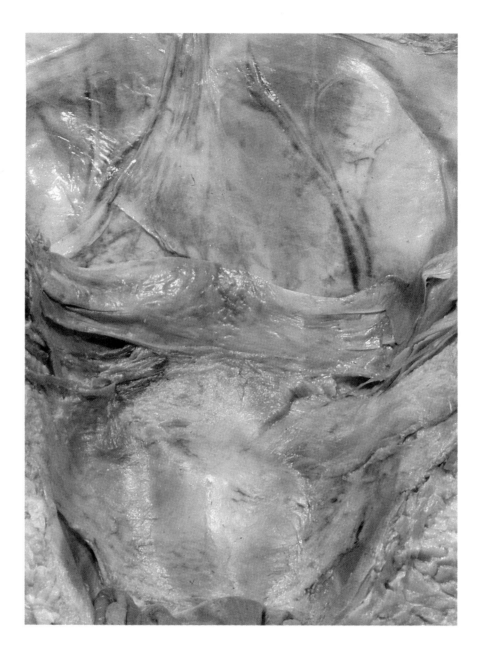

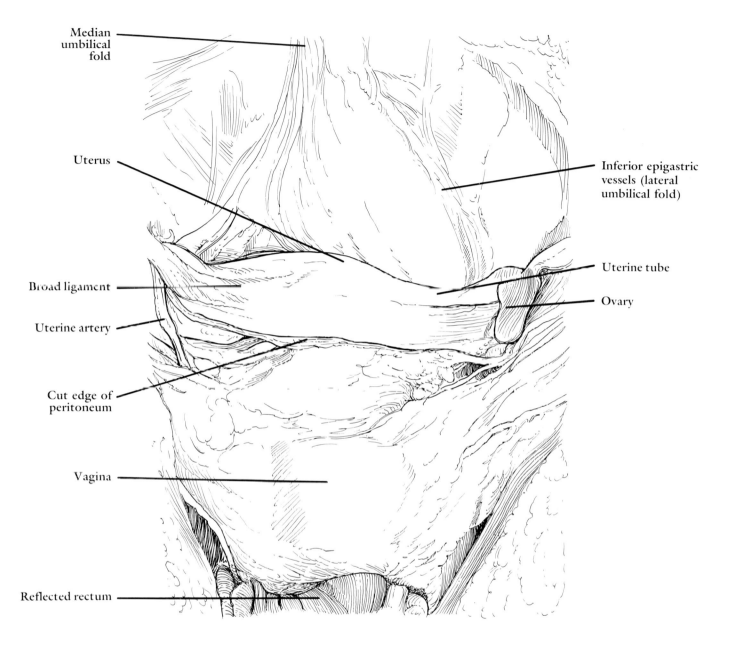

Median umbilical fold

Uterus

Broad ligament

Uterine artery

Cut edge of peritoneum

Vagina

Reflected rectum

Inferior epigastric vessels (lateral umbilical fold)

Uterine tube

Ovary

Specific remarks: Immediately anterior to the *rectum*, which has been reflected inferiorly, and the *rectouterine pouch* are the *vagina, uterus, uterine tube,* and *ovary.* That part of the *parietal peritoneum* which is related to the *uterine fundus,* uterine tube, and ovary is still maintained in situ.

Medial aspect of a sagittal section through the male pelvis, perineum, and external genitalia

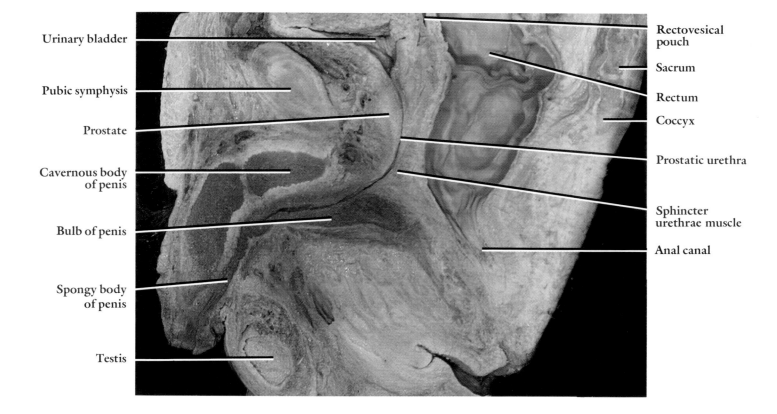

Urinary bladder

Pubic symphysis

Prostate

Cavernous body of penis

Bulb of penis

Spongy body of penis

Testis

Rectovesical pouch

Sacrum

Rectum

Coccyx

Prostatic urethra

Sphincter urethrae muscle

Anal canal

Specific remarks: This section has been made through the *pubic symphysis* and the tip of the *coccyx*. The right face of the section is presented.

General remarks: The *perineum*, which is well demonstrated in this view, in addition to the *pelvic diaphragm*, is an important supporting layer to the *pelvic viscera*.

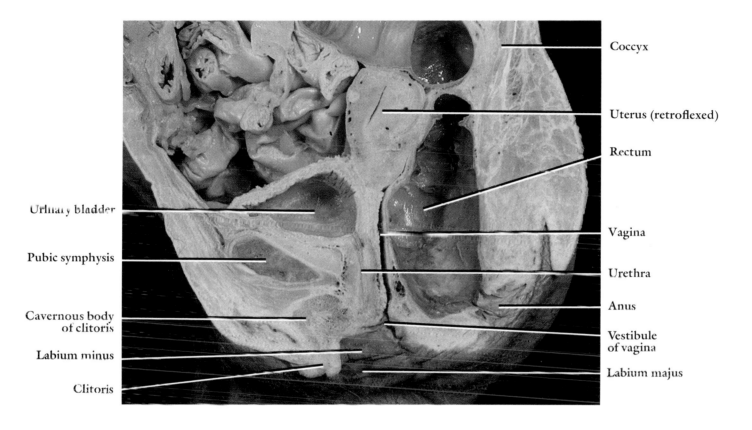

Coccyx

Uterus (retroflexed)

Rectum

Vagina

Urethra

Anus

Vestibule of vagina

Labium majus

Urinary bladder

Pubic symphysis

Cavernous body of clitoris

Labium minus

Clitoris

Specific remarks: This section has been made through the *pubic symphysis* and the tip of *coccyx*. The right face of the section is presented.

General remarks: The *perineum*, which is well demonstrated in this sectional view, in addition to the *pelvic diaphragm*, is an important supporting layer to the *pelvic viscera*. The long axis of the uterus is usually anteverted in relation to the long axis of the vagina. Furthermore, the angle (170 degrees) between the axes of the uterine body and cervical canal is opened anteriorly (anteflexed uterus). In this individual the uterus appears retroflexed with the axes of the uterus and vagina being parallel.

References

201

Tanagho, E.A., and Pugh, R.C.B.: The anatomy and function of the uterovesical junction, Br. J. Urol. **35**:151, 1963.

202

Wendell-Smith, C.P.: Studies on the morphology of the pelvic floor, Doctoral thesis, 1967, University of London.

204

Frobin, W., and Hierholzer, E.: Analysis of human back shape using surface curvatures, J. Biomech. **15**:379, 1982.

205

Joseph, J., and Williams, P.L.: Electromyography of certain hip muscles, J. Anat. **91**:286, 1957.

207

Floyd, F.W., and Silver, P.H.S.: The function of the erector spinae muscle in certain movements and postures in man, J. Physiol. (Lond.) **129**:184, 1955.

209

Batson, O.V.: The vertebral vein system, Am. J. Roentgenol. **78**:195, 1957.

210

Eccles, J.C., and Schade, J.P., editors: Organisation of the spinal cord, Prog. Brain Res., vol. II, 1964.

211

Nakanishi, T.: Studies on the pudendal nerve. I. Macroscopic observations on the pudendal nerve in humans, Acta Anat. Nippon. **42**:223, 1967.

213

Uhlenhuth, E., Hunter, D.W.T., and Loechel, W.E.: Problems in the anatomy of the pelvis, Philadelphia, 1952, J.B. Lippincott Co.

215

Bengmark, S.: The prostatic urethra and prostatic glands, London, England, 1958, Steerup.

Glenister, T.W.: The development of the utricle and of the so-called 'middle' or 'median' lobe of the human prostate, J. Anat. **96**:443, 1962.

Hutch, J.A., and Rambo, O.S., Jr.: A study of the anatomy of the prostate, prostatic urethra, and urinary sphincter system, J. Urol. **104**:443, 1970.

216

Farrer-Brown, G., Beilby, J.W., and Tarbit, M.M.: The blood supply of the uterus. I. Arterial vasculature, J. Obstet. Gynaec. Br. Commonw. **77**:673; II. Venous pattern, J. Obstet. Gynaec. Br. Commonw. **77**:682, 1970.

Koritké, J.G., Gillet, J.Y., and Pietri, J.: Les artères de la trompe uterine chez les femmes, Arch. Anat. Histol. Embryol. **50**:47, 1967.

Mastroianni, L.: The structure and function of the fallopian tube: a correlative review, Clin. Obstet. Gynecol. **5**:781, 1962.

Owman, C., Rosenbren, E., and Sjöberg, N.O.: Adrenergic innervation of the human female reproductive organs: a histochemical and chemical investigation, Obstet. Gynecol. **30**:763, 1967.

Woodruff, J.D., and Pauerstein, C.J.: The fallopian tube, Baltimore, 1969, The Williams & Wilkins Co.

217

Tanagho, E.A., and Miller, F.R.: Initiation of voiding, Br. J. Urol. **42**:175, 1970.

218

Smout, C.F.V., Jacoby, F., and Lillie, E.W.: Gynecological and obstetrical anatomy and functional histology, London, England, 1969, Arnold Publishers.

Part Six
PERINEUM

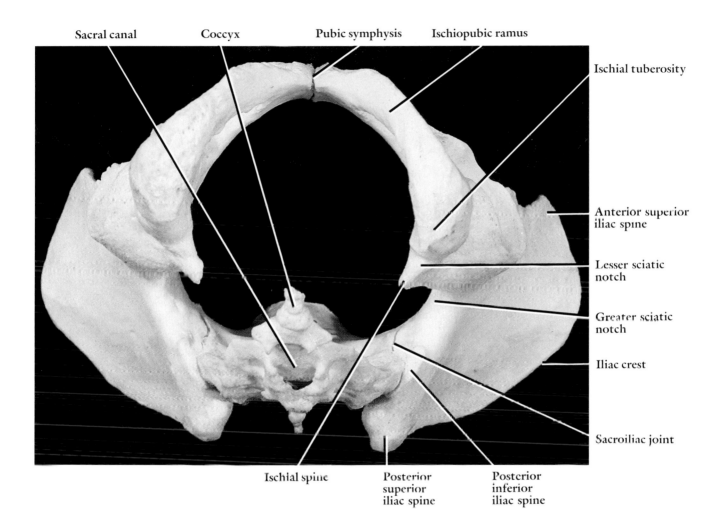

Sacral canal   Coccyx   Pubic symphysis   Ischiopubic ramus

Ischial tuberosity

Anterior superior iliac spine

Lesser sciatic notch

Greater sciatic notch

Iliac crest

Sacroiliac joint

Ischial spine   Posterior superior iliac spine   Posterior inferior iliac spine

Inferior aspect of the external genitalia and perineal region in a living male subject

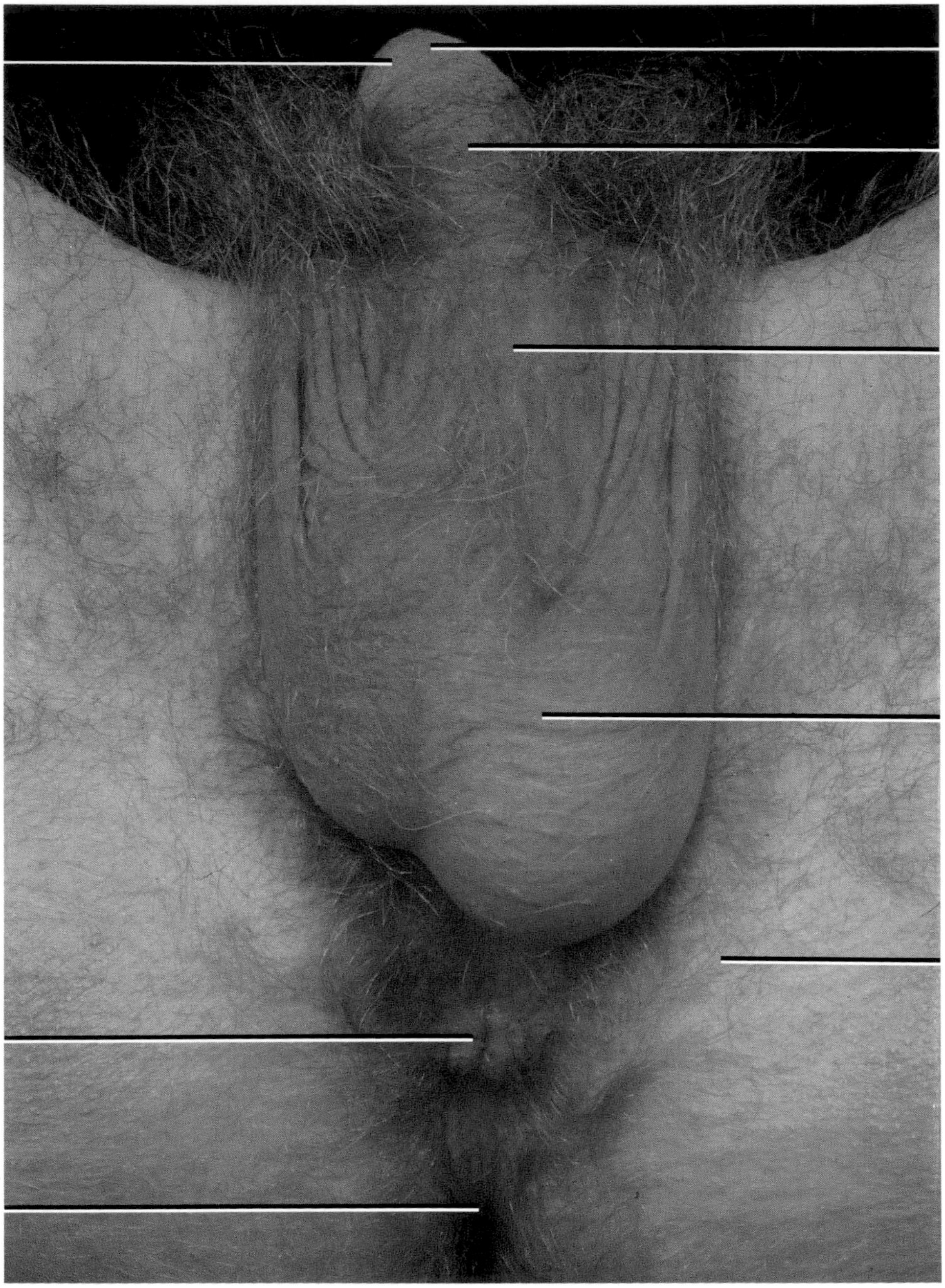

Glans penis

Prepuce

Body of penis

Pubic symphysis

Scrotum

Ischial tuberosity

Anus

Coccyx

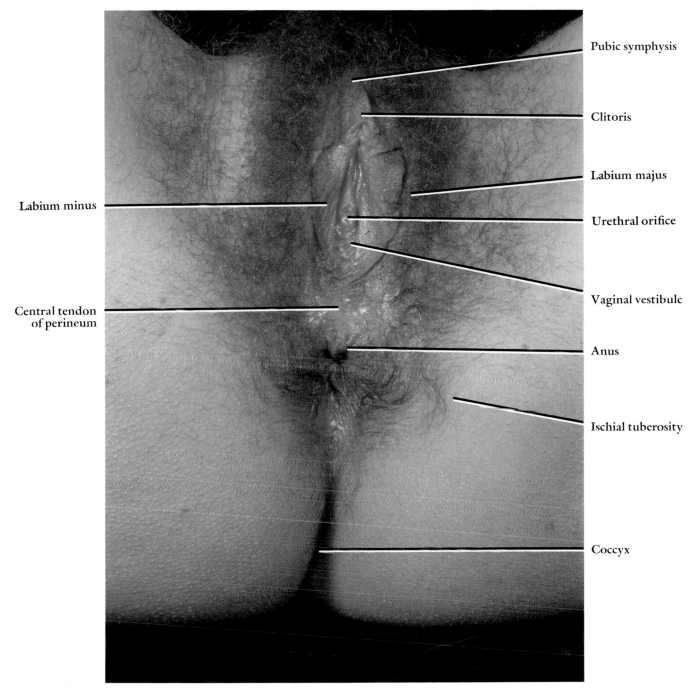

Pubic symphysis

Clitoris

Labium majus

Urethral orifice

Vaginal vestibule

Anus

Ischial tuberosity

Coccyx

Labium minus

Central tendon of perineum

General remarks: Parturition and deliveries that require some surgical assistance make it important to be familiar with the anatomy of this region. The bony boundaries of the *urogenital* and *anal triangles*, the *pubic symphysis*, the *ischiopubic rami*, the *ischial tuberosities*, the *sacrotuberous liga-* *ments*, and the *coccyx* are readily palpable. Some of these landmarks are also used in administering local anesthetics to the region. In an intact *vagina* the orifice is partially covered by a thin fold of mucous membrane, the *hymen*.

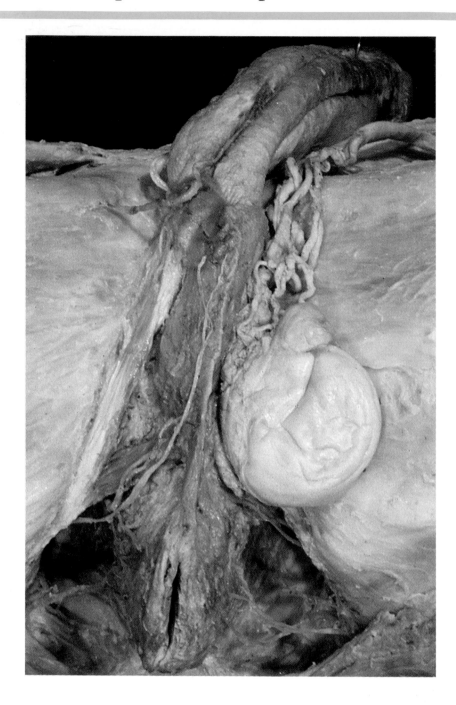

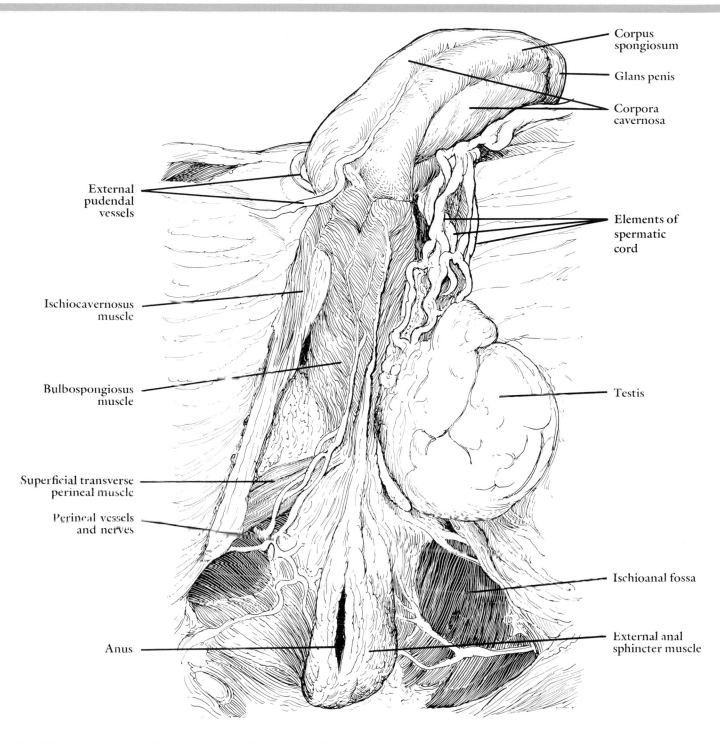

Corpus
spongiosum

Glans penis

Corpora
cavernosa

External
pudendal
vessels

Elements of
spermatic
cord

Ischiocavernosus
muscle

Bulbospongiosus
muscle

Testis

Superficial transverse
perineal muscle

Perineal vessels
and nerves

Ischioanal fossa

External anal
sphincter muscle

Anus

Specific remarks: Muscles of the *urogenital* and *anal triangles,* together with the *erectile bodies,* blood vessels, and nerves, are exposed after skin, subcutaneous tissue, right *testis* with *spermatic cord,* and the superficial regional fascia have been removed. The left *testis* and structures in the spermatic cord, on the other hand, are kept it situ as a point of topographical reference.

General remarks: The *rectoanal lumen* is separated from that of the *ischioanal fossa* only by the intestinal wall and the thickness of the *sphincter* and *levator ani muscles.* Because numerous veins are contained within this intestinal wall, their varicosities, which are caused mostly by an impairment of portal circulation, may protrude either into the intestine, or into the ischioanal fossa.

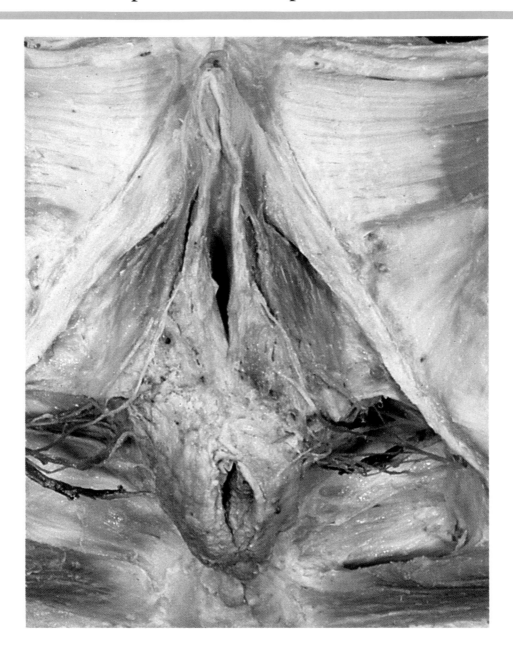

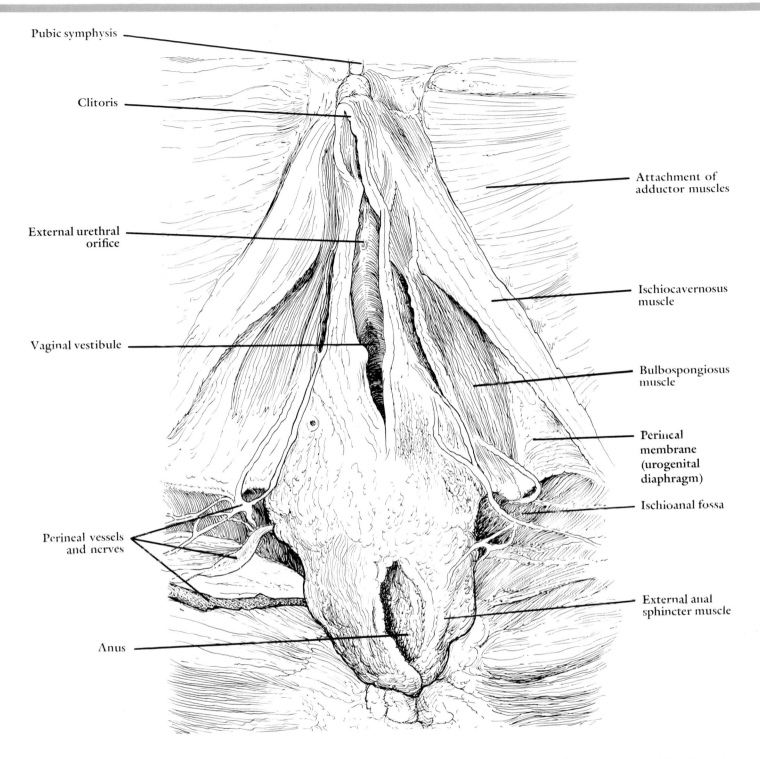

Pubic symphysis

Clitoris

External urethral orifice

Vaginal vestibule

Perineal vessels and nerves

Anus

Attachment of adductor muscles

Ischiocavernosus muscle

Bulbospongiosus muscle

Perineal membrane (urogenital diaphragm)

Ischioanal fossa

External anal sphincter muscle

Specific remarks: Muscles of the *urogenital* and *anal triangles,* together with the *erectile bodies,* blood vessels, and nerves, are exposed after skin, subcutaneous tissue, and the superficial regional fascia have been removed.

General remarks: Because of the gap created in the *urogenital diaphragm* by the passage of the *vagina,* the structure of the female perineum, compared with that of a male subject, provides a less resistant support to the *pelvic viscera.* Since the *central tendon of the perineum (perineal body)* contributes significantly to this resistance, its integrity is strictly considered during perineal surgery.

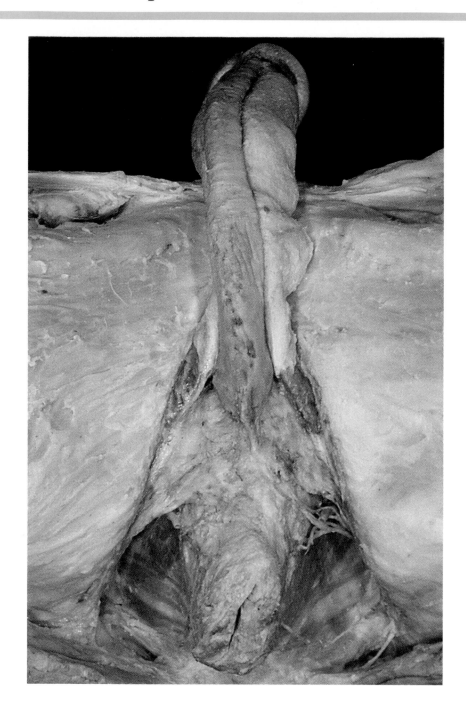

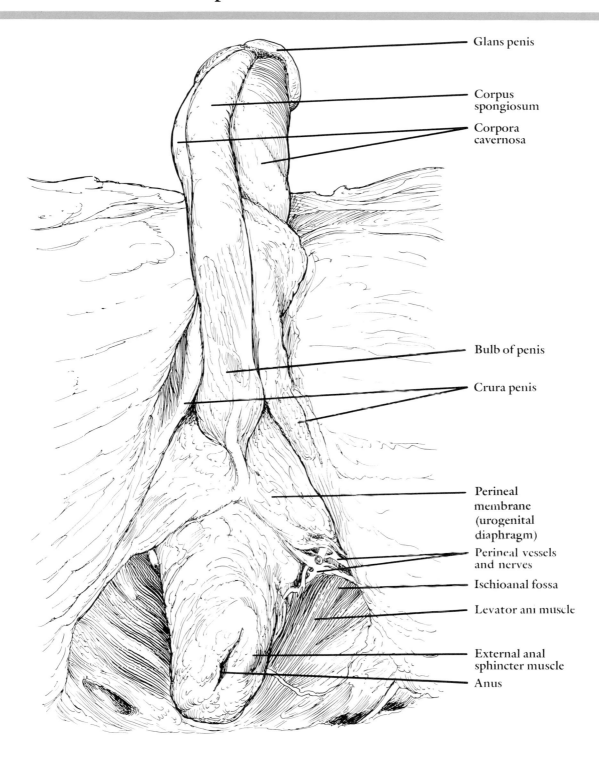

Glans penis

Corpus spongiosum

Corpora cavernosa

Bulb of penis

Crura penis

Perineal membrane (urogenital diaphragm)

Perineal vessels and nerves

Ischioanal fossa

Levator ani muscle

External anal sphincter muscle

Anus

Specific remarks: After the *ischiocavernosus,* the *bulbospongiosus,* and the *superficial transverse perineal* muscles have been removed from the *urogenital triangle,* the *erectile bodies* of the *penis* are revealed. The *crura of the penis* originate from the *ischiopubic rami* to become incorporated into the dorsal structure of the penile shaft. The *bulb of the penis* with the *urethra* in it, extends as the ventral structure of the shaft before it expands to form the *glans penis.* The *perineal membrane layer of the urogenital diaphragm* is demonstrated between the *ischiopubic rami,* immediately superior to the erectile bodies.

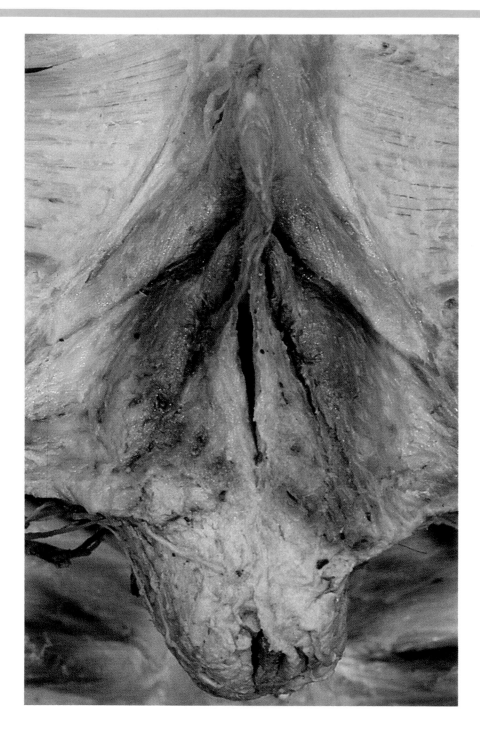

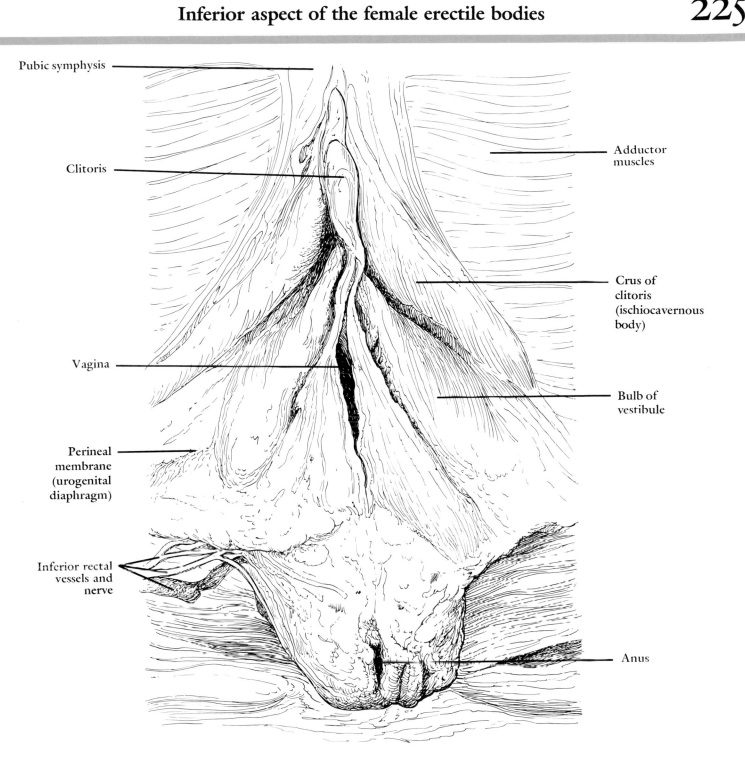

Pubic symphysis

Clitoris

Vagina

Perineal
membrane
(urogenital
diaphragm)

Inferior rectal
vessels and
nerve

Adductor
muscles

Crus of
clitoris
(ischiocavernous
body)

Bulb of
vestibule

Anus

Specific remarks: After the *ischiocavernosus, bulbospongiosus,* and *superficial transverse perineal* muscles have been removed from the *urogenital triangle,* the *erectile bodies* of the *clitoris* are revealed. The *crura of the clitoris* originate from the *ischiopubic rami* to become incorporated into the dorsal structure of the clitoris. The two *bulbs of the vestibule* surround the *vagina* before they together constitute the ventral clitoral structure. The *perineal membrane* is demonstrated between the ischiopubic rami, immediately superior to the erectile bodies.

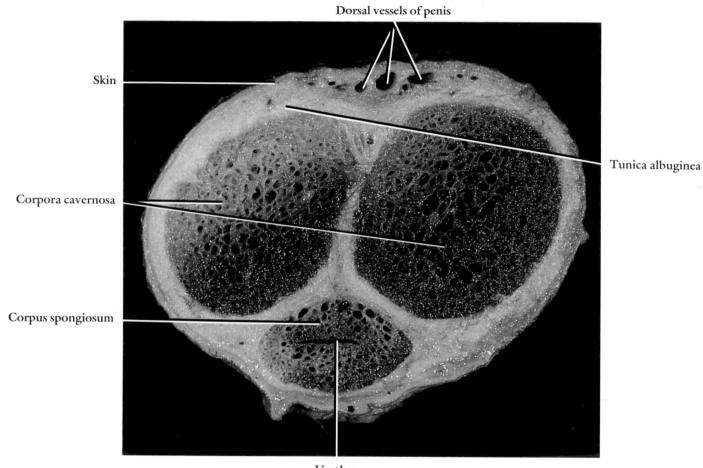

Dorsal vessels of penis

Skin

Tunica albuginea

Corpora cavernosa

Corpus spongiosum

Urethra

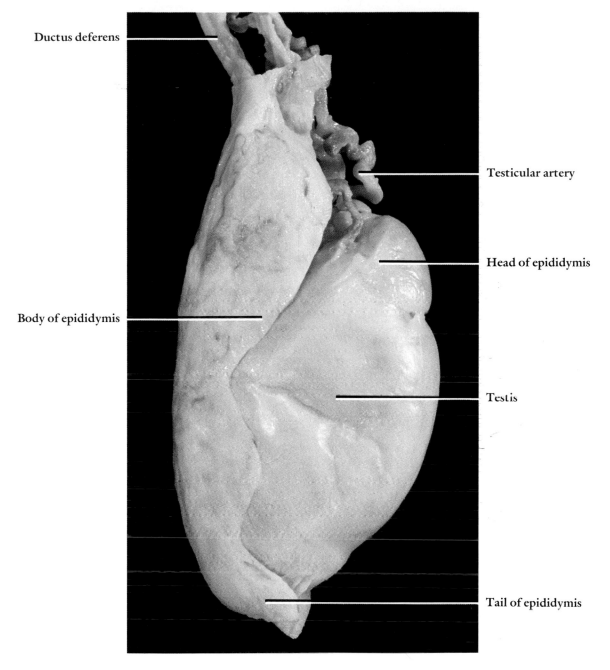

Ductus deferens

Testicular artery

Head of epididymis

Body of epididymis

Testis

Tail of epididymis

Specific remarks: The right *testis, epididymis,* and *spermatic cord* have been removed from the *scrotum* and the *cremasteric fascia* and *tunica vaginalis* dissected away from the lateral aspect.

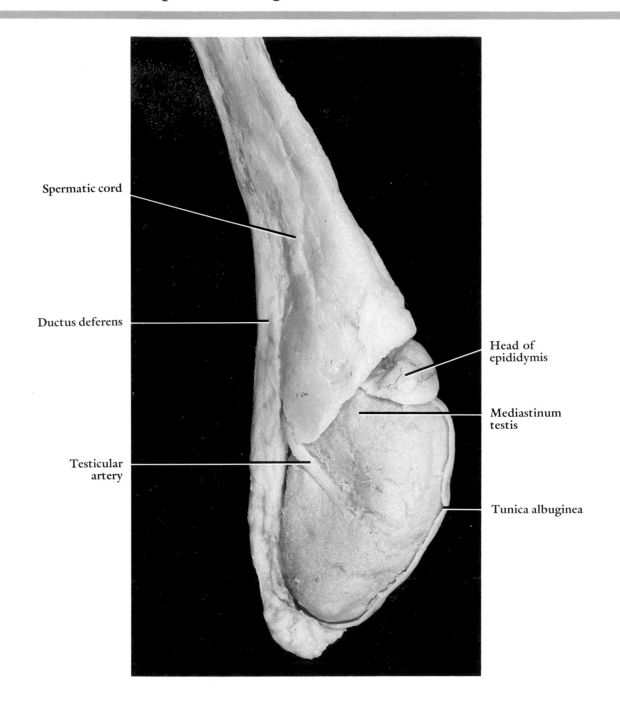

Spermatic cord

Ductus deferens

Testicular
artery

Head of
epididymis

Mediastinum
testis

Tunica albuginea

Specific remarks: The *tunica albuginea*, or *fibrous testicular capsule*, has been incised circularly along the sagittal plane and the right half of it removed to reveal the internal testicular structure.

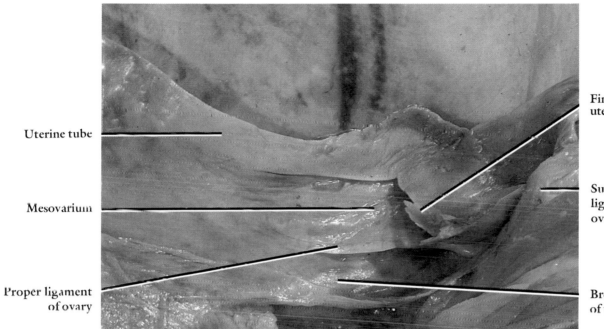

Uterine tube

Mesovarium

Proper ligament
of ovary

Fimbriae of
uterine tube

Suspensory
ligament of
ovary

Broad ligament
of uterus

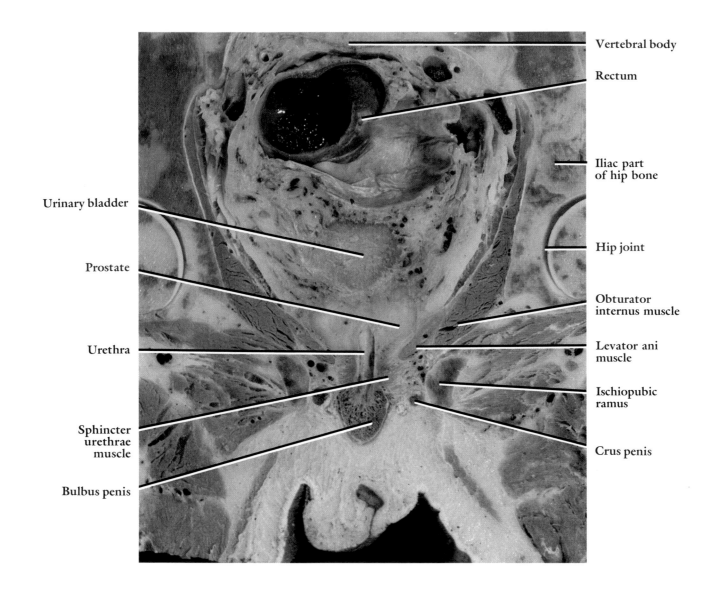

Vertebral body

Rectum

Iliac part
of hip bone

Hip joint

Obturator
internus muscle

Levator ani
muscle

Ischiopubic
ramus

Crus penis

Urinary bladder

Prostate

Urethra

Sphincter
urethrae
muscle

Bulbus penis

Specific remarks: The body has been frontally sectioned at the level of the *obturator foramen,* and the posterior face of the section is presented.

General remarks: This sectional view is especially instructive in ascertaining the disposition of *pelvic* and *urogenital diaphragms* in relation to skeletal elements and *pelvic viscera.*

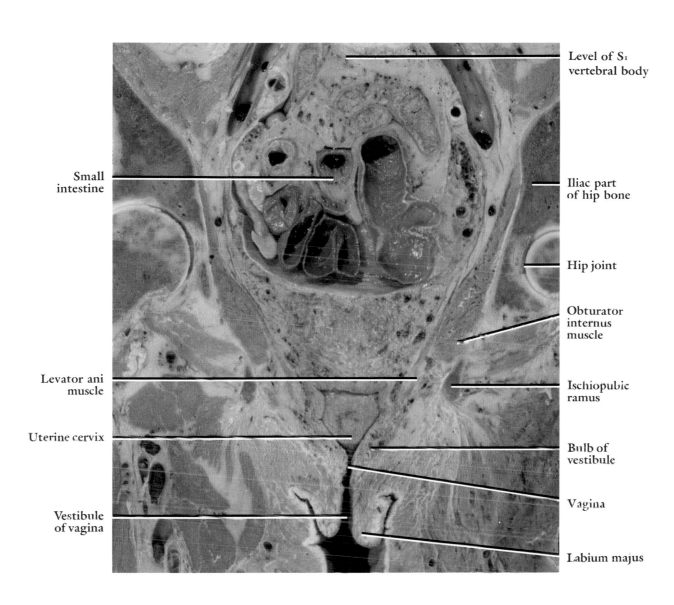

Level of S₁
vertebral body

Small
intestine

Iliac part
of hip bone

Hip joint

Obturator
internus
muscle

Levator ani
muscle

Ischiopubic
ramus

Uterine cervix

Bulb of
vestibule

Vagina

Vestibule
of vagina

Labium majus

Specific remarks: The body has been frontally sectioned at the level of the *obturator foramen,* and the posterior face of the section is presented.

General remarks: This sectional view is especially instructive in ascertaining the disposition of *pelvic* and *urogenital diaphragms* in relation to skeletal elements and *pelvic viscera*.

References

219

Borell, U., and Fernston, I: Radiologic pelvimetry, Acta Radiol. **191**:3, 1960.

221

Huntingford, P.J.: Pudendal nerve block: the results of its routine use, with special reference to trans-vaginal technique, J. Obstet. Gynaec. Br. Commonw. **66**:26, 1959.

223

Curtis, A.H., Anson, B.J., and Ashley, F.L.: Further studies in gynecological anatomy and related clinical problems, Surg. Gynecol. Obstet. **74**:708, 1942.

227

Goldstein, M.B.A., and Meehan, J.P.: A review of the microarchitecture of the corpora cavernosa in man, Anat. Rec. **205**:65A, 1983.

Johnson, A.D., Gomes, W.R., and Vandemark, N.L., editors: The testis, New York, 1970, Academic Press, Inc.

230

Clegg, E.J.: The vascular arrangements within the human prostate gland, Br. J. Urol. **28**:428, 1956.

231

Chiara, F.: Study of the tissue innervation of the female genitalia. I. Uterus, Ann. Ostet. Ginec. **81**:553, 1959.

Part Seven
LOWER LIMB

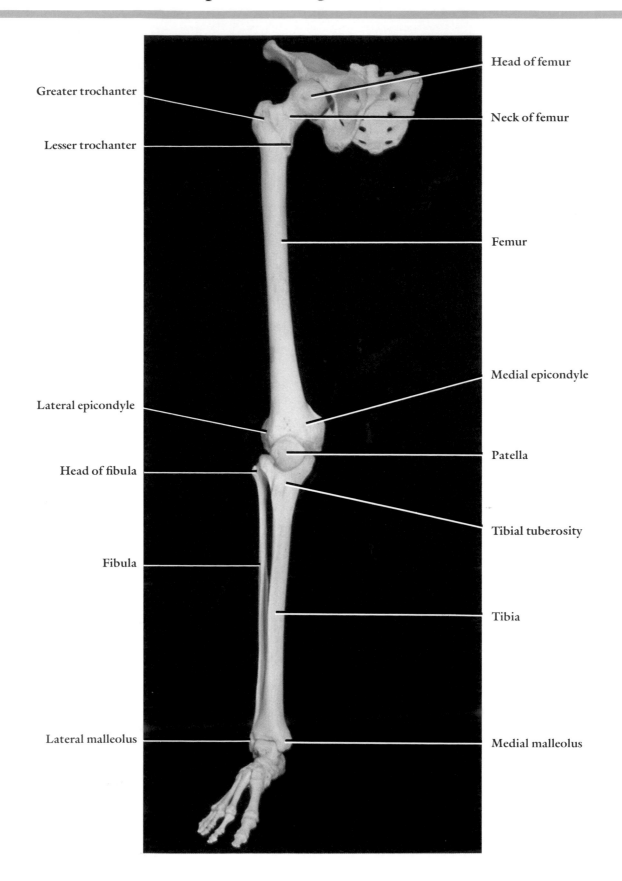

Greater trochanter

Lesser trochanter

Lateral epicondyle

Head of fibula

Fibula

Lateral malleolus

Head of femur

Neck of femur

Femur

Medial epicondyle

Patella

Tibial tuberosity

Tibia

Medial malleolus

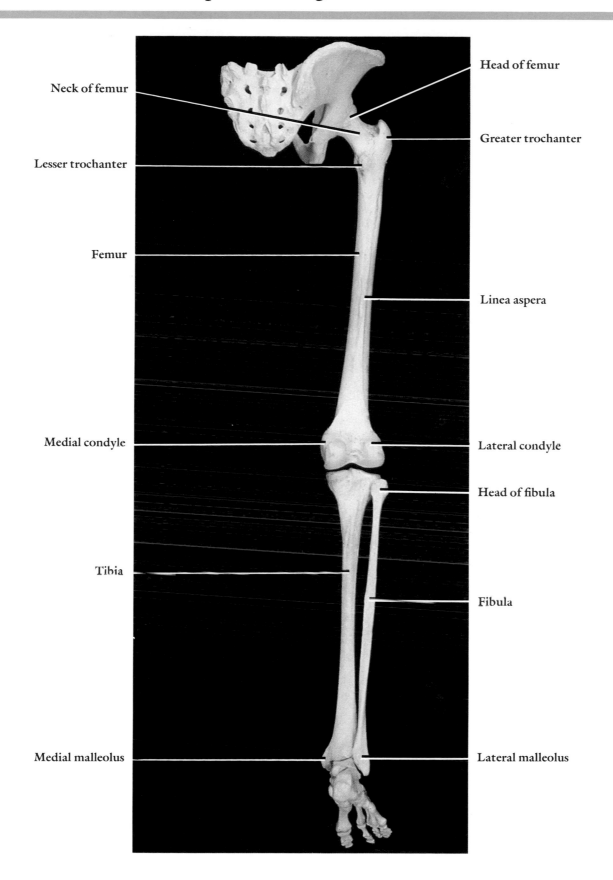

Neck of femur

Head of femur

Lesser trochanter

Greater trochanter

Femur

Linea aspera

Medial condyle

Lateral condyle

Head of fibula

Tibia

Fibula

Medial malleolus

Lateral malleolus

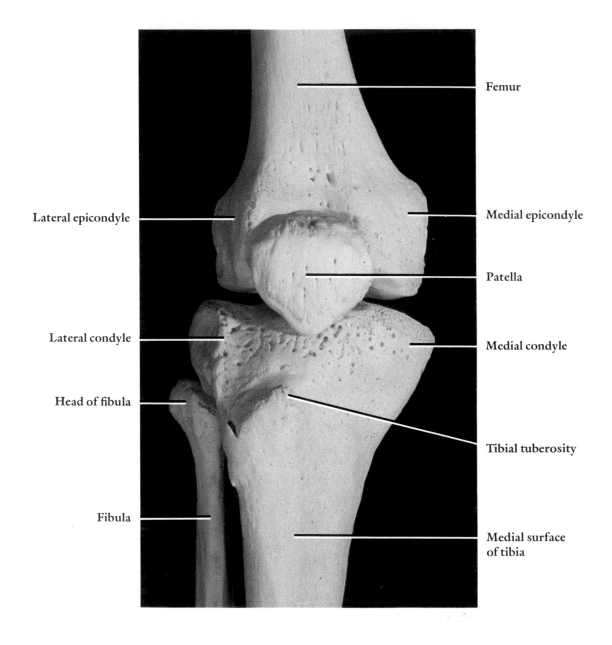

Femur

Lateral epicondyle

Medial epicondyle

Patella

Lateral condyle

Medial condyle

Head of fibula

Tibial tuberosity

Fibula

Medial surface
of tibia

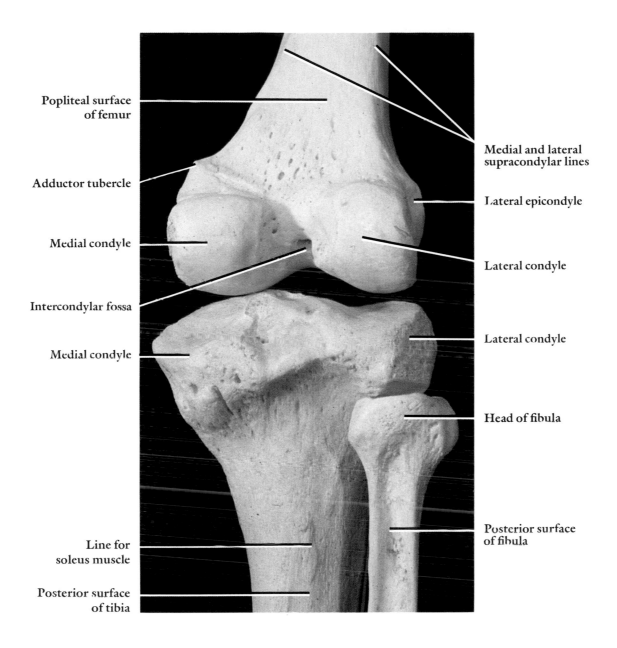

Popliteal surface
of femur

Adductor tubercle

Medial condyle

Intercondylar fossa

Medial condyle

Line for
soleus muscle

Posterior surface
of tibia

Medial and lateral
supracondylar lines

Lateral epicondyle

Lateral condyle

Lateral condyle

Head of fibula

Posterior surface
of fibula

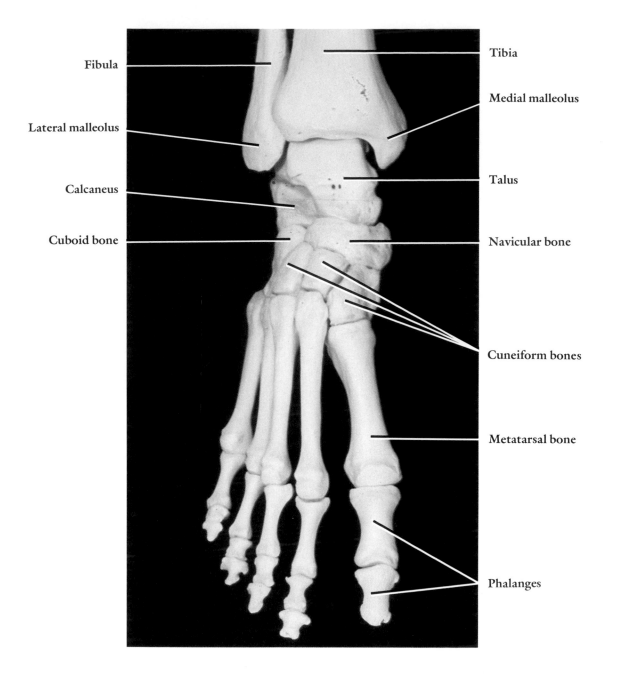

Fibula

Tibia

Lateral malleolus

Medial malleolus

Calcaneus

Talus

Cuboid bone

Navicular bone

Cuneiform bones

Metatarsal bone

Phalanges

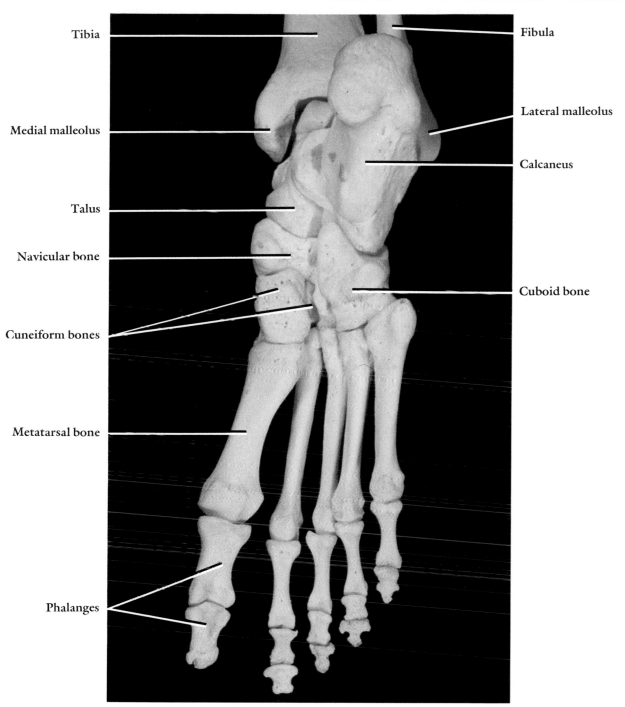

Tibia

Fibula

Medial malleolus

Lateral malleolus

Calcaneus

Talus

Navicular bone

Cuboid bone

Cuneiform bones

Metatarsal bone

Phalanges

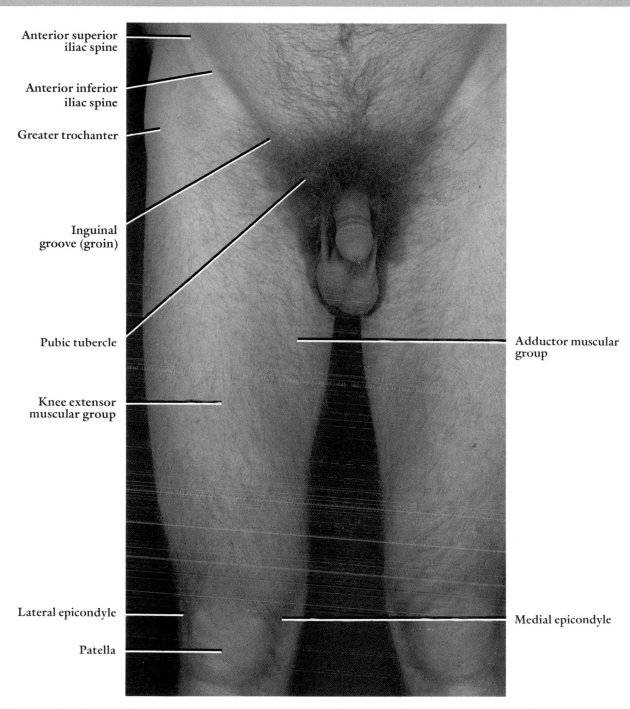

Anterior superior
iliac spine

Anterior inferior
iliac spine

Greater trochanter

Inguinal
groove (groin)

Pubic tubercle

Knee extensor
muscular group

Lateral epicondyle

Patella

Adductor muscular
group

Medial epicondyle

Specific remarks: The configuration of the anterior aspect of the thigh depends mostly on the underlying skeletal and muscular elements. Skeletal elements are visible or palpable at the *anterior superior iliac spine, pubic tubercle, greater tro-* *chanter, medial and lateral epicondyles,* and *patella.* Most pronounced muscular reliefs are those of the *adductors* of the thigh and *extensors* of the leg. The *great saphenous vein* and tributaries are frequently visible through the skin.

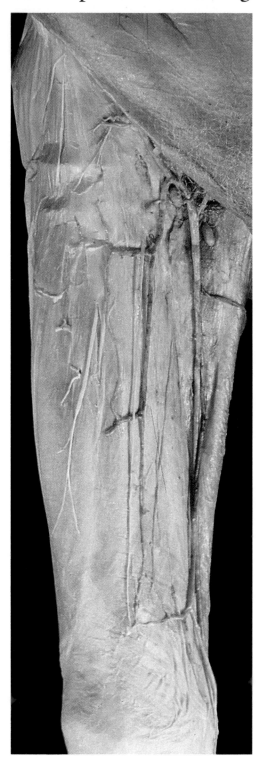

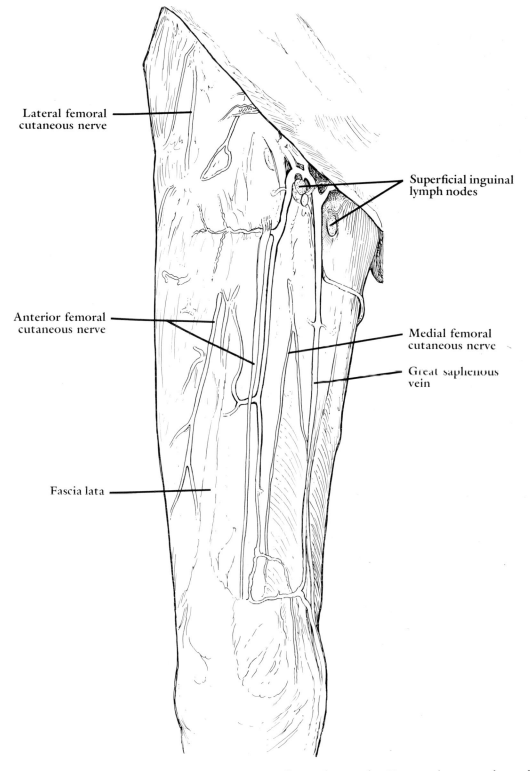

Lateral femoral
cutaneous nerve

Superficial inguinal
lymph nodes

Anterior femoral
cutaneous nerve

Medial femoral
cutaneous nerve

Great saphenous
vein

Fascia lata

Specific remarks: After the skin has been removed, numerous subcutaneous nerves *(lateral femoral cutaneous,* branches of the *femoral and obturator nerves),* the *great saphenous vein* and its tributaries, *superficial inguinal lymph nodes,* and *fascia lata* may be observed.

General remarks: Because it passes through the *fascia lata* the lateral femoral cutaneous nerve is frequently compressed, thus causing various neurological disorders. Lymph nodes around the great saphenous vein drain some parts of the gluteal region, abdominal wall, *external genitalia, anus, perineum,* and the superficial layer of the lower limb.

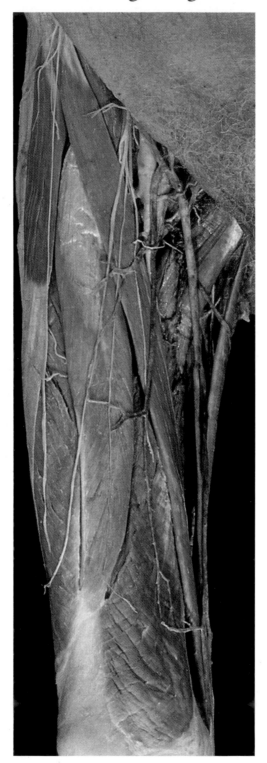

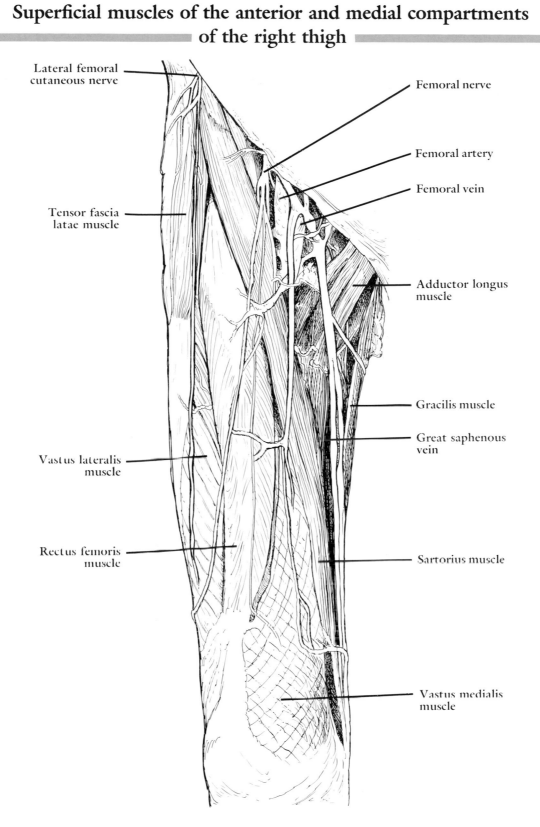

Lateral femoral
cutaneous nerve

Femoral nerve

Femoral artery

Femoral vein

Tensor fascia
latae muscle

Adductor longus
muscle

Gracilis muscle

Great saphenous
vein

Vastus lateralis
muscle

Rectus femoris
muscle

Sartorius muscle

Vastus medialis
muscle

Specific remarks: Deep to the *fascia lata* both muscular groups, the thigh *adductors* and leg *extensors*, are demonstrated. The main neurovascular bundle (*femoral nerve, artery, vein* in that lateromedial order) of these compartments is contained within the *femoral triangle*. The specific borders of the triangle are the *sartorius muscle* laterally, the *adductor longus muscle* medially, and the *inguinal ligament* superiorly.

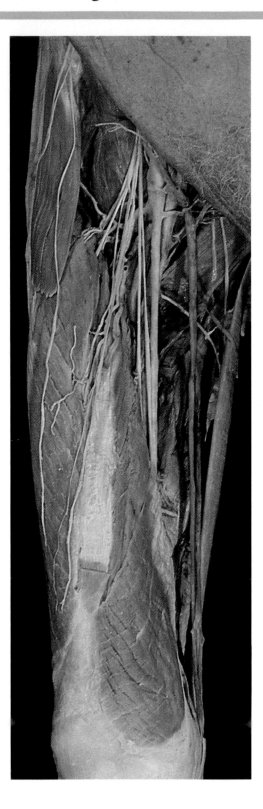

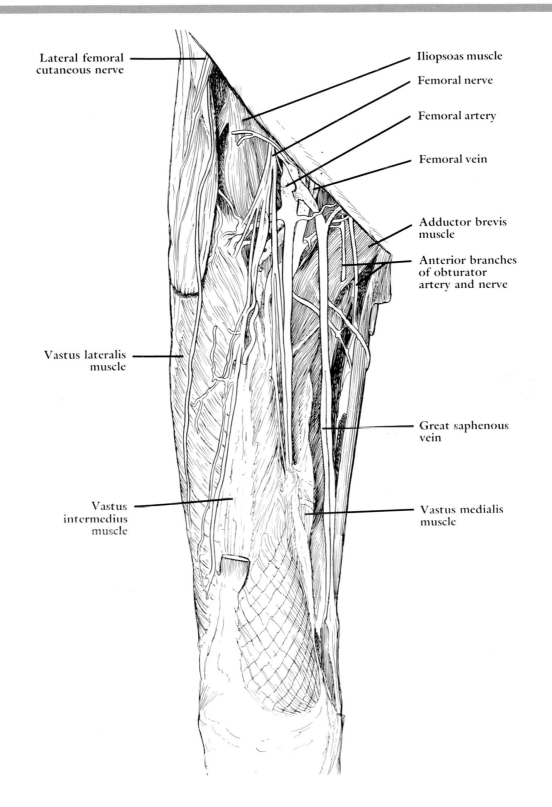

Lateral femoral cutaneous nerve

Iliopsoas muscle

Femoral nerve

Femoral artery

Femoral vein

Adductor brevis muscle

Anterior branches of obturator artery and nerve

Vastus lateralis muscle

Great saphenous vein

Vastus intermedius muscle

Vastus medialis muscle

Specific remarks: At a deeper plane, after the *sartorius* and *rectus femoris muscles* have been removed, the continuing course of *femoral vessels* and the *saphenous nerve* from the *femoral triangle* into the *adductor canal* is demonstrated.

While the vessels are bordered in the canal medially and laterally by the *adductor longus* (removed here) and *vastus medialis muscles* respectively, they are covered anteriorly by a dense membranous part of the *medial intermuscular septum*.

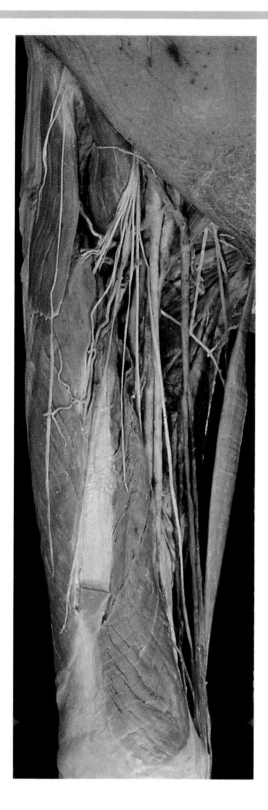

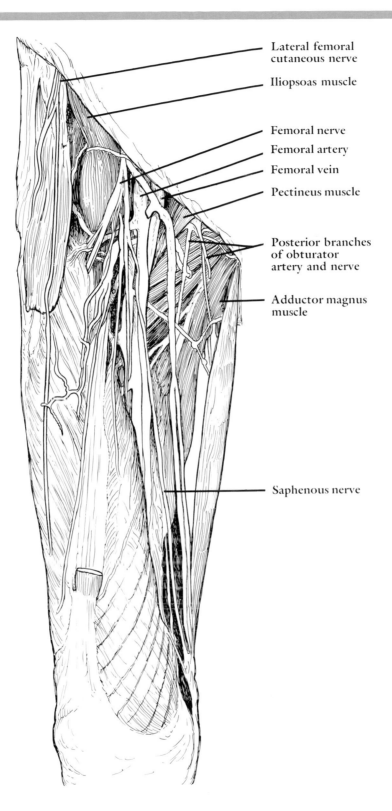

Lateral femoral cutaneous nerve

Iliopsoas muscle

Femoral nerve

Femoral artery

Femoral vein

Pectineus muscle

Posterior branches of obturator artery and nerve

Adductor magnus muscle

Saphenous nerve

Specific remarks: In this dissection the *medial intermuscular septum* and the adductor brevis muscle have been removed. Now the posterior branches of the *obturator neurovascular bundle* are shown.

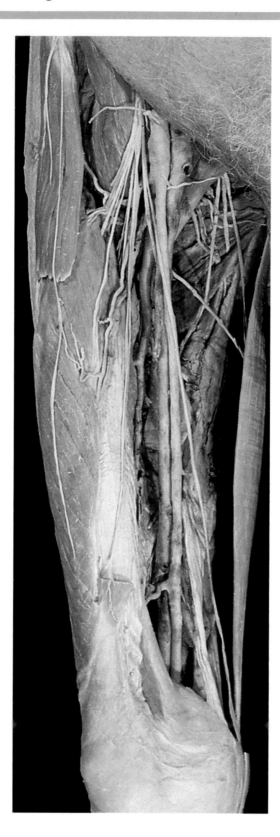

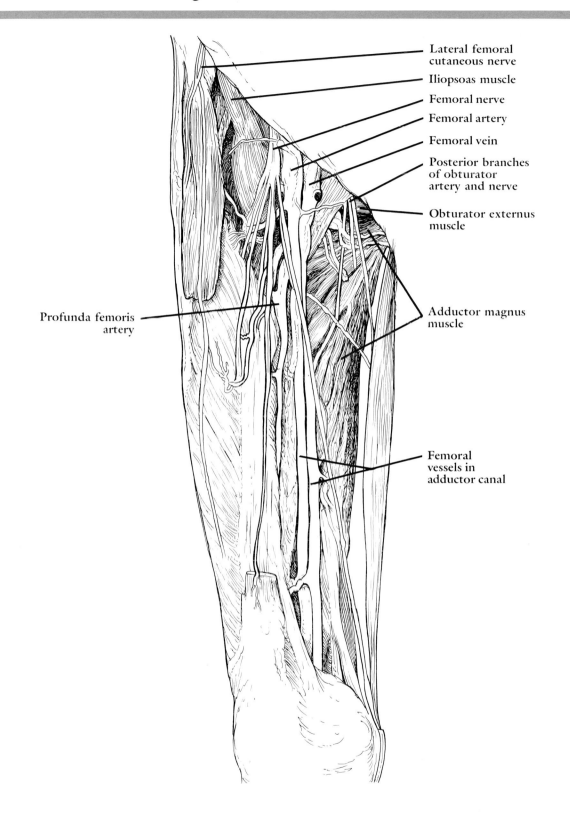

Lateral femoral cutaneous nerve

Iliopsoas muscle

Femoral nerve

Femoral artery

Femoral vein

Posterior branches of obturator artery and nerve

Obturator externus muscle

Profunda femoris artery

Adductor magnus muscle

Femoral vessels in adductor canal

Specific remarks: In the deepest muscular layer, following removal of the *quadriceps femoris* and *adductor brevis muscles,* the relationship of the *femoral blood vessels* with the *adductor magnus muscle* is indicated.

General remarks: Branches of the *profunda femoris artery,* which perforate and pass through the adductor magnus muscle, anastomose with one another in the posterior compartment of the thigh and establish a viable collateral circulation, in addition to one along the *femoral artery proper.*

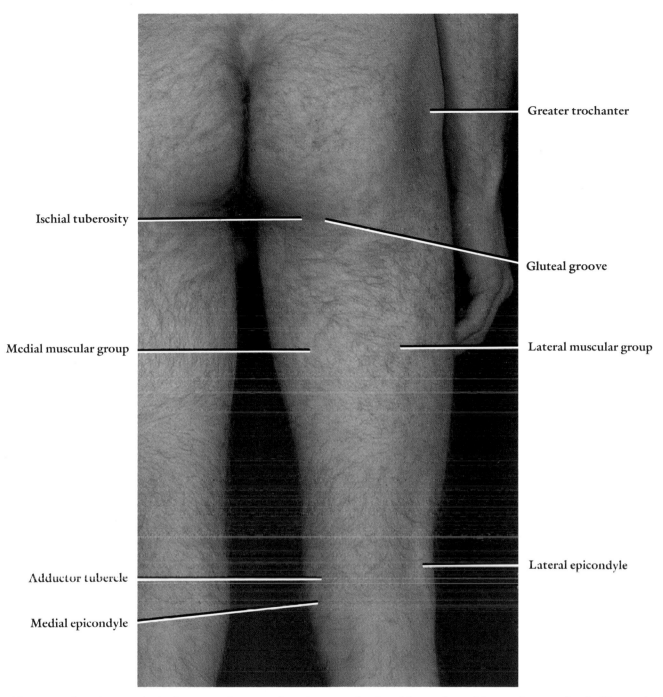

Greater trochanter

Ischial tuberosity

Gluteal groove

Medial muscular group

Lateral muscular group

Lateral epicondyle

Adductor tubercle

Medial epicondyle

Specific remarks: Anatomical elements that can be observed and palpated in the posterior compartment of the thigh include the *ischial tuberosity, greater trochanter, femoral epicondyles and condyles,* and muscular bellies and tendons of the *biceps femoris, semitendinosus,* and *semimembranosus muscles.*

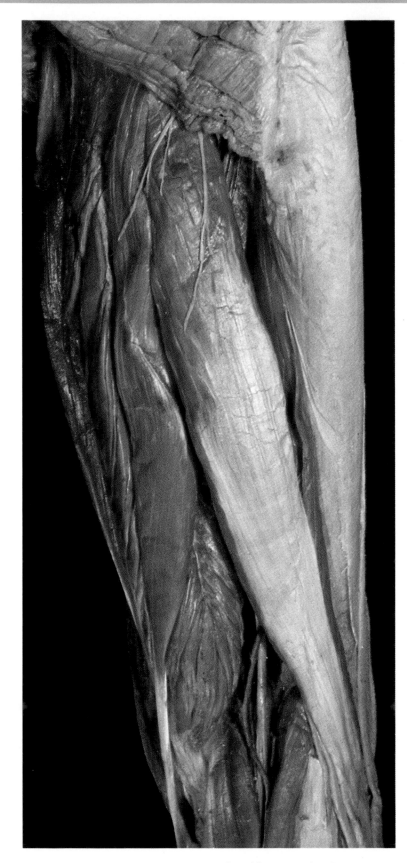

Specific remarks: In contrast to the fascia over the anterior and lateral aspects of the thigh, this regional fascia, which has been dissected away, is relatively thin. Powerful

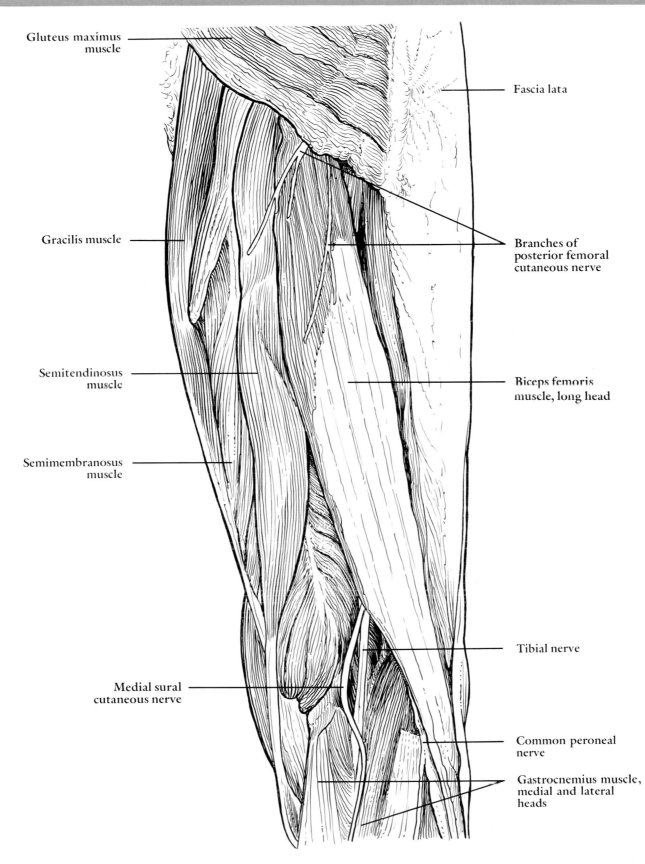

Gluteus maximus
muscle

Gracilis muscle

Semitendinosus
muscle

Semimembranosus
muscle

Medial sural
cutaneous nerve

Fascia lata

Branches of
posterior femoral
cutaneous nerve

Biceps femoris
muscle, long head

Tibial nerve

Common peroneal
nerve

Gastrocnemius muscle,
medial and lateral
heads

flexors of the leg and *extensors* of the thigh, the hamstrings, are arranged in a medial group *(semitendinosus* and *semimembranosus muscles)* and a lateral group *(biceps femoris muscle).* Two muscular groups diverge from one another inferiorly to establish the superomedial and superolateral walls of the *popliteal fossa.*

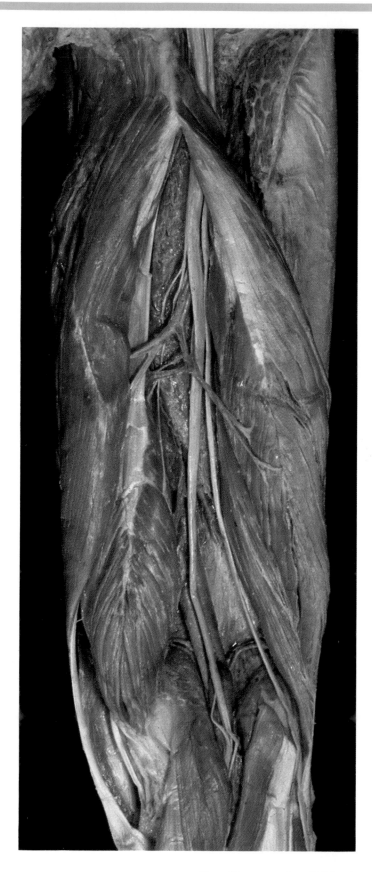

Specific remarks: With the *semitendinosus* and *semimembranosus muscles* reflected medially and the *biceps femoris muscle* reflected laterally, the passage of the *sciatic nerve* through the thigh and its division in the posterior com-

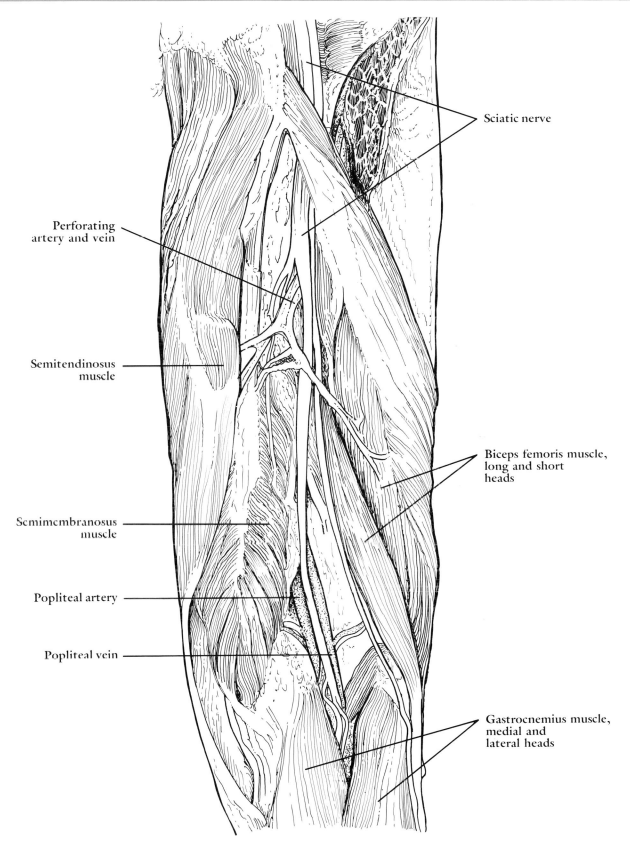

Sciatic nerve

Perforating artery and vein

Semitendinosus muscle

Biceps femoris muscle, long and short heads

Semimembranosus muscle

Popliteal artery

Popliteal vein

Gastrocnemius muscle, medial and lateral heads

partment are seen. Also, the passage of the *femoral blood vessels* and the *perforating arteries* of the *profunda femoris artery* through the *adductor magnus muscle* and the *short head of the biceps femoris muscle* is exposed.

General remarks: The perforating artery demonstrated in this view bifurcates to penetrate into the medial and lateral muscle masses. Inside the muscles the arteries communicate with adjacent similar branches, and finally with the *popliteal artery*, to establish a collateral circulation.

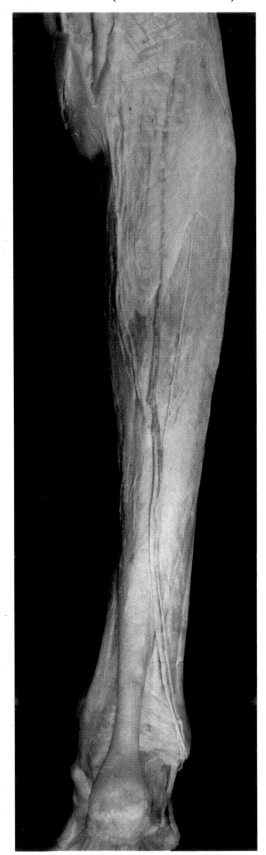

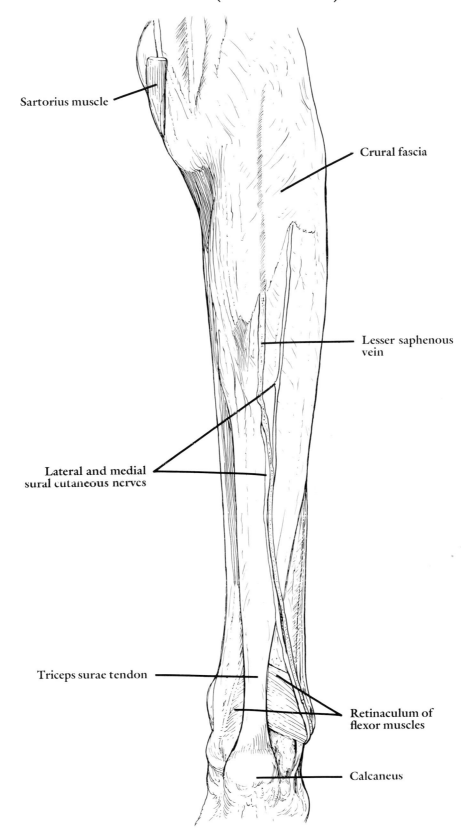

Sartorius muscle

Crural fascia

Lesser saphenous vein

Lateral and medial sural cutaneous nerves

Triceps surae tendon

Retinaculum of flexor muscles

Calcaneus

Gastrocnemius muscle and the contents of the popliteal fossa
(fascia removed)

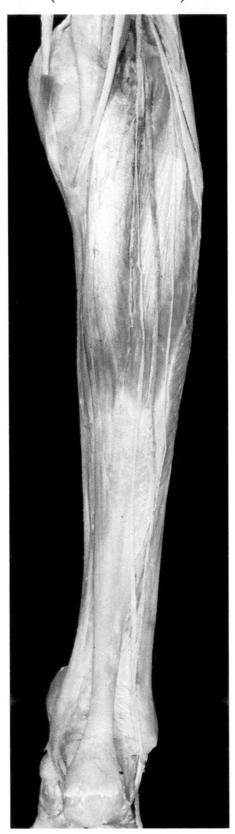

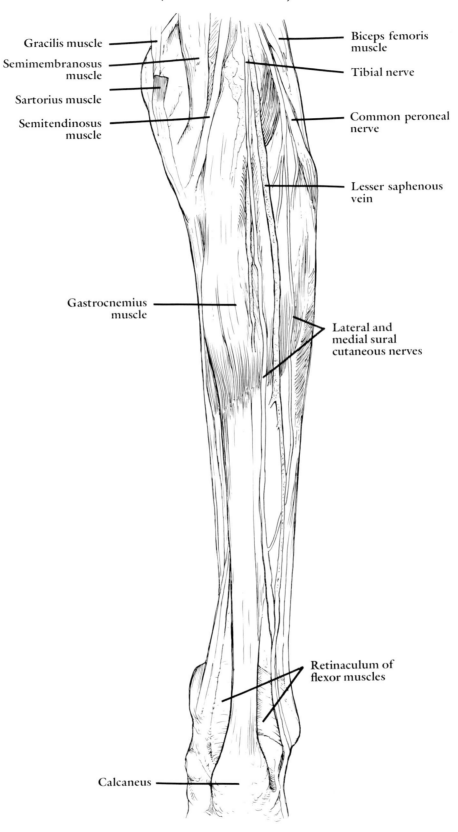

Gracilis muscle

Semimembranosus muscle

Sartorius muscle

Semitendinosus muscle

Biceps femoris muscle

Tibial nerve

Common peroneal nerve

Lesser saphenous vein

Gastrocnemius muscle

Lateral and medial sural cutaneous nerves

Retinaculum of flexor muscles

Calcaneus

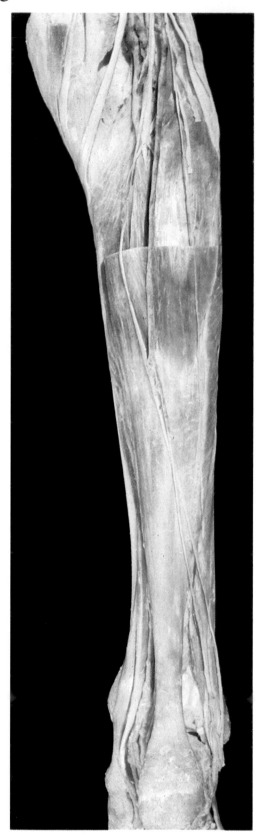

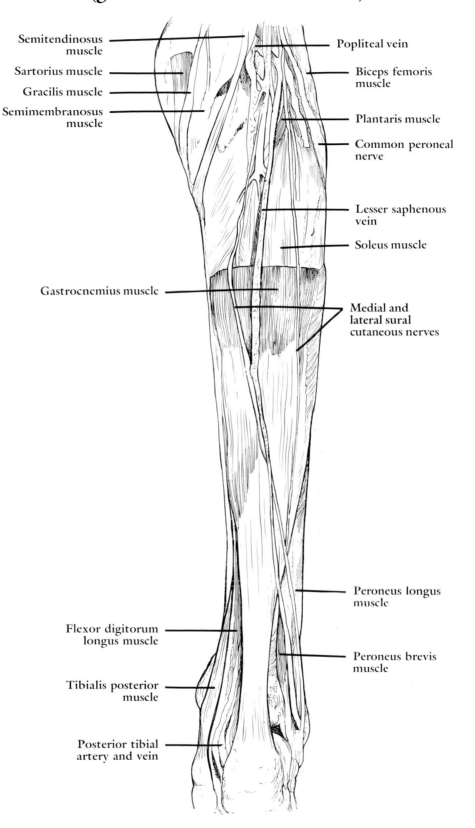

Semitendinosus muscle

Sartorius muscle

Gracilis muscle

Semimembranosus muscle

Popliteal vein

Biceps femoris muscle

Plantaris muscle

Common peroneal nerve

Lesser saphenous vein

Soleus muscle

Gastrocnemius muscle

Medial and lateral sural cutaneous nerves

Peroneus longus muscle

Flexor digitorum longus muscle

Peroneus brevis muscle

Tibialis posterior muscle

Posterior tibial artery and vein

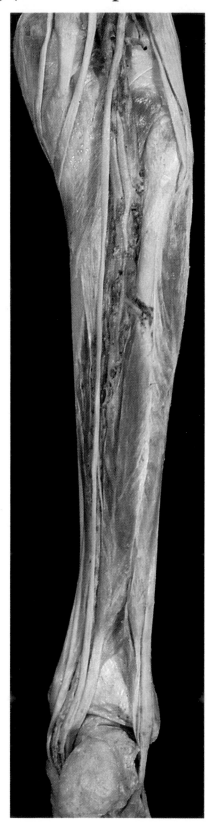

Deep muscles, blood vessels, and nerves in the posterior compartment of the right leg (soleus and plantaris muscles removed)

252

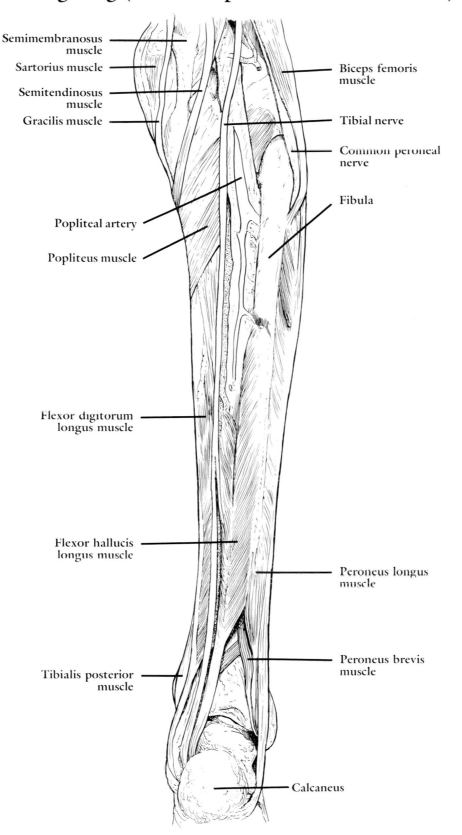

Semimembranosus muscle

Sartorius muscle

Semitendinosus muscle

Gracilis muscle

Biceps femoris muscle

Tibial nerve

Common peroneal nerve

Fibula

Popliteal artery

Popliteus muscle

Flexor digitorum longus muscle

Flexor hallucis longus muscle

Peroneus longus muscle

Peroneus brevis muscle

Tibialis posterior muscle

Calcaneus

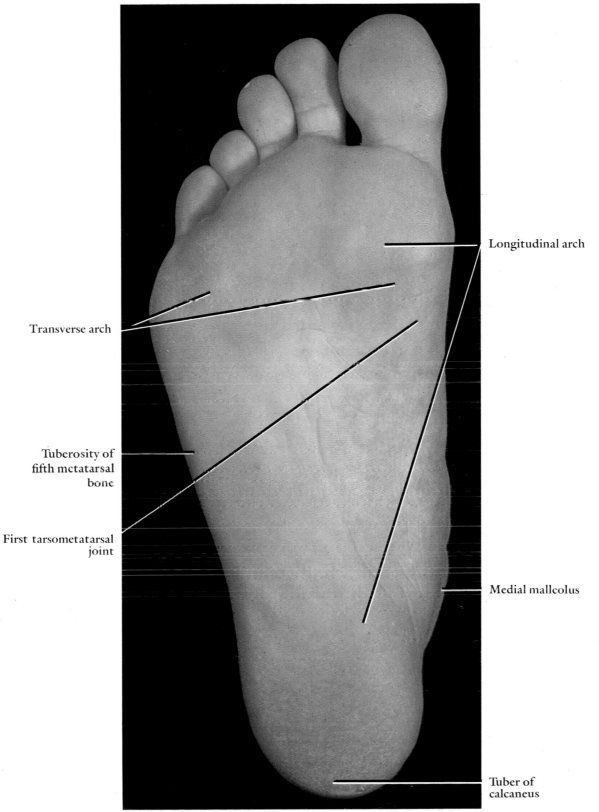

Longitudinal arch

Transverse arch

Tuberosity of
fifth metatarsal
bone

First tarsometatarsal
joint

Medial malleolus

Tuber of
calcaneus

Specific remarks: A typical configuration of this aspect of the foot is characterized by a *longitudinal arch* extending from the *tuber of the calcaneus* to the *metatarsophalangeal line,* and a *transverse arch* crossing the *tarsal* (and somewhat less the *metatarsal*) compartment of the foot.

General remarks: Absence of arches, which is due to the weakness of muscular tone and ligaments, causes a compression over soft tissues and consequently impairs circulation, muscular action, and the stability of the foot. Discomfort and pain can result.

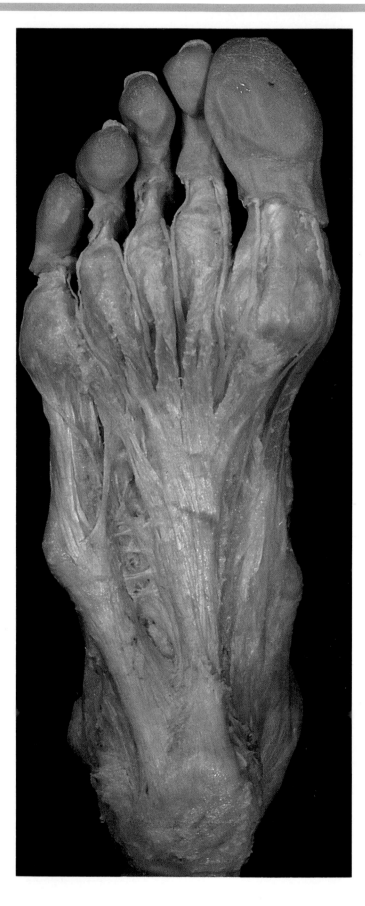

Specific remarks: Fascia over the inferior aspect of the foot is very thick from the *tuber of the calcaneus* to the respective digits. Along the medial and lateral margins of the

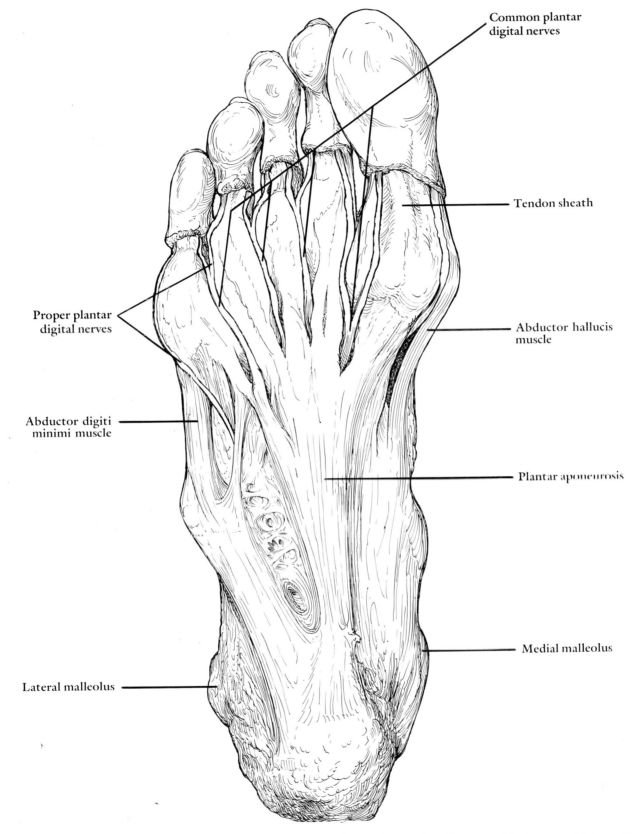

Common plantar
digital nerves

Tendon sheath

Proper plantar
digital nerves

Abductor hallucis
muscle

Abductor digiti
minimi muscle

Plantar aponeurosis

Medial malleolus

Lateral malleolus

region the *abductor hallucis* and *abductor digiti minimi muscles* are respectively present. Digital cutaneous branches from the *medial* and *lateral plantar nerves* pierce the fascia close to the digital roots.

General remarks: Because of their superficial position and a relatively close relationship to the skeletal elements, neurological disorders of digital nerves are frequent.

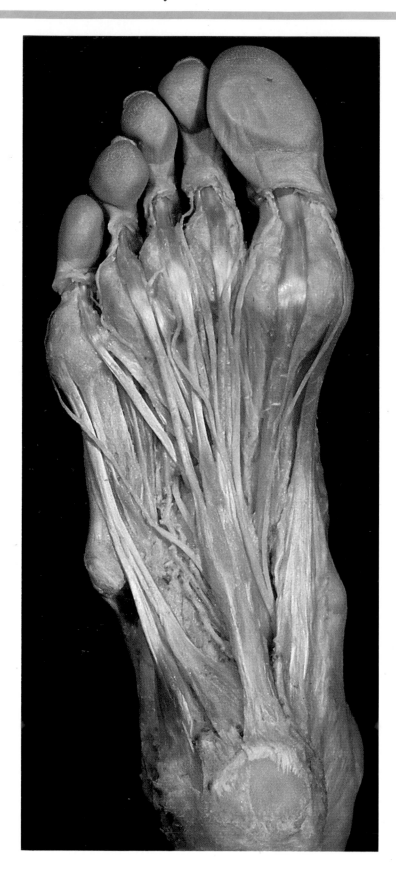

First muscular layer of the sole of the foot

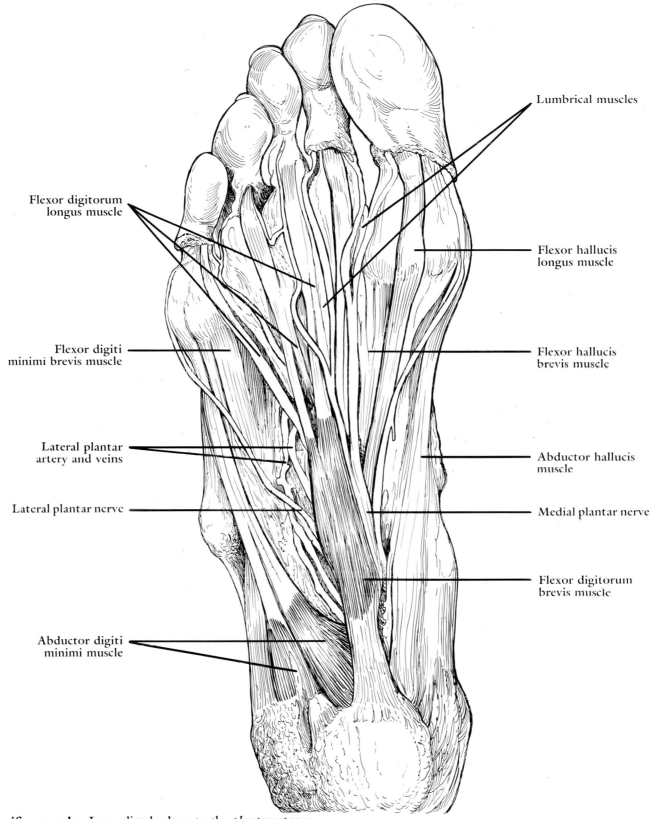

Lumbrical muscles

Flexor digitorum longus muscle

Flexor hallucis longus muscle

Flexor digiti minimi brevis muscle

Flexor hallucis brevis muscle

Lateral plantar artery and veins

Abductor hallucis muscle

Lateral plantar nerve

Medial plantar nerve

Flexor digitorum brevis muscle

Abductor digiti minimi muscle

Specific remarks: Immediately deep to the *plantar aponeurosis* is the *flexor digitorum brevis muscle*. *Medial* and *lateral plantar arteries, veins,* and *nerves* emerge on respective sides from underneath the flexor digitorum brevis muscle.

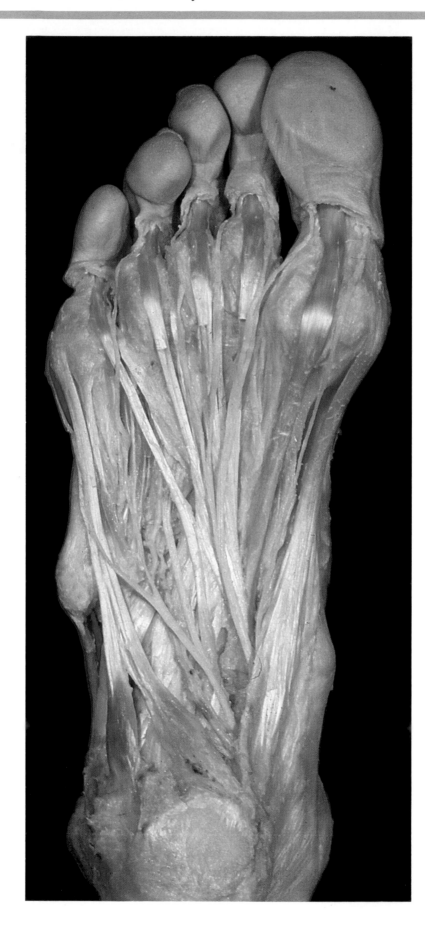

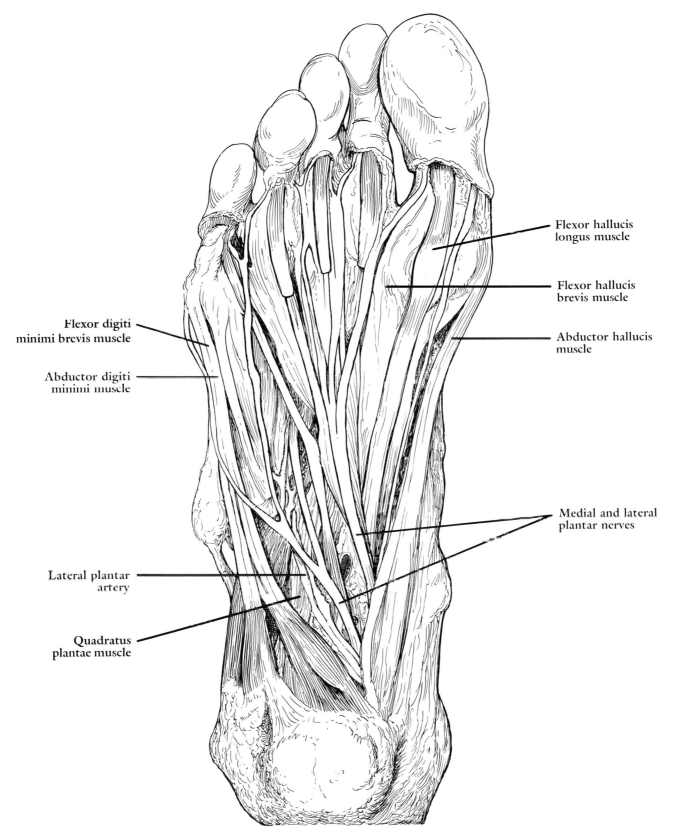

Flexor hallucis
longus muscle

Flexor hallucis
brevis muscle

Abductor hallucis
muscle

Flexor digiti
minimi brevis muscle

Abductor digiti
minimi muscle

Medial and lateral
plantar nerves

Lateral plantar
artery

Quadratus
plantae muscle

Specific remarks: After the *flexor digitorum brevis muscle* is removed, the passage of the *medial* and *lateral plantar arteries, veins,* and *nerves* between this muscle and the *quadratus plantae muscle* can be appreciated. Tendons of the *flexor digitorum longus* and *flexor hallucis longus muscles,* as well as the *lumbrical muscles,* are evident.

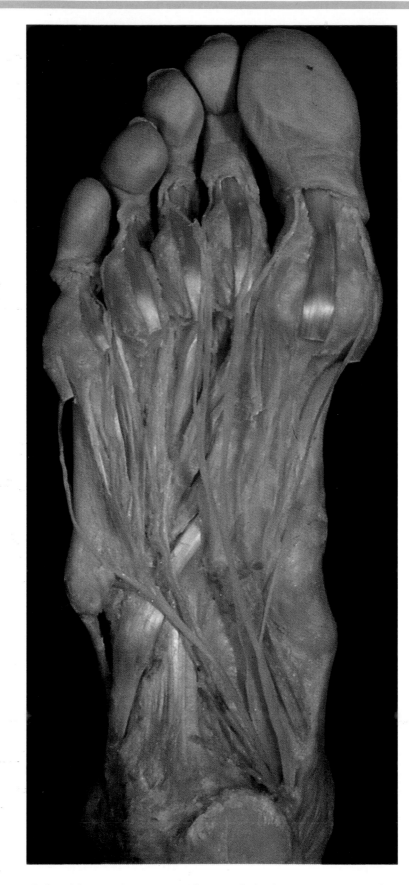

Specific remarks: *Plantar* and *dorsal interossei* are arranged in their respective *intermetatarsal spaces*. Both the muscles and the bones are crossed by the *plantar arch*, which is a continuation of the *lateral plantar artery*.

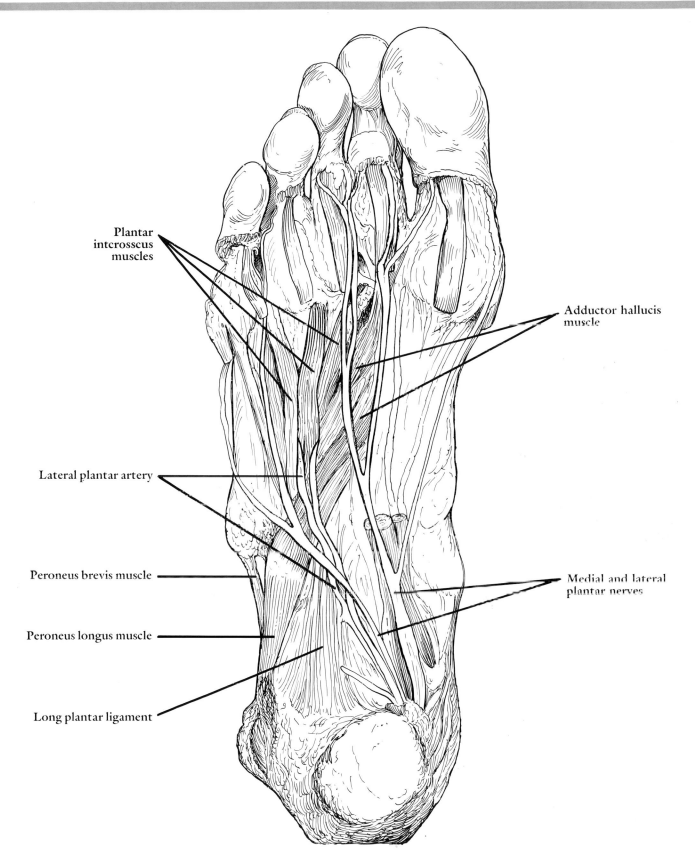

Plantar interosseus muscles

Adductor hallucis muscle

Lateral plantar artery

Peroneus brevis muscle

Peroneus longus muscle

Medial and lateral plantar nerves

Long plantar ligament

General remarks: The plantar arch passes through the contents of the first intermetatarsal space to make a connection between the lateral plantar artery, from the *posterior tibial system,* and the *dorsalis pedis artery,* from the *anterior tibial system.* This is an important arterial anastomosis of the leg and foot circulation.

258   Retinacula and superficial muscular layer of the anterior
and lateral compartments of the leg and the dorsal aspect
of the foot (skin and fascia removed)

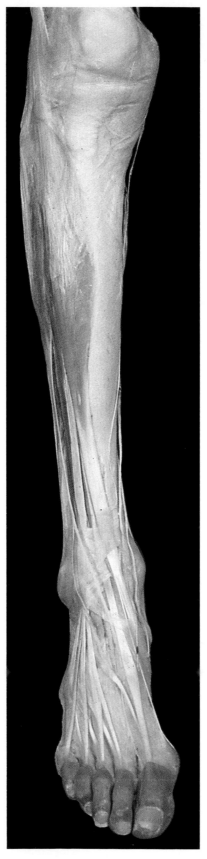

Retinacula and superficial muscular layer of the anterior
and lateral compartments of the leg and the dorsal aspect
of the foot (skin and fascia removed)

258

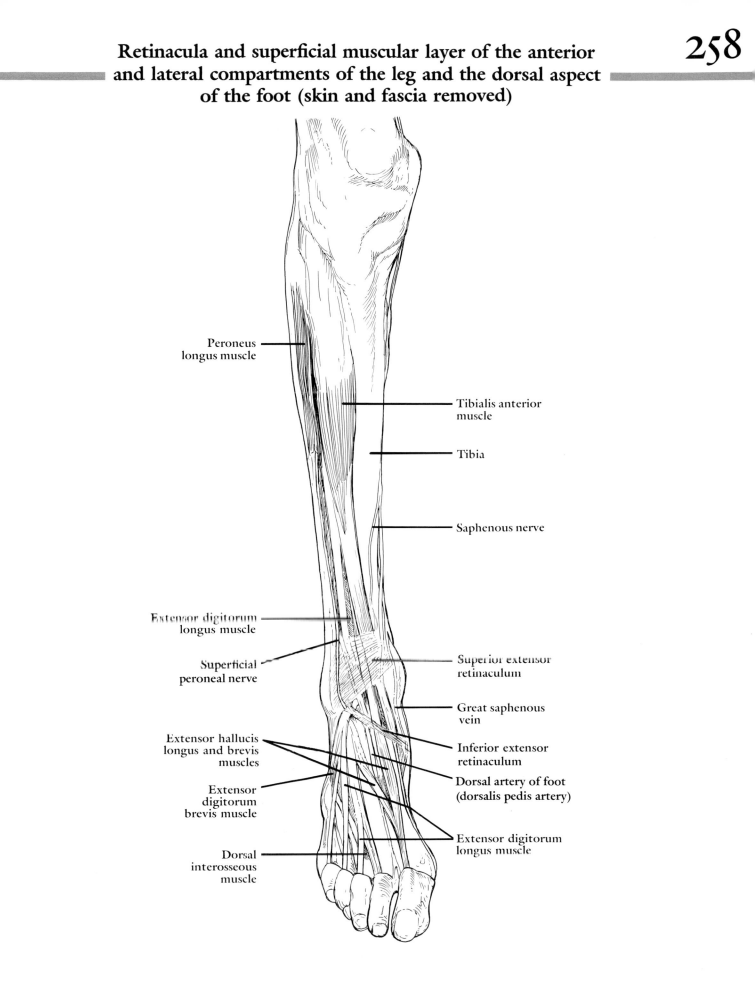

Peroneus
longus muscle

Tibialis anterior
muscle

Tibia

Saphenous nerve

Extensor digitorum
longus muscle

Superficial
peroneal nerve

Superior extensor
retinaculum

Great saphenous
vein

Extensor hallucis
longus and brevis
muscles

Inferior extensor
retinaculum

Extensor
digitorum
brevis muscle

Dorsal artery of foot
(dorsalis pedis artery)

Extensor digitorum
longus muscle

Dorsal
interosseous
muscle

Deep muscular layer of the anterior and lateral compartments of the leg and the dorsal aspect of the foot (extensor digitorum muscle removed)

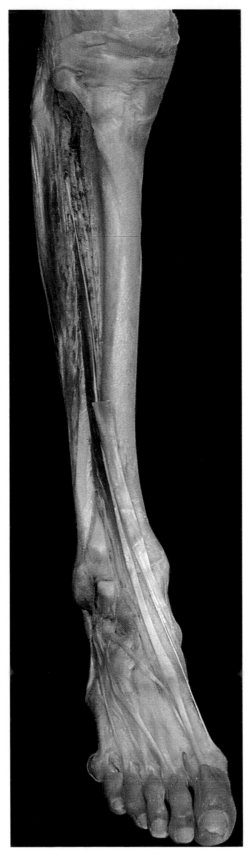

259

Deep muscular layer of the anterior and lateral compartments of the leg and the dorsal aspect of the foot (extensor digitorum muscle removed)

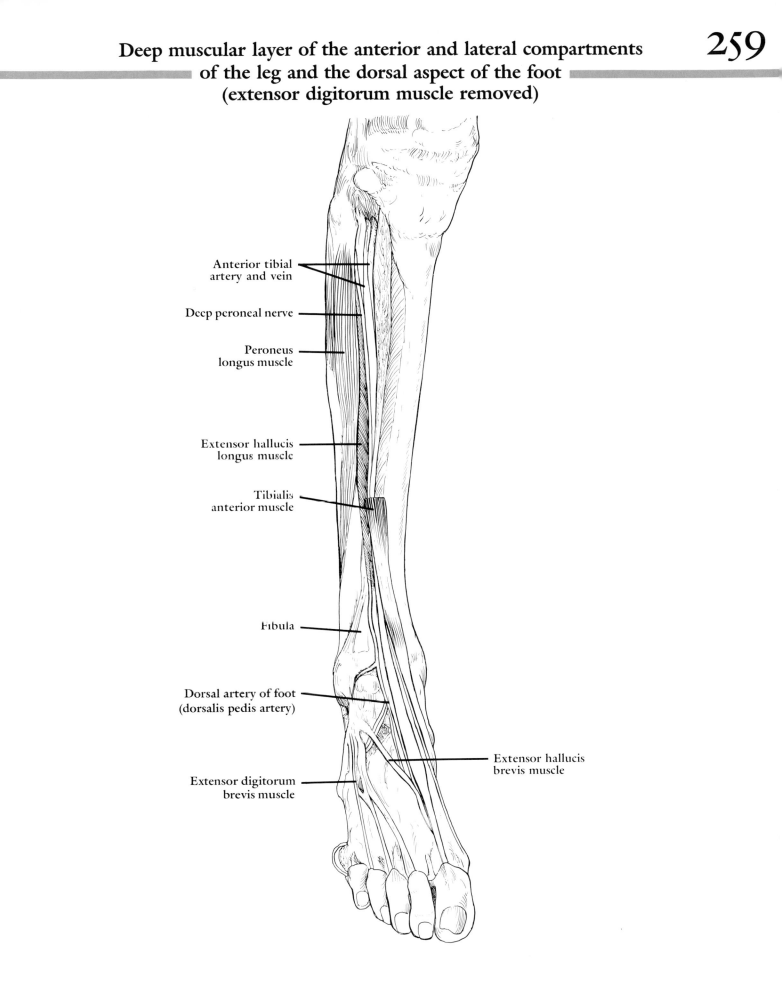

Anterior tibial artery and vein

Deep peroneal nerve

Peroneus longus muscle

Extensor hallucis longus muscle

Tibialis anterior muscle

Fibula

Dorsal artery of foot (dorsalis pedis artery)

Extensor digitorum brevis muscle

Extensor hallucis brevis muscle

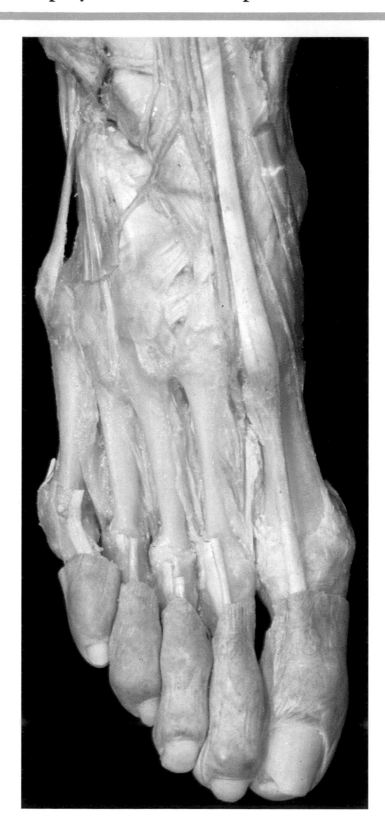

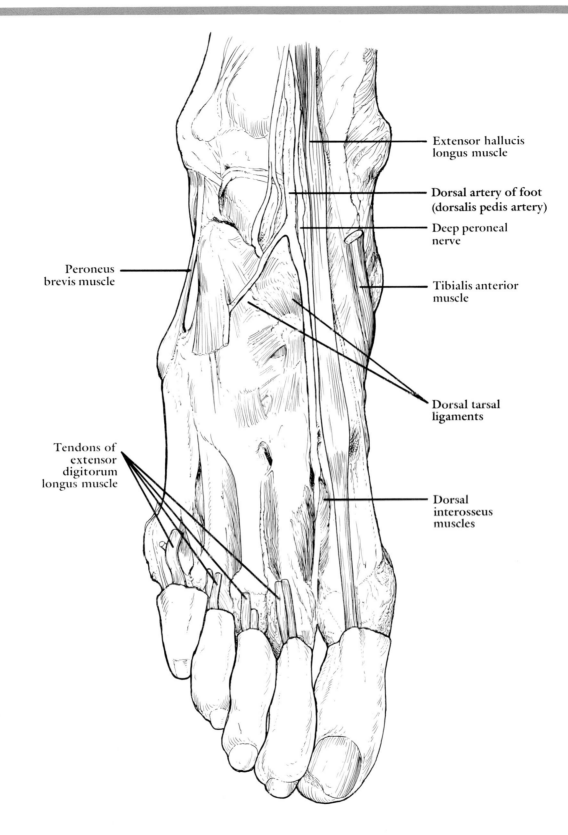

Extensor hallucis
longus muscle

Dorsal artery of foot
(dorsalis pedis artery)

Deep peroneal
nerve

Peroneus
brevis muscle

Tibialis anterior
muscle

Dorsal tarsal
ligaments

Tendons of
extensor
digitorum
longus muscle

Dorsal
interosseus
muscles

Specific remarks: The *anterior tibial artery* crosses anteriorly close to the skeleton of the *ankle joint* to become continuous with the *dorsalis pedis artery*.

General remarks: In addition to forming an anastomosis with the *plantar arch*, the *dorsalis pedis artery* is accessible for taking the pulse and digital compression because of a relatively superficial position and a close relationship to the skeleton.

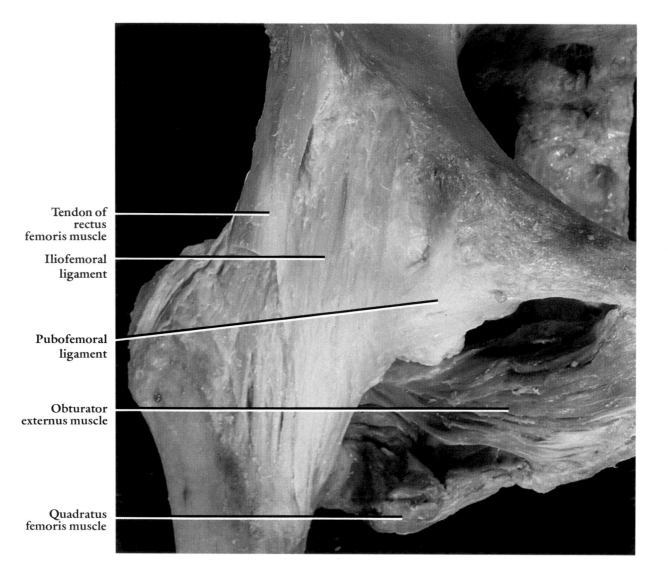

Tendon of
rectus
femoris muscle

Iliofemoral
ligament

Pubofemoral
ligament

Obturator
externus muscle

Quadratus
femoris muscle

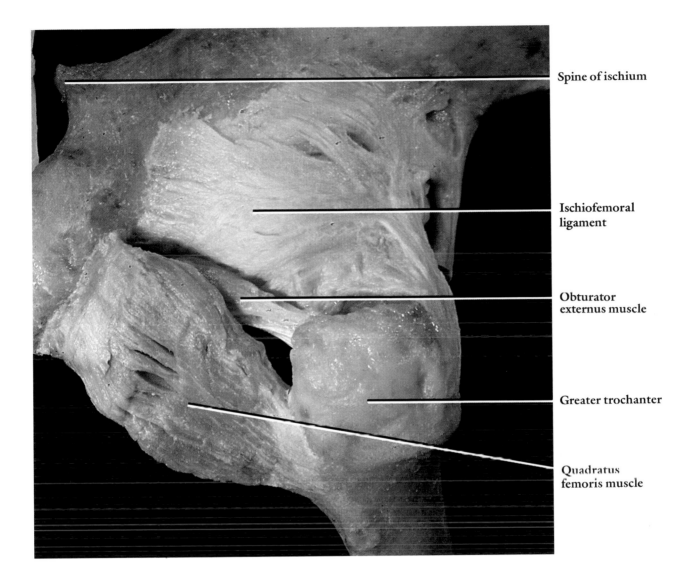

Spine of ischium

Ischiofemoral
ligament

Obturator
externus muscle

Greater trochanter

Quadratus
femoris muscle

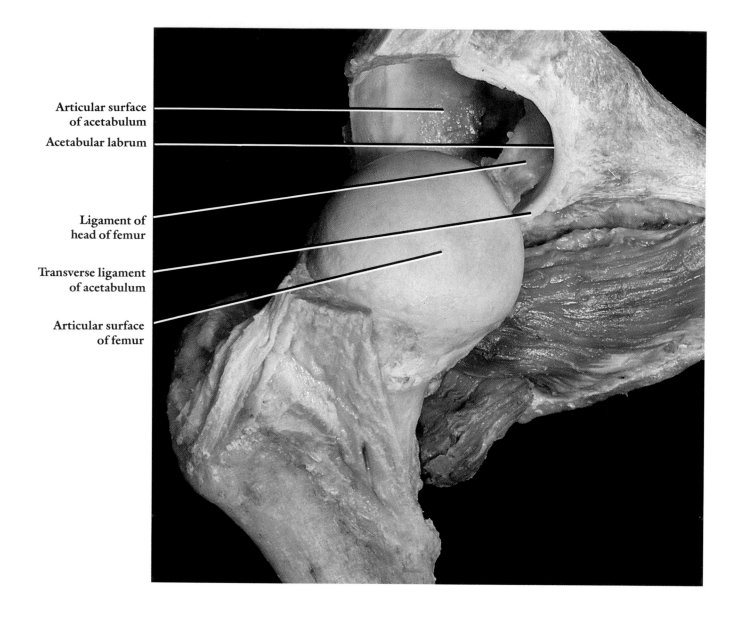

Articular surface
of acetabulum

Acetabular labrum

Ligament of
head of femur

Transverse ligament
of acetabulum

Articular surface
of femur

Specific remarks: The anterior ligaments and the articular
capsule have been cut longitudinally and the *femur* rotated
laterally to open the joint.

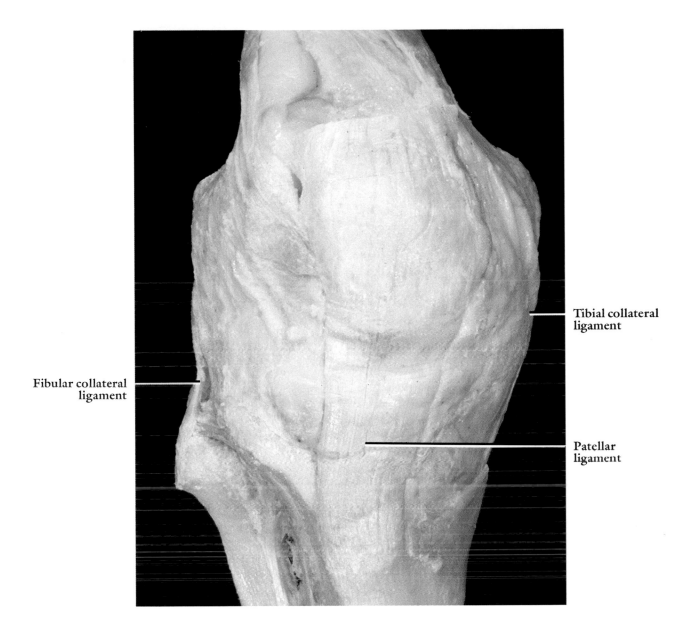

Fibular collateral
ligament

Tibial collateral
ligament

Patellar
ligament

Specific remarks: The *patellar ligament* is protected against the tibial surface by a fat pad, which is especially important during flexion of the leg.

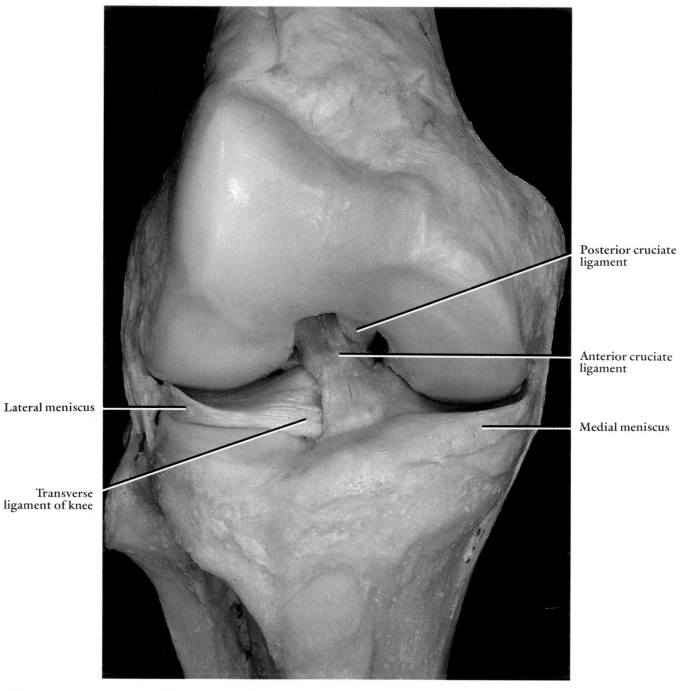

Posterior cruciate ligament

Anterior cruciate ligament

Medial meniscus

Lateral meniscus

Transverse ligament of knee

Specific remarks: The articular capsule and ligaments have been cut horizontally and the knee flexed to demonstrate the interior structures of the joint.

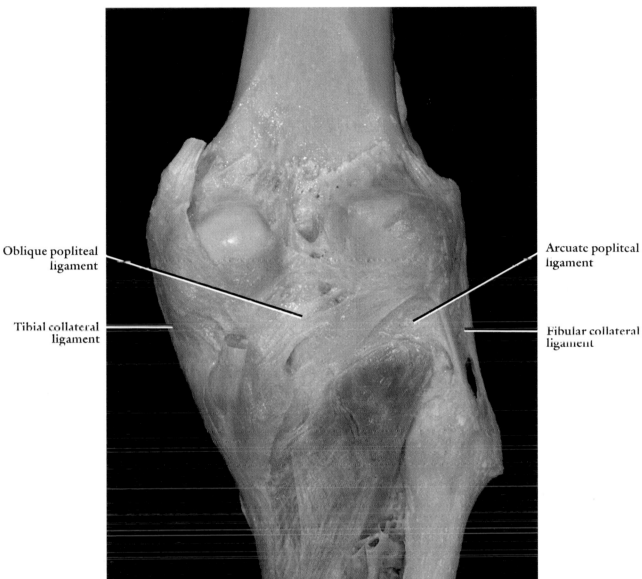

Oblique popliteal ligament

Arcuate popliteal ligament

Tibial collateral ligament

Fibular collateral ligament

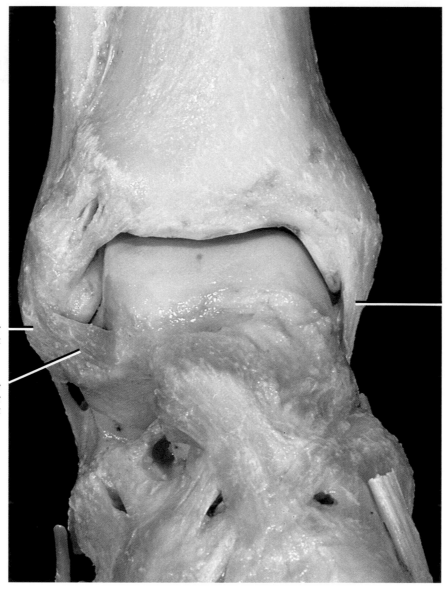

Medial (deltoid) ligament

Calcaneofibular ligament

Anterior talofibular ligament

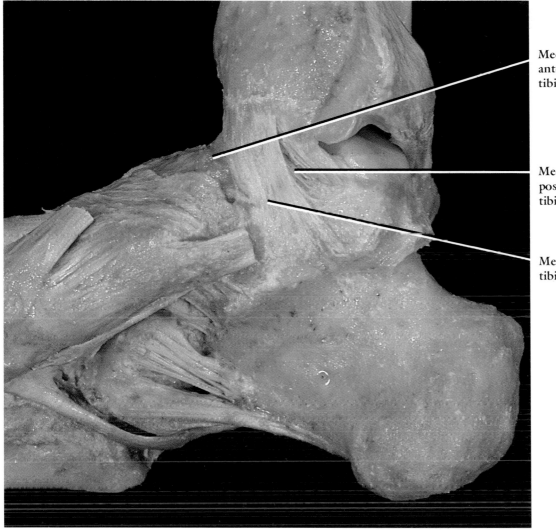

Medial ligament,
anterior
tibiotalar part

Medial ligament,
posterior
tibiotalar part

Medial ligament,
tibiocalcaneal part

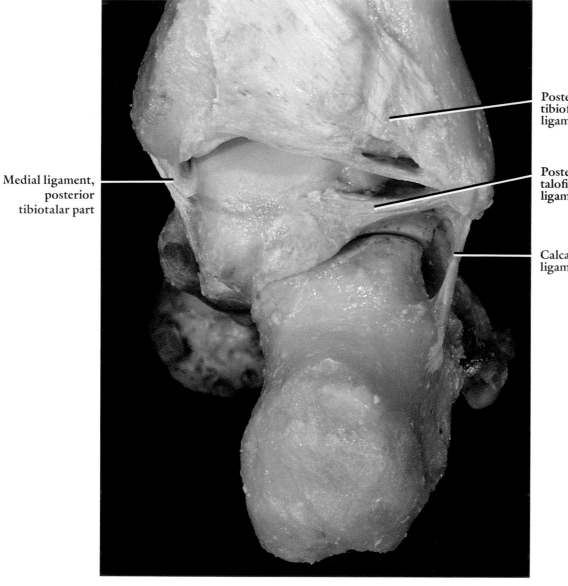

Medial ligament, posterior tibiotalar part

Posterior tibiofibular ligament

Posterior talofibular ligament

Calcaneofibular ligament

Anterior
tibiofibular
ligament

Anterior
talofibular
ligament

Calcaneofibular
ligament

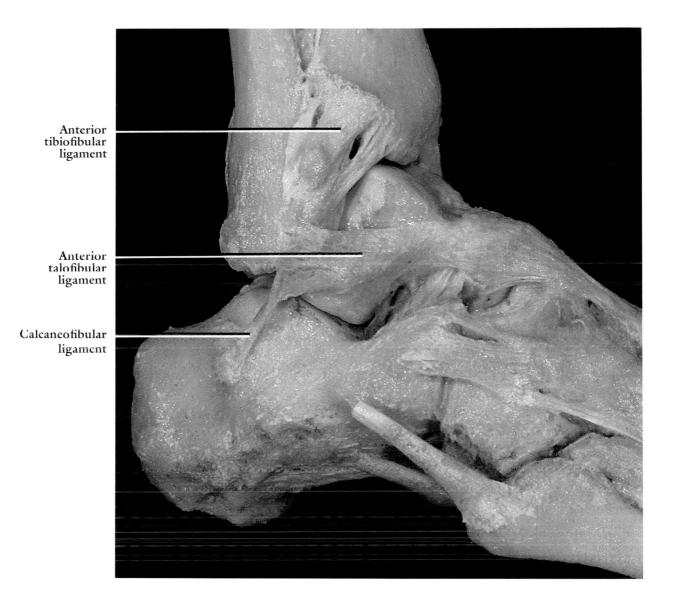

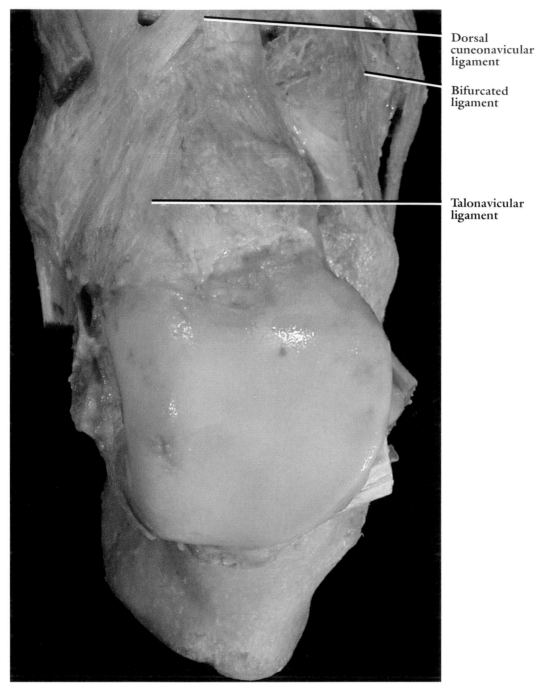

Dorsal
cuneonavicular
ligament

Bifurcated
ligament

Talonavicular
ligament

Specific remarks: For this view the *ankle joint* has been
disarticulated to show the *talar articular surface*.

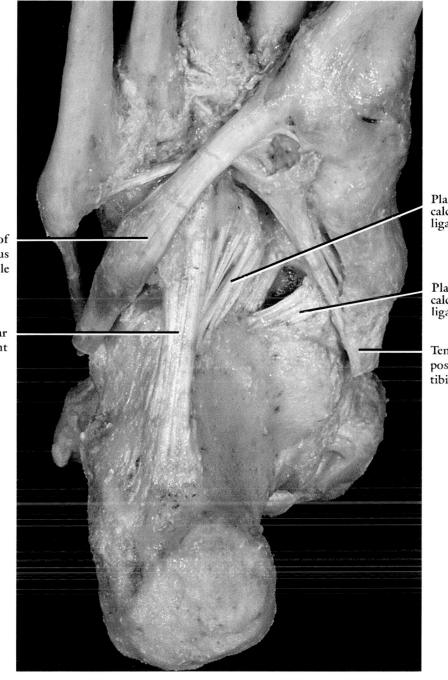

Tendon of
peroneus
longus muscle

Long plantar
ligament

Plantar
calcaneocuboid
ligament

Plantar
calcanconavicular
ligament

Tendon of
posterior
tibial muscle

References

233

Crock, H.V.: A revision of the anatomy of the arteries supplying the upper end of the human femur, J. Anat. **99**:77, 1965.

235

Lewis, O.J.: The tubercle of the tibia, J. Anat. **92**:587, 1958.

237

Hicks, J.H.: The mechanics of the foot. I. The joints, J. Anat. **87**:345, 1953.

Shepard, E.: Tarsal movements, J. Bone Joint Surg., **33B**:258, 1951.

Trolle, D.: Accessory bones of the human foot, Copenhagen, 1948, Munskgaard.

Wood Jones, F.: The foot, London, 1949, Baillière, Tindall & Cox.

239

Dodd, H.R., and Cocket, F.B.: The pathology and surgery of the veins of the lower limb, Edinburgh, 1956, Churchill Livingstone.

Kaplan, E.B.: The iliotibial tract: clinical and morphological significance, J. Bone Joint Surg. **40A**:817, 1958.

Kosinski, C.: Observations on the superficial venous system of the lower extremity, J. Anat. **60**:131, 1926.

240

Janda, V., and Stará, V.: The role of thigh adductors in movement patterns of the hip and knee joints, Courrier Centre Inter. L'enfance **15**:1, 1965.

245

Sneath, R.S.: The insertion of the biceps femoris, J. Anat. **89**:550, 1955.

246

Cave, A.J.E., and Porteous, C.J.: A note on the semimembranosus muscle, Ann. R. Coll. Surg. **24**:251, 1959.

249

Ochoa, J., and Mair, W.E.P.: The normal sural nerve in man. II. Changes in the axons and Schwann cells due to aging, Acta Neuropathol. **13**:217, 1969.

250

Cummins, B., et al.: The structure of calcaneal tendon (of Achilles) in relation to orthopedic surgery: with additional observations on the plantaris muscle, Surg. Gynecol. Obstet. **83**:107, 1946.

White, J.W.: Torsion of achilles tendon: its surgical significance, Arch. Surg. **46**:784, 1943.

251

Joseph, J., Nightingale, A., and Williams, P.L.: Detailed study of electric potentials recorded over some postural muscles while relaxed and standing, J. Physiol. (Lond.) **127**:617, 1955.

252

Last, R.J.: The popliteus muscle and the lateral meniscus, J. Bone Joint Surg. **32B**:93, 1950.

Lewis, O.J.: The tibialis posterior tendon in the primate foot, J. Anat. **98**:209, 1964.

253

Elftman, H.: Biomechanics of muscle with particular application to studies of gait, J. Bone Joint Surg. **48A**:363, 1966.

Feingold, M.L., et al.: The plantar compartments of the foot: a roentgen approach. I. Experimental observations, Invest. Radiol. **12**:281, 1977.

Gray, E.G., and Basmaijan, J.V.: Electromyography and cinematography of leg and foot ("normal" and flat) during walking, Anat. Rec. **161**:1, 1968.

Jones, R.L.: The human foot: an experimental study of its mechanics, and the role of its muscles and ligaments in the support of the arch, Am. J. Anat. **68**:1, 1941.

254

Hicks, J.H.: The mechanics of the foot: the plantar aponeurosis and the arch, J. Anat. **88**:25, 1953.

256

Lewis, O.J.: The comparative morphology of M. flexor accessorius and the associated long flexor tendons, J. Anat. **96**:321, 1962.

262

Joseph, J.: Man's posture, Springfield, Ill., 1960, Charles C Thomas, Publisher.

264

Barnett, C.H.: Locking at the knee joint, J. Anat. **86**:485P, 1952.

Brantigan, O.C., and Voshell, A.F.: Tibial collateral ligament: its function, its bursae, and its relation to medial meniscus, J. Bone Joint Surg. **25**:121, 1943.

266

Cameron, H.V., and MacNab, I.: The structure of the meniscus of the human knee joint, Clin. Orthop. Relat. Res. **89**:215, 1972.

Gardner, E.D.: The innervation of the knee joint, Anat. Rec. **101**:109, 1948.

Last, R.J.: Some anatomical details of the knee joint, J. Bone Joint Surg. **30B**:683, 1948.

Last, R.J.: Specimens from Hunterian collection: synovial cavity of knee joint (specimen S110A); ligaments of knee (specimen S95A), J. Bone Joint Surg. **33B**:442, 1951.

268

Champetier, J., and Descoors, C.: The branches of the posterior tibial nerve in the tibiotalar joint, C.R. Assoc. Anat. **141**:677, 1968.

270

Barnett, C.H., and Napier, J.R.: The axis of rotation at the ankle joint in man: its influence upon the form of the talus and the mobility of the fibula, J. Anat. **86**:1, 1952.

272

Bunning, P.S.C., and Barnett, C.H.: Variations in talocalcaneal articulation, J. Anat. **97**:643P, 1963.

Bunning, P.S.C., and Barnett, C.H.: A comparison of adult and foetal talocalcaneal articulations, J. Anat. **99**:71, 1965.

Hicks, J.H.: The mechanics of the foot. I. The joints, J. Anat. **87**:345, 1953.

Hicks, J.H.: The foot as a support, Acta Anat. **25**:34, 1955.

MacConaill, M.A.: The postural mechanism of the human foot, Proc. R. Ir. Acad. [B] **14**:265, 1945.

McKenzie, J.: The foot as a half-dome, Br. Med. J. **1**:1068, 1955.

Smith, J.W.: The ligamentous structures in the canalis and sinus tarsi, J. Anat. **92**:616, 1958.

Alphabetical index

Groove for transverse sinus, 7
Gyri, 80

H

Hamate bone, 178, 179
Hand, 192-194, 204, 206, 208
Handle of malleus, 93, 95
Hard palate, 8, 123, 141, 145
Head of epididymis, 375, 376
Head of femur, 382, 383
Head of fibula, 382-385, 406, 407
Head of humerus, 168
Head of malleus, 87, 89
Head of pancreas, 285, 287, 291
Head of rib, 174
Head of stapes, 97
Heart, 246, 248, 250, 252, 254, 256, 258, 259, 261, 273
Helix, 27, 91
Hemiazygos vein, 275
Hepatic artery, 289, 301
Hepatic veins, 300
Hiatus for greater petrosal nerve, 18, 85
Hiatus for lesser petrosal nerve, 18, 85
Hilum (lung), 264
Hip bone 168-171
Hip joint, 378, 379, 432-434
Hook of hamate bone, 178
Horizontal fissure (right lung), 264, 269
Horizontal plate of palatine bone, 8
Humeral shaft, 57, 187, 189, 213
Hymen, 365
Hyoglossus muscle, 53, 55, 145
Hyoid bone, 45, 49, 53, 137, 149, 151, 157
Hypoglossal canal, 7, 9, 113
Hypoglossal nerve, 51, 53, 55, 79, 83, 117, 119, 145
Hypothenar eminence, 192, 205, 209
Hypotympanic recess, 89

I

Ileocecal valve, 296
Ileocolic artery, 285, 287
Ileocolic junction, 287
Ileum, 245, 281, 285, 294, 296
Iliac crest, 168, 180, 335, 337, 363
Iliac part of hip bone, 378, 379
Iliacus muscle, 315
Iliocostalis muscle, 215, 341
Iliofemoral ligament, 432
Iliopectineal eminence, 315
Iliopsoas muscle, 395, 397, 399
Impression of azygos arch (right lung), 266
Incisive fossa, 8
Incisors, 8, 143
Incudomalleolar joint, 87
Incus, 87, 89, 95, 97
Index finger, 199
Inferior alveolar artery, 43
Inferior alveolar nerve, 41, 43
Inferior angle of scapula, 335
Inferior articular process of vertebra, 20, 174
Inferior border of spleen, 302
Inferior concha, 9, 125, 127, 129
Inferior epigastric artery, 241, 243, 247
Inferior epigastric vein, 357
Inferior extensor retinaculum, 427
Inferior fascia of pelvic diaphragm, 353

Inferior fornix (conjunctiva), 111
Inferior glenohumeral ligament, 224
Inferior gluteal artery, 339
Inferior gluteal nerve, 339
Inferior gluteal vein, 339
Inferior horn of thyroid cartilage, 149, 153, 158-160
Inferior labial artery, 37
Inferior lobe of lung, 264-267, 269, 271
Inferior lung margin, 264-267
Inferior meatus, 125, 127
Inferior mesenteric artery, 287, 305, 307
Inferior oblique muscle, 105, 111
Inferior orbital fissure, 2, 4
Inferior pancreaticoduodenal artery, 289
Inferior pharyngeal constrictor muscle, 117, 149
Inferior phrenic artery, 305
Inferior rectal artery, 373
Inferior rectal nerve, 373
Inferior rectal vein, 351, 373
Inferior rectus muscle, 105, 111
Inferior sagittal sinus, 75
Inferior scapular angle, 57
Inferior vena cava, 247, 249, 253, 305, 307, 308
Infraglenoid tubercle of scapula, 215
Infrahyoid muscles, 53
Infrahyoid region, 49, 51
Infraorbital artery, 37, 109, 111, 135
Infraorbital canal, 135
Infraorbital foramen, 2, 10, 23, 37, 135
Infraorbital groove, 135
Infraorbital nerve, 37, 109, 111, 135
Infraorbital vein, 37, 109, 111
Infrapiriform compartment of greater sciatic foramen, 349
Infraspinatus muscle, 59, 61, 211, 213, 215
Infraspinous fossa, 173, 225
Infratemporal crest of sphenoid bone, 15
Infratemporal fossa (space), 2-4, 37-43
Infratemporal surface of greater wing of sphenoid bone, 4
Infratrochlear artery, 105, 109
Infratrochlear nerve, 103, 109, 111
Infratrochlear vein, 109
Inguinal canal, 327
Inguinal folds, 281
Inguinal fossae, 281
Inguinal groove, 180, 181, 189
Inguinal ligament, 393
Innermost intercostal muscle, 191
Interarytenoid fold, 119
Interatrial septum, 257
Intercondylar fossa (femur), 385
Intercostal nerve, 277, 345, 347
Intercostal space, 180, 191, 277
Intercostobrachial nerve, 185
Interdigital arteries, 195
Interdigital nerves, 195
Interdigital veins, 195
Intermetatarsal space, 425
Internal acoustic meatus, 9
Internal branch of superior laryngeal nerve, 53, 149, 151
Internal carotid artery, 77, 79, 83, 87, 89
Internal carotid plexus, 103
Internal iliac artery, 351

Internal intercostal membrane, 277
Internal intercostal muscle, 185, 187, 189, 191
Internal jugular vein, 51, 117
Internal oblique muscle of abdomen, 239, 337, 339, 341
Internal occipital protuberance, 7
Internal opening of urethra, 333, 354
Internal pudendal artery, 341, 349, 351
Internal pudendal vein, 341, 349
Internal terminal filament, 347
Internal thoracic artery, 53, 55, 237
Internal thoracic vein, 237
Interosseous membrane, 203, 228, 230
Interthalamic adhesion, 74
Intertubercular groove (humerus), 168
Intertubercular tendon sheath, 224
Interventricular foramen, 75, 81
Interventricular septum, 255
Intervertebral disc, 232
Intervertebral foramen, 21, 69
Intervertebral joint, 232
Intestinal wall (small intestine), 298
Intrarenal vessels, 311
Iris, 107
Ischial spine, 169, 349, 363, 433
Ischial tuberosity, 169, 335, 363-365, 401
Ischioanal fossa, 337, 339, 341, 343, 345, 347, 349, 367, 369, 371
Ischiocavernosus muscle, 367, 369, 371, 373
Ischiofemoral ligament, 433
Ischiopubic ramus, 363, 365, 371, 373, 378, 379
Isthmus faucium, 119

J

Jejunum, 285, 295
Jugular foramen, 5, 7, 8
Jugular notch, 45
Jugulodigastric lymph node, 51
Juguloomohyoid lymph node, 51
Junction of cystic and common hepatic ducts, 301

K

Kidney, 305, 307, 308
Knee joint, 435-437

L

Labium majus, 359, 365, 379
Labium minus, 359, 365
Labyrinth of ethmoid bone, 12, 13
Lacrimal apparatus, 35
Lacrimal artery, 109
Lacrimal canaliculus, 107
Lacrimal caruncle, 107
Lacrimal gland, 101, 103, 109, 111, 131
Lacrimal lake, 107
Lacrimal nerve, 101, 103, 109
Lacrimal papilla, 107
Lacrimal puncta, 107
Lacrimal sac, 107, 111, 133
Lacrimal vein, 109
Lactiferous duct, 181
Lambda, 6
Lambdoid suture, 6
Lamina of cricoid cartilage, 155, 156, 160
Lamina terminalis, 74, 81
Lamina of vertebra, 21, 69, 175, 231

464